T0131003

Pediatric Infectious Disease Around the Globe

Editors

FOUZIA NAEEM
CHOKECHAI RONGKAVILIT

PEDIATRIC CLINICS OF NORTH AMERICA

www.pediatric.theclinics.com

Consulting Editor

BONITA F. STANTON

February 2022 • Volume 69 • Number 1

ELSEVIER

1600 John F. Kennedy Boulevard • Suite 1800 • Philadelphia, Pennsylvania, 19103-2899

http://www.theclinics.com

THE PEDIATRIC CLINICS OF NORTH AMERICA Volume 69, Number 1
February 2022 ISSN 0031-3955, ISBN-13: 978-0-323-84874-9

Editor: Kerry Holland
Developmental Editor: Axell Ivan Jade M. Purificacion

The Pediatric Clinics of North America (ISSN 0031-3955) is published bimonthly by Elsevier Inc., 360 Park Avenue South, New York, NY 10010-1710. Months of issue are February, April, June, August, October, and December. Periodicals postage paid at New York, NY and additional mailing offices. Subscription prices are $263.00 per year (US individuals), $1028.00 per year (US institutions), $331.00 per year (Canadian individuals), $1074.00 per year (Canadian institutions), $395.00 per year (international individuals), $1074.00 per year (international institutions), $100.00 per year (US students and residents), $100.00 per year (Canadian students and residents), and $165.00 per year (international residents and students). To receive students/resident rare, orders must be accompanied by name of affiliated institution, date of term, and the signature of program/residency coordinator on institution letterhead. Orders will be billed at individual rate until proof of status is received. Foreign air speed delivery is included in all *Clinics* subscription prices. All prices are subject to change without notice. **POSTMASTER:** Send address changes to *The Pediatric Clinics of North America*, Elsevier Health Sciences Division, Subscription Customer Service, 3251 Riverport Lane, Maryland Heights, MO 63043. **Customer Service: 1-800-654-2452 (US and Canada). From outside of the US and Canada: 1-314-447-8871. Fax: 1-314-447-8029. For print support, E-mail: JournalsCustomerService-usa@elsevier.com. For online support, E-mail: JournalsOnlineSupport-usa@elsevier.com.**

Reprints. For copies of 100 or more, of articles in this publication, please contact the Commercial Reprints Department, Elsevier Inc., 360 Park Avenue South, New York, NY 10010-1710. Tel.: 212-633-3874; Fax: 212-633-3820; E-mail: reprints@elsevier.com.

The Pediatric Clinics of North America is also published in Spanish by McGraw-Hill Inter-americana Editores S.A., Mexico City, Mexico; in Portuguese by Riechmann and Affonso Editores, Rua Comandante Coelho 1085, CEP 21250, Rio de Janeiro, Brazil; and in Greek by Althayia SA, Athens, Greece.

The Pediatric Clinics of North America is covered in *MEDLINE/PubMed (Index Medicus), Excerpta Medica, Current Contents, Current Contents/Clinical Medicine, Science Citation Index, ASCA, ISI/BIOMED*, and *BIOSIS*.

PROGRAM OBJECTIVE

The goal of the *Pediatric Clinics of North America* is to keep practicing physicians and residents up to date with current clinical practice in pediatrics by providing timely articles reviewing the state-of-the-art in patient care.

TARGET AUDIENCE

All practicing pediatricians, physicians, and healthcare professionals who provide patient care to pediatric patients.

LEARNING OBJECTIVES

Upon completion of this activity, participants will be able to:

1. Review the international aspect of infectious diseases in children.
2. Discuss antimicrobial resistance as an emerging global threat in low and middle-income countries.
3. Recognize the impact of the overuse of antimicrobials.

ACCREDITATIONS

Physician Credit

The Elsevier Office of Continuing Medical Education (EOCME) is accredited by the Accreditation Council for Continuing Medical Education (ACCME) to provide continuing medical education for physicians.

The EOCME designates this journal-based activity for a maximum of 12 *AMA PRA Category 1 Credit*(s)™. Physicians should claim only the credit commensurate with the extent of their participation in the activity.

All other healthcare professionals requesting continuing education credit for this journal-based activity will be issued a certificate of participation.

ABP Maintenance of Certification Credit

Successful completion of this CME activity, which includes participation in the activity and individual assessment of and feedback to the learner, enables the learner to earn up to 12 MOC points in the American Board of Pediatrics' (ABP)

Maintenance of Certification (MOC) program. It is the CME activity provider's responsibility to submit learner completion information to ACCME for the purpose of granting ABP MOC credit.

DISCLOSURE OF CONFLICTS OF INTEREST

The EOCME assesses conflict of interest with its instructors, faculty, planners, and other individuals who are in a position to control the content of CME activities. All relevant conflicts of interest that are identified are thoroughly vetted by EOCME for fair balance, scientific objectivity, and patient care recommendations. EOCME is committed to providing its learners with CME activities that promote improvements or quality in healthcare and not a specific proprietary business or a commercial interest.

The planning committee, staff, authors, and editors listed below have identified no financial relationships or relationships to products or devices they or their spouse/life partner have with commercial interest related to the content of this CME activity:

Aimee Abu-Shamsieh, MD, MPH; Suvaporn Anugulruengkitt, MD, PhD; Michelle Barton, MD, MSc; Hannah M. Brooks, Bsc, MSc; Regina Chavous-Gibson, MSN, RN; Adriana Diakiw, MD; Ella M. E. Forgie, BSc, MA; Samuel Gnanakumar; Shipra Gupta, MD; Michael T. Hawkes, MD, PhD; Jenna Holmen, MD, MPH; Wajid Hussain, MBS FCPS; Watsamon Jantarabenjakul, MD, PhD; Katherine M. Knapp, MD; Soe Maw, MD, MPH; Rajkumar Mayakrishnan, BSc, MBA; Fatima Mir, MBBS, FCPS, MsCR; Fouzia Naeem, MD, MSc; Thanyawee Puthanakit, MD; Farah Naz Qamar, MBBS, FCPS, MSC, FRCP; Sonia Qureshi, MBBS, FCPS, MSC; Chokechai Rongkavilit, MD; Sadia Shakoor, MBBS, FCPS; Prachi Singh, DO; Layne Smith, PharmD; Lunliya Thampratankul, MD; Montida Veeravigrom, MD; Angela F. Veesenmeyer, MD, MPH; Vini Vijayan, MD; Frank Zhu, MD

UNAPPROVED/OFF-LABEL USE DISCLOSURE

The EOCME requires CME faculty to disclose to the participants:

1. When products or procedures being discussed are off-label, unlabelled, experimental, and/or investigational (not US Food and Drug Administration [FDA] approved); and
2. Any limitations on the information presented, such as data that are preliminary or that represent ongoing research, interim analyses, and/or unsupported opinions. Faculty may discuss information about pharmaceutical agents that is outside of FDA-approved labelling. This information is intended solely for CME

and is not intended to promote off-label use of these medications. If you have any questions, contact the medical affairs department of the manufacturer for the most recent prescribing information.

TO ENROLL

To enroll in the *Pediatric Clinics of North America* Continuing Medical Education program, call customer service at 1-800-654-2452 or sign up online at http://www.theclinics.com/home/cme. The CME program is available to subscribers for an additional annual fee of USD 324.00.

METHOD OF PARTICIPATION

In order to claim credit, participants must complete the following:

1. Complete enrolment as indicated above.
2. Read the activity.
3. Complete the CME Test and Evaluation. Participants must achieve a score of 70% on the test. All CME Tests and Evaluations must be completed online.

In order to claim MOC points, participants must complete the following:

1. Complete steps listed above for claiming CME credit
2. Provide your specialty board ID#, birth date (MM/DD), and attestation.
3. Online MOC submission is only available for the American Board of pediatrics' (ABP) Maintenance of Certification (MOC) program

CME INQUIRIES/SPECIAL NEEDS

For all CME inquiries or special needs, please contact elsevierCME@elsevier.com

Contributors

CONSULTING EDITOR

BONITA F. STANTON, MD
Professor of Pediatrics and Founding Dean, Robert C. and Laura C. Garrett Endowed Chair, Hackensack Meridian School of Medicine, President, Academic Enterprise, Hackensack Meridian Health, Nutley, New Jersey, USA

EDITORS

FOUZIA NAEEM, MD, MSc
Clinical Assistant Professor, Division of Pediatric Infectious Diseases, Department of Pediatrics, Valley Children's Healthcare, Stanford University School of Medicine (Affiliated), Madera, California, USA

CHOKECHAI RONGKAVILIT, MD
Clinical Professor, Division of Pediatric Infectious Diseases, Department of Pediatrics, University of California San Francisco, Fresno, California, USA

AUTHORS

AIMEE ABU-SHAMSIEH, MD, MPH
Clinical Professor, Department of Pediatrics, UCSF Fresno Medical Education Program, Fresno, California, USA

SUVAPORN ANUGULRUENGKITT, MD, PhD
Pediatric Infectious Diseases Physician, Division of Pediatric Infectious Diseases, Department of Pediatrics, Faculty of Medicine, Chulalongkorn University, King Chulalongkorn Memorial Hospital, Bangkok, Thailand

MICHELLE BARTON, MD, MSc
Associate Professor, Department of Paediatrics, Chief, Division of Pediatric Infectious Diseases, Schulich School of Medicine, Western University, Associate Scientist, Children's Health Research Institute, Lawson Health Research Institute, London Health Sciences Centre, London, Ontario, Canada

HANNAH M. BROOKS, MSc
Faculty of Nursing, University of Alberta, 5-143 Edmonton Clinic Health Academy, Edmonton, Alberta, Canada

ADRIANA DIAKIW, MD
Assistant Professor of Pediatrics, West Virginia University School of Medicine, Morgantown, West Virginia, USA

SHIPRA GUPTA, MD, FAAP
Assistant Professor of Pediatrics West Virginia University School of Medicine, Morgantown, West Virginia, USA

ELLA M. E. FORGIE, BSc, MA
Department of Anthropology, University of Alberta, Edmonton, Alberta, Canada

MICHAEL T. HAWKES, MD, PhD
Associate Professor; Department of Paediatrics, Department of Medical Microbiology and Immunology, Faculty of Medicine and Dentistry, School of Public Health, University of Alberta, Edmonton Clinic Health Academy; Distinguished Researcher, Stollery Science Lab Member, Women and Children's Health Research Institute, Edmonton, Alberta, Canada

JENNA HOLMEN, MD, MPH
Department of Pediatrics, Division of Pediatric Infectious Diseases and Global Health, UCSF Benioff Children's Hospital, Oakland, Oakland, California, USA

WAJID HUSSAIN, MBBS, FCPS
Fellow, Pediatric Infectious diseases, Department of Paediatrics & Child Health, Aga Khan University, Karachi, Pakistan

WATSAMON JANTARABENJAKUL, MD, PhD
Pediatric Infectious Diseases Physician, Division of Pediatric Infectious Diseases, Department of Pediatrics, Faculty of Medicine, Chulalongkorn University, King Chulalongkorn Memorial Hospital, Bangkok, Thailand

KATHERINE M. KNAPP, MD, FAAP, AAHIVS
Medical Director, Perinatal Program, HIV Prevention and Treatment, Associate Member, Department of Infectious Diseases, St. Jude Children's Research Hospital, Memphis, Tennessee, USA

SOE MAW, MD, MPH
Assistant Clinical Professor, Department of Pediatrics, UCSF Fresno Medical Education Program, Fresno, California, USA

FATIMA MIR, MBBS, FCPS Pediatrics, MsCR
Associate Professor, Department of Pediatrics and Child Health, The Aga Khan University, Karachi, Pakistan

THANYAWEE PUTHANAKIT, MD
Associate Professor, Division of Pediatric Infectious Diseases, Department of Pediatrics, Faculty of Medicine, Chulalongkorn University, King Chulalongkorn Memorial Hospital, Bangkok, Thailand

FARAH NAZ QAMAR, MBBS, FCPS, MSC, FRCP
Associate Professor, Pediatric Infectious diseases, Department of Paediatrics & Child Health, Aga Khan University, Karachi, Pakistan

SONIA QURESHI, MBBS, FCPS, MSC
Assistant Professor, Pediatric Infectious Diseases, Department of Paediatrics & Child Health, Aga Khan University, Karachi, Pakistan

SADIA SHAKOOR, MBBS, FCPS Microbiology
Associate Professor, Department of Pathology, Aga Khan University, Section of Microbiology, The Aga Khan University, Karachi, Pakistan

PRACHI SINGH, DO
Department of Pediatrics, Division of Pediatric Infectious Diseases and Global Health, UCSF Benioff Children's Hospital, Oakland, Oakland, California, USA

LAYNE SMITH, PharmD
West Virginia University School of Pharmacy, Morgantown, West Virginia, USA

LUNLIYA THAMPRATANKUL, MD
Associate Professor, Department of Pediatrics, Faculty of Medicine Ramathibodi Hospital, Mahidol University, Bangkok, Thailand

MONTIDA VEERAVIGROM, MD
Assistant Professor, Section of Child Neurology, Department of Pediatrics, The University of Chicago Biological Sciences, Chicago, Illinois, USA

ANGELA F. VEESENMEYER, MD, MPH
Associate Professor, Department of Child Health, University of Arizona College of Medicine-Phoenix, Pediatric Infectious Disease, Valleywise Health Medical Center, Phoenix, Arizona, USA

VINI VIJAYAN, MD, FIDSA
Division of Pediatric Infectious Diseases, Valley Children's Healthcare, Madera; Clinical Associate Professor (Affiliated), Stanford University School of Medicine, Stanford, California, USA

FRANK ZHU, MD
Assistant Professor, Department of Pediatrics, Division of Pediatric Infectious Diseases, Medical College of Wisconsin, Milwaukee, Wisconsin, USA

Contents

Foreword: Revisiting the Need for Vigilance Concerning Children and International Travel **xv**

Bonita F. Stanton

Preface: Exotic Infections Are Only One Plane Away **xvii**

Fouzia Naeem and Chokechai Rongkavilit

Prevention of Mother-to-Child Human Immunodeficiency Virus Transmission in Resource-Limited Countries **1**

Katherine M. Knapp

The first pediatric AIDS cases were reported in 1982. A decade later, the World Health Organization estimated there were more than 500,000 pediatric AIDS cases resulting from mother-to-child transmission, 90% of which were in sub-Saharan Africa. Although the rate of new infections globally has been cut in half since the peak of the pandemic, human immunodeficiency virus (HIV) remains a public health threat, and rates of new infections continue to increase in some regions. Mother-to-child transmission of HIV has now been virtually eliminated in many parts of the world but remains an issue in resource-limited countries.

Updates in Pediatric Tuberculosis in International Settings **19**

Sadia Shakoor and Fatima Mir

Childhood tuberculosis (TB) has been underreported and underrepresented in TB statistics across the globe. Contributing factors include health system barriers, diagnostic barriers, and community barriers leading to an underdetected epidemic of childhood tuberculosis. Despite considerable progress in childhood TB management, there is a concerning gap in policy and practice in high-burden countries leading to missed opportunities for active case detection, early diagnosis and treatment of TB exposure, and infection and disease in children regardless of human immunodeficiency virus status. Bridging this gap requires multisectoral coordination and political commitment along with an eye to research and innovation with potential to scale.

Pediatric Malaria: Global and North American Perspectives **47**

Ella M.E. Forgie, Hannah M. Brooks, Michelle Barton, and Michael T. Hawkes

Malaria is a leading cause of death in children less than 5 years of age globally, and a common cause of fever in the returning North American traveler. New tools in the fight against malaria have been developed over the past decades: potent artemisinin derivatives; rapid diagnostic tests; long-lasting insecticidal bed nets; and a new vaccine, RTS,S/AS01. Thwarting these advances, parasite and *Anopheles* vector resistance are emerging. In the meantime, clinicians will continue to see malaria among febrile travelers from the tropics. Early recognition, diagnosis, and treatment can be lifesaving, but rely on the vigilance of frontline clinicians.

Salmonellosis Including Enteric Fever **65**

Farah Naz Qamar, Wajid Hussain, and Sonia Qureshi

Salmonella is a gram-negative, motile, nonsporulating, facultative anaerobic bacillus, belongs to the family Enterobacteriaceae. The bacteria were first identified in 1884. It is transmitted through direct contact with an infected person or indirect contact by the consumption of contaminated food and water. More than 2500 serotypes of Salmonella enterica have been identified but less than 100 serotypes are known to cause infections in humans. S. enterica serovar typhi (S. typhi) and S. enterica serovar paratyphi (S. paratyphi A B C) cause enteric fever, whereas nontyphoidal Salmonella serotypes (NTS) cause diarrhea. NTS commonly presents with gastroenteritis and is a self-limiting disease. Enteric fever is a potentially life-threatening acute febrile systemic infection and is diagnosed by isolating a pathogen on culture. With the emergence of the extensive drug-resistant (XDR) S. typhi clone, limited treatment options are available. Vaccination of persons at risk, improvement of sanitation, promotion of food hygiene, and detection and control of chronic carriers are essential preventive control measures of enteric fever.

Amebiasis and Amebic Liver Abscess in Children **79**

Shipra Gupta, Layne Smith, and Adriana Diakiw

Although rare in the developed world, amebiasis continues to be a leading cause of diarrhea and illness in developing nations with crowding, poor sanitation, and lack of clean water supply. Recent immigrants or travelers returning from endemic regions after a prolonged stay are at high risk of developing amebiasis. A high index of suspicion for amebiasis should be maintained for other high-risk groups like men having sex with men, people with AIDS/HIV, immunocompromised hosts, residents of mental health facility or group homes. Clinical presentation of intestinal amebiasis varies from diarrhea to colitis and dysentery. Amebic liver abscess (ALA) is the most common form of extraintestinal amebiasis. Various diagnostic tools are available and when amebiasis is suspected, a combination of stool tests and serology should be sent to maximize the yield of testing. Treatment with an amebicidal drug such as metronidazole/tinidazole and a luminal cysticidal agent such as paromomycin for clinical disease is indicated. However, for asymptomatic disease treatment with a luminal cysticidal agent to decrease chances of invasive disease and transmission is recommended.

Evaluation and Management of Traveler's Diarrhea in Children **99**

Frank Zhu

Traveler's diarrhea is the most common travel disease in both children and adults. Adult guidelines for traveler's diarrhea have been established, but significant gaps persist in guidance for the evaluation and management of pediatric traveler's diarrhea. Adult guidelines are not necessarily applicable in children, and it is essential for clinicians to account for the differences in pediatric pathophysiology, clinical presentations, and treatment recommendations when evaluating and managing pediatric traveler's diarrhea.

Neurocysticercosis in Children **115**

Montida Veeravigrom and Lunliya Thampratankul

Neurocysticercosis is one of the most common parasitic infections in the central nervous system in children. The usual clinical manifestation is new-onset focal seizure. However, there are other multiple clinical manifestations, such as increased intracranial pressure, meningoencephalitis, spinal cord syndrome, and blindness. The diagnosis needs high index of suspicion with clinical history, physical examination, neuroimaging, and immunologic studies. Recent advances in neuroimaging and serology facilitate the accurate diagnosis. Management of neurocysticercosis should focus on critical symptoms first, such as the use of antiepileptic drugs and medical or surgical therapy for increased intracranial pressure.

Important Nematodes in Children **129**

Angela F. Veesenmeyer

Intestinal nematode infections caused by soil-transmitted helminths (STH), such as the roundworm *Ascaris lumbricoides,* the whipworm *Trichuris trichiura,* and the hookworms *Ancylostoma duodenale,* and *Necator americanus*, infect more than 1 billion people throughout the world. School-aged children tend to harbor the greatest numbers of intestinal worms, and as a result, experience more adverse health consequences, such as poor growth, anemia, and cognitive decline. Clinicians should maintain a high degree of suspicion in endemic areas when patients present with surgical abdomens, particularly children. Current antihelminthic drugs are moderately effective, but reinfection is possible. Global efforts are needed to eradicate STH infections.

Multidrug-Resistant Infections in the Developing World **141**

Prachi Singh and Jenna Holmen

Antimicrobials are essential in reducing morbidity and mortality from infectious diseases globally. However, due to the lack of effective surveillance measures and widespread overuse, there is an increasing threat to the effectiveness of antimicrobials. Although there is a global increase in antimicrobial resistance, low- and middle-income countries share a much higher burden. Antimicrobial stewardship efforts such as effective surveillance and reduction in overuse can help combat the increase in antimicrobial resistance.

Pediatric Care for Immigrant, Refugee, and Internationally Adopted Children **153**

Aimee Abu-Shamsieh and Soe Maw

Immigrant children are a diverse group and include refugees, asylees, and internationally adopted children. They have various infectious disease risk factors, depending on conditions within their country of origin, journey, and current living conditions. Infectious disease screening should take place within the framework of a comprehensive medical evaluation in the medical home. Some screening is recommended for all immigrant children including hepatitis B, syphilis, HIV, tuberculosis, and intestinal parasites; other diseases can be tested for based on individual risks. Although guidelines and resources are available, there is limited evidence supporting much of the care of immigrant children and youth.

Vaccines for International Pediatric Travelers **171**

Vini Vijayan

The pretravel management of the international pediatric traveler is based on provision of preventive education, chemoprophylaxis against malaria and traveler's diarrhea, as well as travel vaccinations. Immunization requirements are determined based on the traveler's pretravel immunization status, age, medical history, and destination. Immunization needs also vary depending on the exposures during the trip. Potential exposure to water, insects, or animals as well as duration of travel will help tailor risk avoidance education and travel immunizations. This review provides clinicians an overview of vaccines recommended for children traveling internationally.

Prevention of Emerging Infections in Children **185**

Thanyawee Puthanakit, Suvaporn Anugulruengkitt, and Watsamon Jantarabenjakul

Prevention of emerging infections in children is a dynamic arena where substantial medical advances have enabled intervention and prevention of infection outbreaks. This article discusses 5 infections causing significant morbidity and mortality across Asia, Latin America, and Africa. Avian influenza and the Middle East respiratory syndrome are highly contagious zoonoses spread through aerosol and droplets, affecting predominantly Asia. Dengue infection and chikungunya are endemic mosquito-borne viruses in tropical regions across Asia, Latin America, and Africa. Ebola is a highly contagious virus spread through human-to-human contact. The latest information in clinical manifestations, infection, prevention control, chemoprophylaxis, vaccination, and public health measures is reviewed.

PEDIATRIC CLINICS OF NORTH AMERICA

FORTHCOMING ISSUES

April 2022
Pediatric Otolaryngology
Huma Quraishi and Michael Chee, *Editors*

June 2022
Pediatric Critical Care
Mary Lieh-Lai and Katherine Cashen, *Editors*

August 2022
Progress in Behavioral Health Interventions for Children and Adolescents
Xiaoming Li and Sayward Harrison, *Editors*

RECENT ISSUES

December 2021
Pediatric Gastroenterology
Harpreet Pall, *Editor*

October 2021
Covid-19 in Children
Elizabeth Secord and Eric John McGrath, *Editors*

August 2021
Pediatric Neurosurgery in Primary Care
Jonathan Martin and Greg Olavarria, *Editors*

SERIES OF RELATED INTEREST
Infectious Disease Clinics of North America
www.id.theclinics.com/

THE CLINICS ARE AVAILABLE ONLINE!
Access your subscription at:
www.theclinics.com

Foreword

Revisiting the Need for Vigilance Concerning Children and International Travel

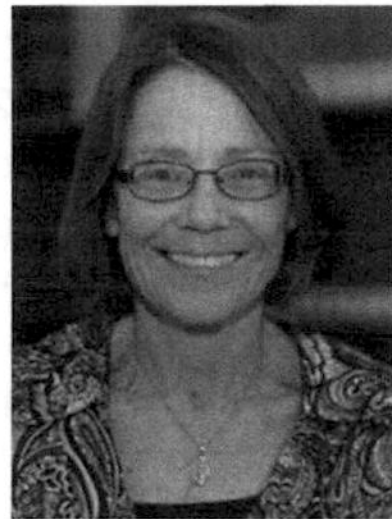

Bonita F. Stanton, MD
Consulting Editor

This issue of *Pediatric Clinics of North America* addresses international travel. It was commissioned before 2020, the year that COVID-19 roared across our globe. While the global infectious diseases landscape has changed dramatically since January 2020, there is every reason to believe that once the pandemic is under control, international travel will again surge, probably surpassing the numbers to which it had climbed through 2019. Therefore, as important as it is now to restrict international travel to and from areas with immunization rates and/or high rates of COVID-19, it is also important to recognize that travel is already increasing, and thus, we must remain vigilant about preventing other, travel-familiar diseases at the same time we are concerned about COVID-19.

Even the modern world has only recently become consumed by international travel. In 1959, only 25 million tourist arrivals were registered globally. However, by 2018, this number had increased 58-fold to 1.4 billion international travelers. Initially, over two-thirds of this travel was to or within Europe, although by 2018, this proportion had declined (somewhat) to 50%. Notable increases were seen among Asia and the Pacific nations, with less than 1% of global travelers visiting these nations in 1950, but nearly a quarter doing so since the early twenty-first century—until the pandemic. Interestingly, international travel involving the United States was almost 30% in 1950 but has slowly declined to about 15% by 2018. Interestingly, Africa and the Middle East each accounted for less than 1% of international travel in 1950 but had both increased to nearly 5% by 2018.[1]

Travel rates by specific forms of travel and deaths due to specific forms of travel have changed markedly since 1950. For example, commercial aviation as the most common means of travel has increased dramatically since 1950; however, the rate

Pediatr Clin N Am 69 (2022) xv–xvi
https://doi.org/10.1016/j.pcl.2021.09.010

of deaths per million flights has decreased even more so. Thus, while in the 1950s there was an average of five to six deaths per million flights, since 2010, there has been less than one death per million flights.[1]

However, this substantial decrease in aviation-caused deaths during international travel has been obliterated by the even more substantial decline in tourism-related flights. Indeed, the impact of COVID-19 on aviation has been dramatic. From 2019 (pre-COVID) through 2021, there has been a 73% decline in tourism-aviation. That means there were one billion fewer international travelers in 2020 compared with 2019.[2] Specifically, there were 1.461 *billion* international tourist-travelers in 2020 compared with 381 *million* in 2019.[3]

So, what does this have to do with pediatric infectious diseases? Frankly, at this point, we are not certain. The good news is children—including those under the age of 12 years who cannot be vaccinated as of the time I am writing this—have experienced significantly lower rates of COVID-19 than adults. The very significant decline during this same timeframe in rates of other readily transmitted diseases, such as influenza, has been well described by many. However, much of that decline was doubtless attributable to the "lock-downs" that many families—parents from work and children from school—endured. I am writing this editorial in September 2021, just as we seem to be beginning to see the decline of yet another surge in COVID-19 infections throughout the United States, approximately 90% of which has been attributed to the Delta variant of COVID-19. This mutant is susceptible to the three approved vaccines against COVID-19 in the United States. But the Delta variant persevered and found the alarmingly high numbers of adults who had elected not to be vaccinated and the children who were too young to be included in the vaccine-approved populations.

In summary, this issue of *Pediatric Clinics of North America* serves us well as the diseases it focuses on are still with us, in all likelihood will remain with us for some time, and will continue to increase in prevalence as our country's population returns to, and our country's governance opens its doors to, international tourism.

Bonita F. Stanton, MD
Hackensack Meridian
School of Medicine
Academic Enterprise
Hackensack Meridian Health
123 Metro Boulevard
Nutley, NJ 07110, USA

E-mail address:
bonita.stanton@hmhn.org

REFERENCES

1. Roser M. Tourism. Our world in data. 2017. Available at: https://ourworldindata.org/tourism. Accessed: September 25, 2021.
2. Milesi-Ferretti GM. The COVID-19 travel shock hit tourism-dependent economies hard. Available at: https://www.brookings.edu/research/the-covid-19-travel-shock-hit-tourism-dependent-economieshard/#:~:text=The%20COVID%20crisis%20has%20led,120%20million%20direct%20tourism%20jobs. Accessed September 26, 2021.
3. Hiltner S, Fisher L. How bad was 2020 for tourism? Look at the numbers. New York Times. July 27. 2021. Available at: https://www.nytimes.com/2021/03/08/travel/tourism-2020-coronavirus.html. Accessed May 25, 2021.

Preface

Exotic Infections Are Only One Plane Away

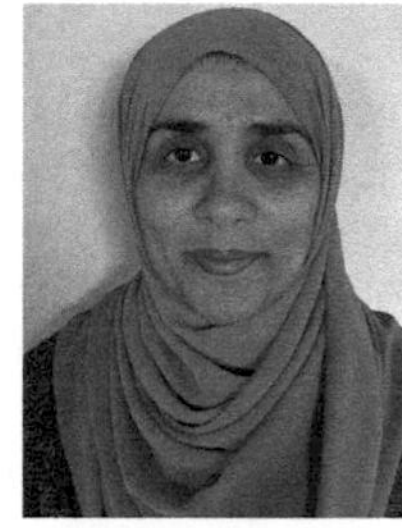

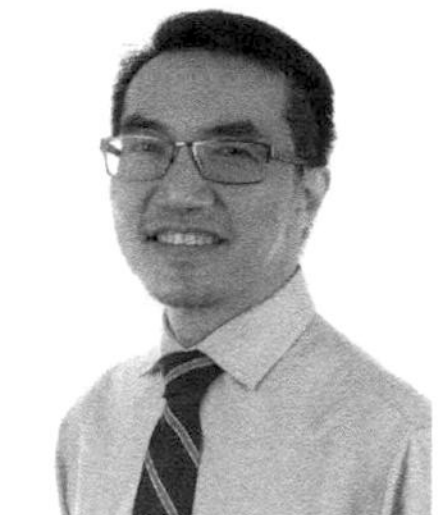

Fouzia Naeem, MD, MSc   Chokechai Rongkavilit, MD
Editors

International travel is increasingly common. Over 93 million US citizens, including children and teens, traveled outside the country for business and leisure purposes in 2018. Travel continued to increase until 2020 when it dropped to 9.8 million due to the COVID-19 pandemic. Travel medicine has become an essential field owing to the rapid growth in international travel, particularly in the developing world. Travel, especially to low- and middle-income countries, is significantly associated with an increased risk of infections, many of which are not seen in high-income countries.

Individuals visiting friends, relatives, and long-stay travelers are at a greater risk of acquiring malaria, enteric fever, hepatitis A, tuberculosis, multidrug-resistant organisms, intestinal parasites, and others. This is likely due to prolonged stays and closer proximity to the local population. Only a minority of international travelers seek pretravel counseling for preventive measures, chemoprophylaxis, and vaccinations before travel. Essential knowledge on travel medicine and specific infections unique to a certain geographic region allows pediatricians to provide proper counseling and implement a timely diagnostic test and management if such an infection is encountered.

This issue of *Pediatric Clinics of North America* is a collaborative work of various pediatric specialists from all over the world to provide a comprehensive review on the international aspect of infectious diseases in children. The content offers up-to-date information on distinct infections as well as antimicrobial resistance. Antimicrobial resistance is an emerging global threat in low- and middle-income countries with limited access to appropriate medical care. One reason for this increase is the overuse of antimicrobials, which is likely worsened by the COVID-19 pandemic. Our focus is to create awareness among pediatricians about the increasing threat of antimicrobial

Pediatr Clin N Am 69 (2022) xvii–xviii
https://doi.org/10.1016/j.pcl.2021.09.009

resistance and the dynamic change of various infections, with a consideration being prioritized for those practicing in resource-limited settings.

Fouzia Naeem, MD, MSc
Division of Pediatric Infectious Diseases
Department of Pediatrics
Valley Children's Healthcare
Stanford University School of Medicine (Affiliated)
Madera, CA 93636, USA

Chokechai Rongkavilit, MD
Division of Pediatric Infectious Diseases
Department of Pediatrics
University of California San Francisco
Fresno Branch Campus
155 North Fresno Street
Fresno, CA 93701, USA

E-mail addresses:
fnaeem@valleychildrens.org (F. Naeem)
chokechai.rongkavilit@ucsf.edu (C. Rongkavilit)

Prevention of Mother-to-Child Human Immunodeficiency Virus Transmission in Resource-Limited Countries

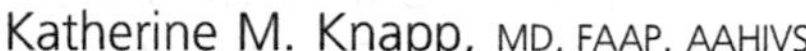

Katherine M. Knapp, MD, FAAP, AAHIVS

KEYWORDS

• Prevention of mother-to-child transmission (PMTCT) • HIV • Resource-limited • Guidelines • Antiretroviral therapy (ART)

KEY POINTS

- Mother-to-child transmission (MTCT) of human immunodeficiency virus (HIV) has been virtually eliminated in resource-rich countries, but in 2018, there were an estimated 160,000 children worldwide newly infected with HIV.
- Sub-Saharan Africa, which has been hardest hit by the HIV epidemic, has seen some of the greatest declines in rates of new infections and in MTCT: in South Africa, where 7.5 million people are living with HIV, the MTCT rate dropped to 3%.
- An estimated 65% of MTCT is at or around the time of delivery, even among breastfed populations.
- Although virologic control is of paramount importance, it is not the sole factor in preventing MTCT of HIV: transmission has occurred even in women with undetectable viral loads.

INTRODUCTION

AIDS, now known to be a sequela of infection with human immunodeficiency virus (HIV), was first recognized in 1981, and the first pediatric cases were reported the following year.[1–3] Soon thereafter, cases began being reported from around the globe. A decade later, the World Health Organization (WHO) estimated there were more than 500,000 pediatric AIDS cases resulting from mother-to-child transmission (MTCT), 90% of which were in sub-Saharan Africa.[4] Although the rate of new infections globally has been cut in half since the peak of the pandemic, HIV remains a public health threat, and rates of new infections continue to increase in Eastern Europe, central Asia, the

Department of Infectious Diseases, St. Jude Children's Research Hospital, 262 Danny Thomas Place, Mail Stop 600, Memphis, TN 38105, USA
E-mail address: katherine.knapp@stjude.org

Pediatr Clin N Am 69 (2022) 1–18
https://doi.org/10.1016/j.pcl.2021.08.007
pediatric.theclinics.com

Middle East, North Africa, and Latin America.[5,6] MTCT of HIV has now been virtually eliminated in many parts of the world but remains an issue in resource-limited countries.

ANTIRETROVIRALS IN THE PREVENTION OF MOTHER-TO-CHILD TRANSMISSION OF HUMAN IMMUNODEFICIENCY VIRUS

Zidovudine (ZDV), also known as 3′-azido-3′-deoxythymidine (AZT), was the first antiretroviral therapy (ART) available, approved by the Food and Drug Administration in 1987. The drug had not then been evaluated in pregnancy and could not be recommended for treatment of pregnant women. In 1990, the AIDS Clinical Trials Group (ACTG) surveyed sites to obtain information about women who were already taking ZDV when they became pregnant.[7] The ACTG received data for 43 women from 17 sites, more than half of whom took ZDV for at least 2 trimesters of pregnancy. ZDV was found to be well tolerated and safe, and not associated with congenital anomalies. Pharmacokinetic studies demonstrated that ZDV crossed the placenta well.[8,9]

Based on available data suggesting ZDV was not associated with adverse effects during the pregnancy or to the fetus, the Pediatric ACTG (PACTG) developed a protocol to assess its efficacy in PMTCT.[10] PACTG protocol 076 was a double-blind, placebo-controlled trial enrolling pregnant women between 14 and 34 weeks' gestation. Of note, these women were at most only mildly symptomatic; the inclusion criteria specified that they have a $CD4^+$ count greater than 200 cells/mm^3 and not otherwise meet criteria for antiretroviral treatment. PACTG 076 enrolled women at 59 centers in the United States and in France, beginning in April 1991. The treatment regimen consisted of ZDV administration to the mother antepartum (AP) and intrapartum (IP; 2 mg/kg intravenously [IV] over 1 hour, then 1 mg/kg/h until delivery), and to the newborn for 6 weeks after birth. At the first interim analysis in December 1993, it was determined that 8.3% of the infants in the ZDV group was infected, compared with 25.5% in the placebo group. With this evidence that ZDV reduced the transmission rate by two-thirds, the study was stopped early, and all participants were offered treatment. This was the landmark study demonstrating antiretrovirals could prevent MTCT of HIV.

The results of the 076 study were announced in early 1994 and quickly adopted in the United States and other resource-abundant countries, leading to marked declines in the rate of perinatal HIV transmission.[11,12] However, the findings of the 076 study did have some limitations: eligible women were relatively healthy, had not previously been treated, and were not enrolled until after the first trimester. It remained to be seen if these results could translate to all pregnant women living with HIV. Furthermore, the cost of this long treatment course could limit its feasibility in resource-limited settings.

Following demonstrated efficacy of ZDV in PMTCT, several studies evaluated shorter AP courses (ie, beginning at 36 weeks' gestation), in both breastfed and formula-fed populations.[13–17] These short-course ZDV regimens were effective, but longer courses have been demonstrated to be more effective.[18]

The Perinatal HIV Prevention Trial-1 (Thailand) was a randomized, double-blind trial of 4 ZDV regimens with the same IP component but varying AP-postpartum (PP) components: long-long, long-short, short-long, and short-short.[18] The long AP course began at 28 weeks' gestation, and the short AP began at 35 weeks. The long PP arm was a 6-week course for the infant, and the short PP course was for only 3 days. At the first interim analysis, the short-short arm was discontinued. The long-long arm was similar to the 076 regimen but used oral rather than IV IP administration and was as effective. However, the long-long arm was significantly less expensive than the 076 regimen (less than one-fourth the cost), making it a viable option in resource-limited countries.

The availability of nevirapine (NVP) offered an attractive alternative to ZDV in PMTCT. NVP is rapidly absorbed after oral administration, quickly crosses the placenta, and has a long half-life. The HIVNET 012 study in Uganda compared ZDV to NVP when given IP to the women and PP to the infants only.[19] In the NVP arm, women received a single dose (sd) at the onset of labor, and infants received sdNVP within 72 hours of birth. This regimen was found to be efficacious and was quickly adopted as a simple, inexpensive, viable option for PMTCT in resource-limited countries.[20]

Table 1 provides a summary of selected studies of antiretroviral prophylaxis for PMTCT in resource-limited settings.[13–19,21,22]

ANTIRETROVIRAL THERAPY FOR MATERNAL HEALTH AND PREVENTION OF MOTHER-TO-CHILD TRANSMISSION OF HUMAN IMMUNODEFICIENCY VIRUS

As ART became more available in resource-limited countries, more pregnant women were meeting criteria for treatment for their own health. In 2006, a $CD4^+$ count $\leq$200 cells/mm^3 was the threshold for which treatment was recommended for all.[23] The 2010 guidelines increased that threshold to $\leq$350 cells/mm^3.[24] **Table 2** provides WHO guidelines for PMTCT through 2013.[23–25]

The Promoting Maternal and Infant Survival Everywhere (PROMISE) study began in 2011 and assessed maternal ART vs prophylaxis for PMTCT in women with $CD4^+$ counts greater than 350 cells/mm^3.[26] This study was conducted in India, Malawi, South Africa, Tanzania, Uganda, Zambia, and Zimbabwe. PROMISE compared the following: (1) ZDV plus sdNVP at delivery followed by tenofovir disoproxil fumarate (TDF) plus emtricitabine (FTC) for 1 to 2 weeks' PP ("zidovudine alone" arm); (2) ZDV plus lamivudine (3TC) plus lopinavir-ritonavir (LPV/r) ("zidovudine-based ART"); and (3) TDF plus FTC plus LPV/r ("tenofovir-based ART"). In that trial, the transmission rate was low for all 3 arms, but significantly lower in the ART arms than in the ZDV alone arm (0.5% vs 1.8%).

The Strategic Timing of Antiretroviral Therapy (START) study was designed to assess risks and benefits of immediate initiation of ART in nonpregnant adults with $CD4^+$ counts $\geq$500 cells/mm^3 compared with deferring treatment until the $CD4^+$ count was $\leq$350 cells/mm^3.[27] The START study was a large international study conducted in 35 countries that began enrolling in 2009. At an interim monitoring analysis in May 2015, it was recommended that the findings be disseminated immediately and that all participants in the deferred-initiation arm be offered ART. The immediate initiation of ART was superior to deferred initiation for both serious AIDS-related and non-AIDS–related events, and there were no safety concerns, providing evidence for immediate initiation of ART in all people living with HIV (PLWH), regardless of $CD4^+$ count.

The START study results support the ambitious goals of the WHO and the Joint United Nations Programme on HIV/AIDS (UNAIDS) to greatly expand access to ART for all with hopes of ending the epidemic by 2030.[28,29]

EFFECT OF INCREASED AVAILABILITY OF ANTIRETROVIRAL THERAPY ON PREVENTION OF MOTHER-TO-CHILD TRANSMISSION IN RESOURCE-LIMITED COUNTRIES

In 2014, UNAIDS/WHO announced new global HIV targets to achieve by 2020: 90% of PLWH will know their HIV status, 90% of PLWH will be receiving ART, and 90% of

Table 1
Summary of selected studies of antiretrovirals for prevention of mother-to-child transmission in resource-limited settings

Study	Antiretrovirals	Antepartum (AP)	Intrapartum (IP)	Postpartum (PP) (Mother)	Infant	Comments
CDC short-course ZDV: Côte d'Ivoire[13,16]	ZDV vs placebo	Short (from 36 wk)	Oral	—	—	Transmission 22.5% (ZDV) vs 30.2% (placebo) at 24 mo (breastfed)
CDC short-course ZDV: Thailand[14]	ZDV vs placebo	Short (from 36 wk)	Oral	—	—	Transmission 9.4% (ZDV) vs 18.9% (placebo) at 6 mo (formula-fed)
PETRA: South Africa, Tanzania, Uganda[15]	ZDV + 3TC vs placebo 4 arms: AP/IP/PP, IP/PP, IP-only, placebo	Short (from 36 wk)	Oral	Short (1 wk)	Short (1 wk)	Transmission at 18 mo by arm: AP/IP/PP: 14.9% IP/PP: 18.1% IP-only: 20% Placebo: 22.2% (breastfed and formula-fed)
DITRAME: Côte d'Ivoire, Burkina Faso[16,17]	ZDV vs placebo	Short (from 36 wk)	Oral	Short (1 wk)	—	Transmission 22.5% (ZDV) vs 30.2% (placebo) at 24 mo (breastfed)
Perinatal HIV Prevention Trial-1: Thailand[18]	ZDV, 4 arms with different lengths of AP and PP treatment: short-short, short-long, long-short, long-long	Short (from 36 wk) or long (from 28 wk)	Oral	—	Short (3 d) or long (6 wk)	Transmission 10.5% in short-short arm: this arm discontinued at first interim analysis Transmission at 6 mo by arm: Long-long: 6.5% Long-short: 4.7% Significantly higher in utero MTCT with short AP: 5.1% vs 1.6% (formula-fed)

HIVNET 012: Uganda[21]	sd NVP vs. ZDV	—	Oral sdNVP vs ZDV	—	sdNVP within 72 h of birth vs ZDV × 1 wk	Transmission 15.7% (NVP) vs 25.8% (ZDV) at 18 mo (breastfed)
SAINT: South Africa[22]	sdNVP vs. ZDV +3TC	—	Oral sdNVP vs ZDV + 3TC	sdNVP within 48 h of delivery vs ZDV + 3TC for 1 wk	sdNVP within 48 h of birth vs ZDV + 3TC for 1 wk	Transmission 12.3% (NVP) vs 9.3% (ZDV) at 8 wk

Table 2
Evolution of World Health Organization guidelines for prevention of mother-to-child transmission (2006–2013 versions)

Year	Population	Antepartum (AP)	Intrapartum (IP)	Postpartum (PP)	Infant
2006[23]	Women meeting criteria for ART: • $CD4^+$ ≤200 cells/mm^3 • WHO clinical stage 3 if $CD4^+$ ≤350 cells/mm^3 • WHO clinical stage 4 (if $CD4^+$ not available, treat for stage 3 or 4)	Recommended regimen: AZT + 3TC + NVP			AZT × 7 d (if mother received <4 wk ART, infant should receive AZT × 4 wk)
	Women not meeting criteria for ART	AZT beginning at 28 wk	sdNVP + AZT + 3TC (If woman received >4 wk AZT during pregnancy, may omit IP/PP prophylaxis)	AZT + 3TC × 7 d	sdNVP + AZT × 7 d (if mother did not receive NVP, infant's dose should be given as soon as possible after birth)
2010[24]	Women meeting criteria for ART: • $CD4^+$ ≤350 cells/mm^3 • WHO clinical stage 3 or 4	Recommended regimens: AZT + 3TC + NVP AZT + 3TC + EFV			AZT or NVP × 4–6 wk
	Women not meeting criteria for ART Option A	AZT beginning at 14 wk	Only if mother received <4 wk AZT: sdNVP + AZT + 3TC	Only if mother received <4 wk AZT: AZT + 3TC × 7 d	Breast-feeding: sdNVP at birth, then daily NVP until 1 wk after cessation of breast-milk feeds Not breast-feeding: sdNVP at birth, then daily AZT or NVP × 4–6 wk
	Option B	ART beginning at 14 wk until 1 week after cessation of breastmilk feeds. Recommended regimens: AZT + 3TC + LPV/r; AZT + 3TC + ABC; AZT + 3TC + EFV; TDF + (3TC or FTC) + EFV			All infants: AZT or NVP × 4–6 wk

2013[25]	All women receive ART during pregnancy and breast-feeding	Option B • Lifelong treatment for women who meet criteria: $CD4^+$ ≤500 cells/mm^3, WHO clinical stage 3 or 4, or per national guidelines. • For women not meeting the above criteria for treatment based on $CD4^+$ count or WHO clinical stage, or not eligible per national guidelines, discontinue ART after cessation of breast-feeding Option B+ • Lifelong treatment for all	Breast-feeding: NVP × 6 wk Not breast-feeding: AZT or NVP × 4–6 wk

Abbreviations: ABC, abacavir; EFV, efavirenz.

those receiving ART will have viral suppression.[28] Modeling suggested that achieving these targets would mean that at least 73% of all PLWH would be virally suppressed (a 2- to 3-fold increase) and that, if these targets were met, the epidemic would end by 2030. In September 2015, the WHO announced that the 2016 guidelines would recommend lifelong ART for all PLWH.[29] In September 2020, UNAIDS provided an update on the progress toward achieving the 90-90-90 goals.[30] As of the end of 2019, 81% of PLWH knew their HIV status, 67% of PLWH were receiving ART, and almost 59% of those on ART achieved viral suppression. Undoubtedly, the coronavirus disease 2019 (COVID-19) pandemic has affected progress toward achieving these targets.

The most recent WHO guidelines also offer new recommendations about using nucleic acid testing at birth to improve early infant diagnosis and using combination prophylaxis for infants at high risk of acquiring HIV infection.[29] The WHO recommends using ZDV + NVP for 6 weeks in infants at high risk, with consideration for extending infant prophylaxis to 12 weeks (with ZDV + NVP or NVP alone) in breastfed infants at high risk of infection.

The global decrease in new infections is in large part due to decreased incidence in eastern and southern Africa (38% reduction since 2010).[31] This region has also seen the most rapid scale-up in availability of treatment and has seen the most significant decrease in AIDS-related mortality (49% decrease since 2010). Incidence:prevalence ratios have been decreasing in this region as well, reflecting a decrease in new infections and PLWH living longer. The global incidence:prevalence ratio decreased to 4.4% in 2019, and in eastern and southern Africa, the ratio decreased to 3.5%, making it likely to achieve the 3% ratio seen in resource-rich parts of the world. Twenty-five countries have reached the 3% milestone, including countries with large epidemics, such as South Africa and Zimbabwe (**Table 3**). MTCT of HIV also decreased from 2010 to 2019 in all of the countries in eastern and southern Africa for which data were available. In South Africa, which has the highest prevalence of HIV in the world (7.5 million PLWH), the MTCT rate, including during breast-feeding, dropped to 3%. However, although rates are dropping overall, the percentage of new infections among women of child-bearing age is increasing in this region, underscoring the importance of prevention measures targeting young women.

Other regions have not made as much progress in PMTCT and decreasing rates of new HIV infections. **Table 4** describes new HIV infections and measures for PMTCT by global region. In western and central Africa, only 58% of PLWH, including pregnant women, were receiving ART in 2019. It is estimated that 42% of pediatric infections in this region in 2019 was because pregnant women did not receive ART during pregnancy, and 18% was due to women not receiving ART during breast-feeding. Among western and central African nations for which data are available, 3 countries actually showed decreases in the percentage of pregnant women receiving ART: Cameroon (10%), Gambia (49%), and Niger (43%). The MTCT rates in these 3 countries increased (Gambia, 28%; Niger, 24%) or remained the same (Cameroon, 30%).

However, significant progress has been made toward elimination of MTCT (EMTCT) in the Caribbean, where new perinatal infections have decreased by almost half since 2010. In Cuba, all women have access to ART during pregnancy, and the transmission rate there has dropped to 4%. In 2015, Cuba was the first country to meet criteria specified by the WHO to receive their validation for commitment to EMTCT as a public health problem.[32] Twelve other nations, many also in the Caribbean, have since met these criteria: Armenia, Belarus, Thailand, Anguilla, Antigua and Barbuda, Bermuda, Cayman Islands, Montserrat, St. Christopher and Nevis, Malaysia, Sri Lanka, and Maldives.

Table 3
Status of the human immunodeficiency virus epidemic and mother-to-child transmission in Eastern and Southern Africa (regional and country-specific data)[a]

Region/ Country	Incidence: Prevalence Ratio	90-90-90 Goals (Estimated Percentages with Ranges)			Prevention of Mother-to-Child Transmission (Estimated Percentages with Ranges)		
		PLWH Who Know Their HIV Status	PLWH on ART	PLWH on ART Who Are Virally Suppressed	Pregnant Women on ART	Infants Tested by 8 wk of Age	Transmission Rate
Eastern and southern Africa regional data	3.5	87% (77%–97%)	72% (62%–81%)	65% (57%–72%)	95% (71%–100%)	68% (57%–91%)	8% (6%–10%)
Angola	7.56	62% (52%–73%)	27% (23%–32%)	—	63% (47%–79%)	7.4% (5.9%–9.7%)	19% (15%–22%)
Botswana	2.49	92% (82%–99%)	82% (74%–89%)	79% (71%–86%)	100% (86%–100%)	84.6% (74->95%)	2% (2%–2%)
Comoros	4.65	82% (45%–100%)	60% (32%–100%)	51% (28%–92%)	—	—	—
Eritrea	2.60	86% (63%–100%)	62% (45%–84%)	53% (39%–71%)	39% (26%–55%)	21.1% (14.8%–31.6%)	24% (16%–28%)
Eswatini (formerly Swaziland)	2.23	98% (91%–100%)	96% (88%–100%)	92% (85%–100%)	100% (88%–100%)	—	2% (2%–3%)
Ethiopia	2.22	82% (63%–100%)	74% (57%–95%)	66% (51%–85%)	74% (52%–99%)	—	17% (12%–23%)
Kenya	2.77	90% (79%–100%)	74% (65%–86%)	68% (60%–79%)	94% (73%–100%)	68.8% (56.9%–89%)	11% (8%–15%)
Lesotho	3.22	93% (87%–99%)	65% (61%–70%)	61% (57%–65%)	84% (65%–98%)	73.4% (63.1%–94.6%)	9% (6%–11%)
Madagascar	15.14	15% (12%–19%)	13% (11%–17%)	—	24% (20%–32%)	—	35% (32%–39%)
Malawi	3.10	90% (81%–95%)	79% (71%–84%)	72% (65%–77%)	100% (77%–100%)	76.2% (65.6->95%)	6% (5%–8%)
Mauritius	—	69% (59%–80%)	25% (22%–29%)	17% (15%–20%)	100% (100%–100%)	—	13% (12%–14%)
Mozambique	5.92	77% (62%–96%)	60% (48%–74%)	45% (36%–56%)	100% (74%–100%)	70.8% (52.9% to >95%)	14% (11%–18%)

(continued on next page)

Table 3
(continued)

Region/ Country	Incidence: Prevalence Ratio	90-90-90 Goals (Estimated Percentages with Ranges)			Prevention of Mother-to-Child Transmission (Estimated Percentages with Ranges)		
		PLWH Who Know Their HIV Status	PLWH on ART	PLWH on ART Who Are Virally Suppressed	Pregnant Women on ART	Infants Tested by 8 wk of Age	Transmission Rate
Namibia	3.29	95% (88%–100%)	85% (79%–91%)	78% (72%–84%)	100% (94%–100%)	>95% (89.7% to >95%)	4% (3%–5%)
Rwanda	2.30	89% (79%–97%)	87% (77%–95%)	79% (71%–87%)	99% (79%–100%)	86.6% (74.8% to >95%)	6% (5%–9%)
Seychelles	—	—	—	—	—	—	—
South Africa	2.63	92% (85%–98%)	70% (64%–74%)	64% (58%–68%)	97% (69%–100%)	83.3% (69.5% to >95%)	3% (3%–5%)
South Sudan	9.64	27% (20%–33%)	18% (14%–23%)	14% (11%–18%)	44% (31%–57%)	11.8% (9%–16.4%)	27% (24%–31%)
Uganda	3.66	89% (83%–98%)	84% (78%–92%)	75% (70%–83%)	100% (83%–100%)	56.3% (49.7%–68.2%)	6% (5%–8%)
United Republic of Tanzania	4.52	83% (75%–90%)	75% (67%–81%)	69% (62%–74%)	92% (72%–100%)	46.6% (40%–60.1%)	11% (9%–13%)
Zambia	4.08	90% (85%–97%)	85% (80%–92%)	77% (72%–82%)	86% (69%–76%)	70.3% (62.6%–87.3%)	11% (9%–13%)
Zimbabwe	2.92	90% (78%–100%)	85% (74%–97%)	73% (64%–84%)	91% (69%–100%)	55.7% (46.2%–73.1%)	8% (6%–11%)

[a] Data from the UNAIDS Data 2020 Report.[25]

Table 4
Status of the human immunodeficiency virus epidemic and mother-to-child transmission in global regions (where data available, ranges in parentheses)[a]

		New HIV Infections				PLWH on ART		Prevention of Mother-to-Child Transmission		
				Females as % of Total						
Region	Incidence: Prevalence Ratio	Overall Number	% Increase or Decrease Since 2010	15–24 y of Age	25–49 y of Age	PLWH on ART	Who Are Virally Suppressed	Pregnant Women on ART	Infants Tested by 8 wk of Age	Transmission Rate
Eastern and southern Africa	3.5 (2.8–4.5)	730,000 (580,000–940,000)	↓38	30	30	72% (62%–81%)	65% (57%–72%)	95% (71%–100%)	68% (57%–91%)	8% (6%–10%)
Western and central Africa	4.9 (3.1–8)	240,000 (150,000–390,000)	↓25	27	33	58% (44%–75%)	45% (36%–58%)	58% (40%–78%)	33% (25%–47%)	20% (16%–24%)
Middle east and north Africa	8.2 (4.4–15.6)	20,000 (11,000–38,000)	↑22	8	25	38% (25%–63%)	32% (22%–52%)	30% (21%–44%)	—	30% (25%–35%)
Eastern Europe and central Asia	10.1 (8.6–11.7)	170,000 (140,000–190,000)	↑72	6	30	44% (37%–50%)	41% (36%–46%)	—	—	—
Asia and the Pacific	5.1 (3.6–6.7)	300,000 210,000–390,000)	↓12	11	19	60% (43%–75%)	55% (41%–68%)	56% (42%–71%)	37% (30%–45%)	26% 20%–29%)
Latin America	5.7 (3.5–8.3)	120,000 (73,000–180,000)	↑21	6	17	60% (38%–81%)	53% (35%–71%)	74% (49%–98%)	35% (27%–43%)	15% (12%–18%)

(*continued on next page*)

Table 4
(*continued*)

Region	Incidence: Prevalence Ratio	New HIV Infections		Females as % of Total		PLWH on ART		Prevention of Mother-to-Child Transmission		
		Overall Number	% Increase or Decrease Since 2010	15–24 y of Age	25–49 y of Age	PLWH on ART	Who Are Virally Suppressed	Pregnant Women on ART	Infants Tested by 8 wk of Age	Transmission Rate
Caribbean	3.9 (2.6–5.7)	13,000 (8700–19,000)	↓29	16	22	63% (49%–77%)	50% (41%–61%)	86% (67%–100%)	56% (46%–70%)	12% (9%–16%)
Western (WE) and Central (CE) Europe and North America (NA)	3.0 (2.2–4.0)	65,000 (49,000–87,000)	↓30% (WE) ↑45% (CE) —	4	15	81% (62%–98%)	67% (53%–80%)	—	—	—

[a] Data from the UNAIDS Data 2020 Report.[25]

FACTORS INFLUENCING RISK OF MOTHER-TO-CHILD TRANSMISSION

The data above show that in areas where pregnant women have access to ART, the MTCT rates have declined significantly. However, transmission still occurs, even in resource-rich countries, so obviously ensuring access to ART is not enough for EMTCT.[33] Although virologic control is of paramount importance, it is not the sole factor in preventing MTCT. Transmission has occurred even in women with undetectable viral loads.[33–36]

MTCT may occur in utero, during labor and delivery, or PP through breast-feeding. In utero infection has been defined by polymerase chain reaction detection of HIV in an infant during the first 2 days of life and is estimated to account for 35% to 40% of cases of MTCT in non-breast-feeding populations.[37–39] It is thought that most in utero transmission occurs during the third trimester.[39,40] A study in a breast-feeding population estimated 26% of transmission occurred in utero, 65% occurred IP or early PP, and 12% occurred late PP (defined as a first positive test after 3–5 months of age).[41]

COINFECTIONS

Lower genital tract infections (including bacterial vaginosis, vulvovaginal candidiasis, *Trichomonas vaginalis*, and herpes simplex virus [HSV]) are known to increase mucosal expression and facilitate transmission of HIV.[42] Active infections in the IP period increase the infant's exposure to HIV. Breast infections may also increase transmission via breast-feeding, and women should be advised to seek treatment immediately for mastitis.[43]

HSV lesions in HIV-infected persons show high levels of HIV RNA. Several studies have shown HSV infection to be a risk factor for MTCT of HIV.[44–48] In a study in Thailand, stored maternal plasma and cervicovaginal samples were tested for HSV-2 antibodies and DNA.[47] Of 307 women for whom samples were available, 74.3% were HSV-2 seropositive and 7.8% were shedding HSV-2 at the time of delivery. HSV-2 shedding was associated with HIV transmission, independent of HIV RNA levels in the plasma or cervicovaginal samples. In a Zimbabwe study, 82.5% of women were seropositive for HSV-2 at delivery.[48] In that study, the investigators found that HSV-2 coinfection may have accounted for greater than 25% of the IP HIV transmission. Thus, prevention and proper treatment of HSV play a role in prevention of MTCT of HIV.

INTRAPARTUM FACTORS

Several studies have associated prolonged rupture of membranes before delivery with increased risk of MTCT of HIV.[49–51] This observation suggested that cesarean section before the onset of labor might prevent transmission. Cesarean sections are recommended in resource-rich countries for women with viral loads above a threshold level (>1000 in the United States), but this is not a feasible strategy in resource-limited countries.[52]

RISKS ASSOCIATED WITH BREAST-FEEDING

Transmission via breast-feeding is low in women with virologic control who are receiving ART; therefore, plasma viral load may be an indicator of viral load in the breast milk.[53,54] In a study in Kenya, HIV was detected in breast milk samples in 89% of the women, with a viral load range of less than 30 to 426,580 copies/mL.[54] The median viral load was significantly higher in colostrum/early milk (ie, collected within first 10 days of life) than in breast milk samples obtained later. Breast milk viral load did correlate with plasma viral load and MTCT. Each 10-fold increase in viral load in the breast milk increased the risk of transmission 2-fold. Of 138 women for whom more than 1 breast milk sample was available, 56.5% intermittently had detectable HIV. Sixty percent of the women who transmitted infection to their infants were constant shedders, and 40% were intermittent shedders. The WHO recommends that women take ART throughout breast-feeding.

Because of the risk of transmission via breast milk, breast-feeding is not recommended for women living with HIV in resource-rich countries. In resource-poor countries, where limited access to alternative food sources and unsafe water supplies are common, the benefits of breast-feeding outweigh the risks.[54] The WHO recommends either exclusive breast-feeding for at least 6 months while receiving ART or no breast-feeding.[55]

THE PREVENTION OF MOTHER-TO-CHILD TRANSMISSION CASCADE AND OPPORTUNITIES FOR IMPROVED INTERVENTIONS

The PMTCT Cascade defines the opportunities for intervention in the path from identifying HIV-infected pregnant women to final determination of HIV status of their infants.[56] Provision of ART alone is not sufficient to end HIV transmission. The most effective way to prevent MTCT is to prevent infection in the mother. For women who are infected, it is important to identify infection early, preferably before pregnancy. Women should plan for the birth and access a medical facility for delivery if possible. Women identified during pregnancy need to be linked to an HIV care provider and have access to family planning after delivery.

SUMMARY

The number of children infected with HIV each year continues to decline but remains unacceptably high. An estimated 1.5 million new infections in children have been prevented since 2010, but in 2018, there were an estimated 160,000 newly infected children.[57] The success in prevention is a result of lifelong ART becoming increasingly more available in resource-limited settings. There are many factors contributing to continued transmission, including undiagnosed infection, no antenatal care, nonadherence, and new infections during pregnancy or breast-feeding (with implications for need for repeat testing). Also of concern is the growing rate of infections in women of childbearing age in sub-Saharan Africa.

CLINICS CARE POINTS

- All pregnant women living with human immunodeficiency virus (HIV) should receive lifelong antiretroviral therapy for both maternal health and prevention of mother-to-child transmission.
- In resource-poor countries with unsafe water supplies and limited access to alternative food sources, the benefits of breast-feeding outweigh the risks of HIV transmission. Women living with HIV should remain on ART while breast-feeding and should breast-feed exclusively for at least 6 months.
- Adolescent girls and young women account for about a third of new infections in sub-Saharan Africa; targeted efforts are needed for prevention and early detection of HIV infection in these populations.

DISCLOSURE

The author has nothing to disclose.

REFERENCES

1. Centers for Disease Control (CDC). Pneumocystis pneumonia–Los Angeles. MMWR Morb Mortal Wkly Rep 1981;30(21):250–2.
2. Centers for Disease Control (CDC). A cluster of Kaposi's sarcoma and Pneumocystis carinii pneumonia among homosexual male residents of Los Angeles and Orange Counties, California. MMWR Morb Mortal Wkly Rep 1982;31(23):305–7.
3. Centers for Disease Control (CDC). Unexplained immunodeficiency and opportunistic infections in infants–New York, New Jersey, California. MMWR Morb Mortal Wkly Rep 1982;31(49):665–7.
4. World Health Organization Global Programme on AIDS. Current and future dimensions of the HIV/AIDS pandemic: a capsule summary. 1991. Available at: https://apps.who.int/iris/handle/10665/60567. Accessed June 10, 2021.
5. Joint United Nations Programme on HIV/AIDS (UNAIDS). Global HIV & AIDS statistics fact sheet. Available at: https://www.unaids.org/en/resources/fact-sheet. Accessed June 10, 2021.
6. Joint United Nations Programme on HIV/AIDS (UNAIDS). UNAIDS data 2020. Available at: https://www.unaids.org/en/resources/documents/2020/unaids-data. Accessed June 10, 2021.
7. Sperling RS, Stratton P, O'Sullivan MJ, et al. A survey of zidovudine use in pregnant women with human immunodeficiency virus infection. N Engl J Med 1992; 326(13):857–61.
8. Watts DH, Brown ZA, Tartaglione T, et al. Pharmacokinetic disposition of zidovudine during pregnancy. J Infect Dis 1991;163(2):226–32.
9. O'Sullivan MJ, Boyer PJ, Scott GB, et al. The pharmacokinetics and safety of zidovudine in the third trimester of pregnancy for women infected with human immunodeficiency virus and their infants: phase I acquired immunodeficiency syndrome clinical trials group study (protocol 082). Zidovudine Collaborative Working Group. Am J Obstet Gynecol 1993;168(5):1510–6.
10. Connor EM, Sperling RS, Gelber R, et al. Reduction of maternal-infant transmission of human immunodeficiency virus type 1 with zidovudine treatment. Pediatric AIDS Clinical Trials Group Protocol 076 Study Group. N Engl J Med 1994;331(18): 1173–80.
11. Centers for Disease Control and Prevention (CDC). Zidovudine for the prevention of HIV transmission from mother to infant. MMWR Morb Mortal Wkly Rep 1994; 43(16):285–7.
12. Cooper ER, Nugent RP, Diaz C, et al. After AIDS clinical trial 076: the changing pattern of zidovudine use during pregnancy, and the subsequent reduction in the vertical transmission of human immunodeficiency virus in a cohort of infected women and their infants. Women and Infants Transmission Study Group. J Infect Dis 1996;174(6):1207–11.
13. Wiktor SZ, Ekpini E, Karon JM, et al. Short-course oral zidovudine for prevention of mother-to-child transmission of HIV-1 in Abidjan, Côte d'Ivoire: a randomised trial. Lancet 1999;353(9155):781–5.
14. Shaffer N, Chuachoowong R, Mock PA, et al. Short-course zidovudine for perinatal HIV-1 transmission in Bangkok, Thailand: a randomised controlled trial. Bangkok Collaborative Perinatal HIV Transmission Study Group. Lancet 1999; 353(9155):773–80.

15. Petra Study Team. Efficacy of three short-course regimens of zidovudine and lamivudine in preventing early and late transmission of HIV-1 from mother to child in Tanzania, South Africa, and Uganda (Petra study): a randomised, double-blind, placebo-controlled trial. Lancet 2002;359(9313):1178–86.
16. Leroy V, Karon JM, Alioum A, et al. Twenty-four month efficacy of a maternal short-course zidovudine regimen to prevent mother-to-child transmission of HIV-1 in West Africa. AIDS 2002;16(4):631–41.
17. Dabis F, Msellati P, Meda N, et al. 6-month efficacy, tolerance, and acceptability of a short regimen of oral zidovudine to reduce vertical transmission of HIV in breastfed children in Côte d'Ivoire and Burkina Faso: a double-blind placebo-controlled multicentre trial. DITRAME Study Group. DIminution de la Transmission Mère-Enfant. Lancet 1999;353(9155):786–92.
18. Lallemant M, Jourdain G, Le Coeur S, et al. A trial of shortened zidovudine regimens to prevent mother-to-child transmission of human immunodeficiency virus type 1. Perinatal HIV Prevention Trial (Thailand) Investigators. N Engl J Med 2000; 343(14):982–91.
19. Guay LA, Musoke P, Fleming T, et al. Intrapartum and neonatal single-dose nevirapine compared with zidovudine for prevention of mother-to-child transmission of HIV-1 in Kampala, Uganda: HIVNET 012 randomised trial. Lancet 1999; 354(9181):795–802.
20. World Health Organization. Antiretroviral drugs for treating pregnant women and preventing HIV infections in infants. Guidelines on care, treatment and support for women living with HIV/AIDS and their children in resource-constrained settings. Available at: https://www.who.int/hiv/pub/mtct/en/arvdrugsguidelines.pdf. Accessed June 13, 2021.
21. Moodley D, Moodley J, Coovadia H, et al. A multicenter randomized controlled trial of nevirapine versus a combination of zidovudine and lamivudine to reduce intrapartum and early postpartum mother-to-child transmission of human immunodeficiency virus type 1. J Infect Dis 2003;187(5):725–35.
22. Dabis F, Bequet L, Ekouevi DK, et al. Field efficacy of zidovudine, lamivudine and single-dose nevirapine to prevent peripartum HIV transmission. AIDS 2005;19(3): 309–18.
23. World Health Organization. Antiretroviral drugs for treating pregnant women and preventing HIV infection in infants: towards universal access. Recommendations for a public health approach. 2006. Available at: https://www.who.int/hiv/pub/guidelines/pmtctguidelines3.pdf?ua=1. Accessed June 12, 2021.
24. World Health Organization. Rapid advice: use of antiretroviral drugs for treating pregnant women and preventing HIV infection in infants. Available at: https://apps.who.int/iris/handle/10665/44249. Accessed June 12, 2021.
25. Consolidated guidelines on the use of antiretroviral drugs for treating and preventing HIV infection: recommendations for a public health approach. Geneva: World Health Organization; 2013. Available at: https://pubmed.ncbi.nlm.nih.gov/24716260/. Accessed June 15, 2021.
26. Fowler MG, Qin M, Fiscus SA, et al. Benefits and risks of antiretroviral therapy for perinatal HIV prevention. N Engl J Med 2016;375(18):1726–37.
27. INSIGHT START Study Group, Lundgren JD, Babiker AG, Gordin F, et al. Initiation of antiretroviral therapy in early asymptomatic HIV infection. N Engl J Med 2015; 373(9):795–807.
28. Joint United Nations Programme on HIV/AIDS (UNAIDS). 90-90-90: an ambitious treatment target to help end the AIDS epidemic. Available at: https://www.unaids.org/en/resources/909090. Accessed June 10, 2021.

29. World Health Organization. Consolidated guidelines on the use of antiretroviral drugs for treating and preventing HIV infection. In: Recommendations for a public health approach. 2nd edition; 2016. Available at: https://apps.who.int/iris/bitstream/handle/10665/208825/9789241549684_eng.pdf?sequence=1. Accessed June 15, 2021.
30. Joint United Nations Programme on HIV/AIDS (UNAIDS). Update: 90-90-90: good progress, but the world is off-track for hitting the 2020 targets. Available at: https://www.unaids.org/en/resources/presscentre/featurestories/2020/september/20200921_90-90-90. Accessed June 10, 2021.
31. Joint United Nations Programme on HIV/AIDS (UNAIDS). UNAIDS DATA 2020. Available at: https://www.unaids.org/sites/default/files/media_asset/2020_aids-data-book_en.pdf. Accessed June 20, 2021.
32. World Health Organization. WHO validation for the elimination of mother-to-child transmission of HIV and/or syphilis. Available at: https://www.who.int/reproductivehealth/congenital-syphilis/WHO-validation-EMTCT/en/. Accessed June 11, 2021.
33. Townsend CL, Byrne L, Cortina-Borja M, et al. Earlier initiation of ART and further decline in mother-to-child HIV transmission rates, 2000-2011. AIDS 2014;28(7):1049–57.
34. Mayaux MJ, Dussaix E, Isopet J, et al. Maternal virus load during pregnancy and mother-to-child transmission of human immunodeficiency virus type 1: the French perinatal cohort studies. SEROGEST Cohort Group. J Infect Dis 1997;175(1):172–5.
35. Sperling RS, Shapiro DE, Coombs RW, et al. Maternal viral load, zidovudine treatment, and the risk of transmission of human immunodeficiency virus type 1 from mother to infant. Pediatric AIDS Clinical Trials Group Protocol 076 Study Group. N Engl J Med 1996;335(22):1621–9.
36. Maternal viral load and vertical transmission of HIV-1: an important factor but not the only one. The European Collaborative Study. AIDS 1999;13(11):1377–85.
37. Bryson YJ, Luzuriaga K, Sullivan JL, et al. Proposed definitions for in utero versus intrapartum transmission of HIV-1. N Engl J Med 1992;327(17):1246–7.
38. Dunn DT, Brandt CD, Krivine A, et al. The sensitivity of HIV-1 DNA polymerase chain reaction in the neonatal period and the relative contributions of intra-uterine and intra-partum transmission. AIDS 1995;9(9):F7–11.
39. Rouzioux C, Costagliola D, Burgard M, et al. Estimated timing of mother-to-child human immunodeficiency virus type 1 (HIV-1) transmission by use of a Markov model. The HIV Infection in Newborns French Collaborative Study Group. Am J Epidemiol 1995;142(12):1330–7.
40. Ehrnst A, Lindgren S, Dictor M, et al. HIV in pregnant women and their offspring: evidence for late transmission. Lancet 1991;338(8761):203–7.
41. Bertolli J, St Louis ME, Simonds RJ, et al. Estimating the timing of mother-to-child transmission of human immunodeficiency virus in a breast-feeding population in Kinshasa, Zaire. J Infect Dis 1996;174(4):722–6.
42. King CC, Ellington SR, Kourtis AP. The role of co-infections in mother-to-child transmission of HIV. Curr HIV Res 2013;11(1):10–23.
43. Semba RD, Kumwenda N, Hoover DR, et al. Human immunodeficiency virus load in breast milk, mastitis, and mother-to-child transmission of human immunodeficiency virus type 1. J Infect Dis 1999;180(1):93–8.
44. Corey L, Wald A, Celum CL, et al. The effects of herpes simplex virus-2 on HIV-1 acquisition and transmission: a review of two overlapping epidemics. J Acquir Immune Defic Syndr 2004;35(5):435–45.

45. Chen KT, Segú M, Lumey LH, et al. Genital herpes simplex virus infection and perinatal transmission of human immunodeficiency virus. Obstet Gynecol 2005; 106(6):1341–8.
46. Drake AL, John-Stewart GC, Wald A, et al. Herpes simplex virus type 2 and risk of intrapartum human immunodeficiency virus transmission [published correction appears in Obstet Gynecol. 2007 Apr;109(4):1002-3]. Obstet Gynecol 2007; 109(2 Pt 1):403–9.
47. Bollen LJ, Whitehead SJ, Mock PA, et al. Maternal herpes simplex virus type 2 coinfection increases the risk of perinatal HIV transmission: possibility to further decrease transmission? AIDS 2008;22(10):1169–76.
48. Cowan FM, Humphrey JH, Ntozini R, et al. Maternal herpes simplex virus type 2 infection, syphilis and risk of intra-partum transmission of HIV-1: results of a case control study. AIDS 2008;22(2):193–201.
49. Mandelbrot L, Mayaux MJ, Bongain A, et al. Obstetric factors and mother-to-child transmission of human immunodeficiency virus type 1: the French perinatal cohorts. SEROGEST French Pediatric HIV Infection Study Group. Am J Obstet Gynecol 1996;175(3 Pt 1):661–7.
50. Landesman SH, Kalish LA, Burns DN, et al. Obstetrical factors and the transmission of human immunodeficiency virus type 1 from mother to child. The Women and Infants Transmission Study. N Engl J Med 1996;334(25):1617–23.
51. Minkoff H, Burns DN, Landesman S, et al. The relationship of the duration of ruptured membranes to vertical transmission of human immunodeficiency virus. Am J Obstet Gynecol 1995;173(2):585–9.
52. Jamieson DJ, Read JS, Kourtis AP, et al. Cesarean delivery for HIV-infected women: recommendations and controversies. Am J Obstet Gynecol 2007;197(3 Suppl):S96–100.
53. Shapiro RL, Kitch D, Ogwu A, et al. HIV transmission and 24-month survival in a randomized trial of HAART to prevent MTCT during pregnancy and breastfeeding in Botswana. AIDS 2013;27(12):1911–20.
54. Rousseau CM, Nduati RW, Richardson BA, et al. Longitudinal analysis of human immunodeficiency virus type 1 RNA in breast milk and of its relationship to infant infection and maternal disease. J Infect Dis 2003;187(5):741–7.
55. Effect of breastfeeding on infant and child mortality due to infectious diseases in less developed countries: a pooled analysis. WHO Collaborative Study Team on the Role of Breastfeeding on the Prevention of Infant Mortality [published correction appears in Lancet 2000 Mar 25;355(9209):1104]. Lancet 2000;355(9202): 451–5.
56. Hamilton E, Bossiky B, Ditekemena J, et al. Using the PMTCT cascade to accelerate achievement of the global plan goals. J Acquir Immune Defic Syndr 2017; 75(Suppl 1):S27–35.
57. Joint United Nations Programme on HIV/AIDS (UNAIDS). Start Free. Stay Free. AIDS Free. 2019 Report. Available at: https://www.unaids.org/sites/default/files/media_asset/20190722_UNAIDS_SFSFAF_2019_en.pdf. Accessed June 15, 2021.

Updates in Pediatric Tuberculosis in International Settings

Sadia Shakoor, MBBS, FCPS Microbiology[a],
Fatima Mir, MBBS, FCPS Pediatrics, MsCR[b,*]

KEYWORDS

• Childhood TB • LTBI in children • Policy-practice gaps • LMICs • HBCs
• Paucibacillary • TB diagnostics • DS-TB

KEY POINTS

- Poor surveillance in international settings, especially resource-poor high-burden settings, due largely to health system barriers, variations in case definitions and difficulty in diagnosis, and standardization and reporting, lead to an underdetected epidemic of childhood tuberculosis (TB).
- Considerable progress has been made in consolidated guidelines on appropriate dosing and safe and effective regimens for treating childhood TB. However, gaps in implementing treatment completion in high-burden countries (HBCs) remain.
- New drugs in pipeline have yet to permeate national TB programs in low- and middle-income countries.
- BCG vaccination at birth is implemented in most HBCs. However, efficacy against TB is higher when coupled with stringent tuberculin skin test screening, which is missing in most HBCs.
- Policy-practice gaps stem from poor integration of TB services for children with other maternal and children health programs such as reproductive health, integrated management of childhood illness, HIV, and nutrition support and immunization, resulting in inadequate detection of TB exposures, infections and cases among children.

INTRODUCTION

Over 1 million children are diagnosed with tuberculosis (TB) each year.[1] Many more in high-burden countries (HBCs) are exposed to tuberculous adult contacts and are never evaluated for exposure or preventive therapy,[2] thus maintaining a vulnerable

[a] Department of Pathology, Section of Microbiology, Aga Khan University, Supariwala Building, PO Box 3500, Karachi, Pakistan; [b] Department of Pediatrics and Child Health, The Aga Khan University, Faculty Office Building, PO Box 3500, Stadium Road, Karachi 74800, Pakistan
* Corresponding author.
E-mail address: Fatima.mir@aku.edu

Pediatr Clin N Am 69 (2022) 19–45
https://doi.org/10.1016/j.pcl.2021.09.004

pool of children and weakening any existing control measures. The current vaccine is not effective enough to prevent TB. The epidemic of pediatric TB in low- and middle-income countries (LMICs) therefore continues unabated and is complicated by emerging infectious and noninfectious epidemics, viz, human immunodeficiency virus (HIV), malnutrition, coronavirus disease 2019 (COVID-19), and diabetes.

Advances in the science, diagnosis, and management of TB in children have continued, and this review presents the existing situation in international settings and focuses on recent advances with the potential to improve outcomes of pediatric TB.

EPIDEMIOLOGY OF PEDIATRIC TUBERCULOSIS IN INTERNATIONAL SETTINGS

TB continues to afflict several populations across the globe in different socioeconomic settings. The highest burden of disease is typically seen in countries with weakened health systems,[3,4] which characteristically also marginalize vulnerable pediatric populations. Prevention of spread and control as well as adequate individual management of TB therefore requires political will and a strategic system approach, with ambitious targets and rigorous monitoring and evaluation framework.

Programmatic Approach

The World Health Organization (WHO) announced an End TB strategy in 2015, with overarching targets to reduce TB incidence and mortality by 90% and 95%, respectively, by 2035.[1] The goals and performance targets for subpopulations were revised at the United Nations high-level meeting in September 2018. A new strategy and roadmap were released jointly by the StopTB Partnership and WHO with special emphasis on prevention and control of pediatric TB.

Global Situation and Gaps

In 2019 children accounted for 12% of the global estimated TB cases and 16.5% of the total deaths. Children, however, are disproportionate to their estimated share of incident cases in regard to having poor access to health care, late diagnosis, and poor management.

Fig. 1 shows target attainment gaps in case detection and treatment of rifampin-resistant (RR) TB and multidrug-resistant (MDR) TB (ie, resistant to both isoniazid and rifampin). Of the estimated 1.2 million cases, only half a million were diagnosed and notified in 2019.[1] Less than 10% of the estimated RR TB cases were diagnosed in children in 2019.[1] Although improved from previous years, these fell short of the required 5-year targets, and the future notifications are expected to fall in 2020 onward owing to the impact of the ongoing COVID-19 pandemic and interruption in health services.[5]

Of note, children comprised less than 5% of total notified cases in 8 of 30 HBCs, a figure that highlights underdetection and underreporting of pediatric disease and raises pertinent concerns about health care access and equality.

Regional Incidence of Childhood Tuberculosis: Where are the Gaps?

Driven by the HBCs within regions, the estimated incidence of TB among children 0 to 14 years of age was highest in the WHO Southeast Asia region, followed by Africa, Western Pacific, and Eastern Mediterranean region (**Fig. 2**).[1] Both the estimated and reported female to male ratio in children 0 to 14 years of age remained 0.9 in HBCs.

Fig. 3 is a snapshot of the case detection gaps in children 0 to 14 years of age in the 20 highest burden countries that shared 84% of the overall incident cases in all age

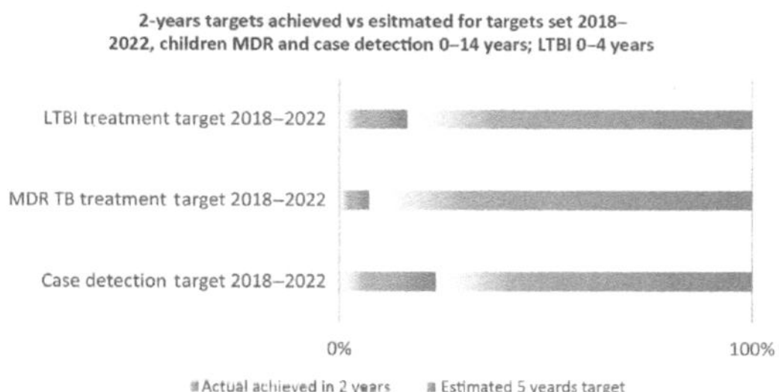

Fig. 1. Progress in pediatric TB 2018 to 2022 target achievements; targets were set by WHO. Achieved targets in 2018 and 2019 for case detection fell short by 10% (1.04 million cases detected in 2 years vs an estimated 2-year target of 1.4 million), whereas those for multidrug-resistant (MDR) TB fell short by 32.2% (8986 children treated vs an estimated requirement of 46,000 in 2 years). Latent TB infection (LTBI) treatment targets for children aged 0 to 4 years also lagged annually by 10%. (Source of data: Global Tuberculosis Report, WHO, 2020.)

groups in 2019.[1] Greatest gaps exist in low-resource settings with severely reduced health care budget allocations in Africa and Asia. Although many of these countries have TB programs supported by the Global Fund to Fight AIDS, TB, and Malaria, the lack of a coordinated health system and weaknesses of horizontal programs such as Integrated Management of Childhood Illnesses and lack of integration result in unmet gaps in access and management.

Age-disaggregated data were not available for MDR and RR TB for all the 20 HBCs and for none of the WHO member states before 2018. The practice of age-disaggregated surveillance of TB is recent, and expected to give impetus to pediatric TB monitoring, evaluation, and service improvement. However, this will only be possible with removal of existing health system barriers that impact coverage, access, and affordability of pediatric services in high-burden settings.

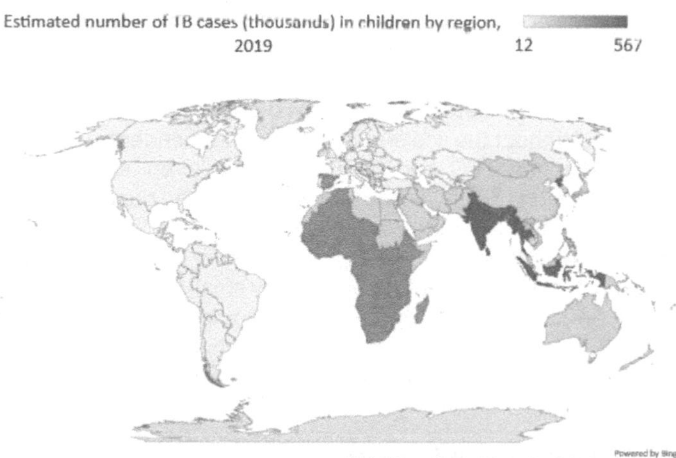

Fig. 2. Regional estimates of burden of TB in children 0 to 14 years of age, data from Global TB report 2020. Regional estimates are driven by data in high-burden countries (HBCs). (Source of data: Global Tuberculosis Report, WHO, 2020.)

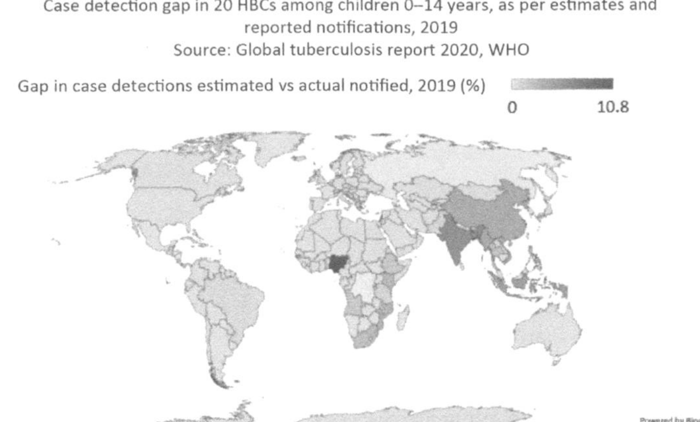

Fig. 3. Map with pediatric TB incidence (number reported in 2019) as per 2020 Global TB Report in 20 HBCs with 84% of total reported case burden in 2019. Despite a high burden of TB, childhood cases (0–14 years) only comprise 0% to 5% of total notified cases, highlighting gaps in case detection and diagnosis. (Source of data: Global Tuberculosis Report, WHO, 2020.)

Drug-Resistant Tuberculosis in Children

The challenges of TB surveillance, reporting and diagnosis are even more pronounced for MDR TB in children. Age-disaggregated data on MDR TB treatment (number of cases treated as notified by country programs) for WHO member states is only available after 2018. Data on incidence are sparse and inaccurate.

Dodd and colleagues6 estimated through a modeling approach that in 2014, of 850,000 new infections in children, 25,000 were MDR and 1200 were extensively drug resistant ([XDR] currently defined as an MDR TB strain that is resistant to fluoroquinolones).[6] Other modeling estimates have concluded that at least 30,000 MDR TB infections occur in children every year (3.2% of incident cases in children).[7] Children with bacteriologically confirmed MDR TB are sicker and more likely to have comorbid conditions such as HIV and malnutrition,[8] making TB surveillance a priority in HIV and undernourished populations.

One of the challenges in determining MDR TB rates is the requirement of bacteriologic confirmation. Without the scale-up of culture-independent rapid molecular diagnostic tools to diagnose RR and MDR TB in children and the adaptation of epidemiologic definitions,[9] prevalence statistics and incidence estimations based on modeling with unreliable inputs will remain inadequate.

The impact of underdetection is clearly perceived in the lag in MDR TB treatment target achievement (see **Fig. 1**), where only a very small proportion of children are reported as being treated for MDR TB. Owing to incomplete vital registries and incomplete mortality reporting especially in HBCs and high MDR burden settings, the disease outcomes of children with MDR TB are unavailable but are expected to be dire.

Pulmonary Tuberculosis Versus Extrapulmonary Tuberculosis and Disseminated Tuberculosis in Children

Extrapulmonary sites of infection are more likely to occur in children than in adults owing to more efficient lymphatic spread. However, because many children will also have pulmonary disease, surveillance data may misclassify them as pulmonary TB cases. Moreover, if clinicians also fail to identify signs of extrapulmonary TB, cases will be undertreated. The challenges therefore are multifold and exist at both macrolevels and microlevels.

Of note, for specific forms of extrapulmonary TB, viz, TB meningitis, outcomes are significantly poorer especially in children younger than 5 years.[10] Disaggregated data reporting for specific types of extrapulmonary TB is therefore critical in estimating its burden especially in HBCs to divert resources to develop and sustain specific strategies in the detection and management more effectively.

Arguably defined as TB involving the hematopoietic system or 2 or more noncontiguous body sites,[11] disseminated TB is common in children. No data on disseminated TB are reported by TB programs in HBCs. Disseminated TB is estimated to occur in up to 5% of TB cases in adults[12]; however, children are at greater risk because they are disproportionately affected by specific risk factors such as malnutrition. In HBCs therefore it is likely that a significant proportion of undetected burden of both extrapulmonary and disseminated TB exists with proportionately high mortality in children.

Congenital and Neonatal tuberculosis

There are no incidence estimates available for perinatal or neonatal TB. Congenital TB is a result of exposure in utero or during birth. Exposure to maternal respiratory droplets after birth can lead to neonatal TB. Although TB in pregnancy was estimated to occur in more than 200,000 women in 2014 alone, the actual incidence of maternal TB resulting in neonatal TB is likely higher in HBCs owing to increased susceptibility to TB in late pregnancy.[13] Congenital and neonatal TB have high mortality, but data are not available to inform the true burden in HBCs.

Because little scientific evidence is available for the impact of various strategies for diagnosis, management, and prevention of congenital and neonatal TB, this is an area requiring attention and further research. Studies in high-prevalence areas, viz, the 30 high TB and HIV burden settings, in pregnant women and neonates can be highly informative in the planning of successful diagnostic, treatment, and preventive strategies.

Tuberculosis Mortality

Owing to limitations in national vital registration data availability in HBCs, TB mortality data reported by HBCs remain inaccurate. Estimates of TB deaths (based on incidence and case fatality data) for the 0- to 14-year age group for both HIV-positive and HIV-negative children were 16% of total TB deaths across all regions and slightly higher for male children.[1] Most deaths occurred in Africa and South East Asia, however, the ratio of under-14 mortality to the overall mortality did not vary significantly, with the exception of higher mortality estimate among HIV-infected children in Africa.[1] Dodd and colleagues[14] performed a global mortality burden estimate for children aged 0 to 14 years in 2015 and reported an average case fatality rate of 24%, with higher rates among HIV-infected children in Africa. Data also suggested that mortality would be reduced by half if case detection rates were improved in children.

Prevalent and Emerging Risk Factors

To effectively reduce the transmission of TB, it is important to focus on pediatric subpopulations with predisposing risk factors. Active TB disease in children is at least a 2-step process: first, an exposure leading to infection, and second, infection progressing to active disease. Risk factors for initial infection are socioeconomic and lifestyle associated. Owing to the impact of socioeconomic factors on initial infection, screening and treatment of latent TB infection (LTBI) is an effective strategy to reduce the incidence of TB in migrant children. In contrast, progression to disease depends on biological and host-specific risk factors. Among known host characteristics that are risk factors for active TB in children are HIV, primary immune deficiency disorders, and undernutrition.[1] Undernutrition is prevalent in HBCs, with prevalence ranging from 2.5% in Brazil and Russia to as high as 40% in Congo and 60% in Central African Republic.[1] The prevalence of HIV varies in different settings; 14 of the 20 highest burden countries also have high HIV prevalence, and additional 16 countries are also included in the WHO list of high TB and HIV burden countries.[1] Of note, data on estimates for children living with HIV for the period 2015 to 2019 were only available for 10 of these countries, with a rising trend in 3 countries.[15] Only 53% children accessed antiretroviral treatment in 2019,[16] which is a mere 5% increase from 2015 reports.[17] Rising incidence and marginalization leading to limited access to antiretroviral treatment increases the risk of active TB in children.

Contribution of other known risk factors such as childhood diabetes and parental smoking is less well defined. Exposure to parental smoking is associated with a 2-fold increased risk of TB infection and 4-fold increased risk for active TB in children.[18] Prevalence of TB in one study among type 1 diabetic children was 5-fold higher than in children without diabetes.[19] Other issues such as illicit drug use among children also seem to be common in HBCs[20] but is underdetected among marginalized children in LMICs.[21]

Major Issues and Barriers in Delineating Tuberculosis Epidemiology Among Children in International Settings

Childhood TB epidemiology remains difficult to address. Health system as well as social and diagnostic issues serve as barriers against pediatric TB case finding in HBCs. Systematic issues of data capture and reporting are underlined in the global TB report as major obstacles in detecting children with TB[1]; inventory studies and capture-recapture surveys are important to highlight the inadequacy of current notification systems in HBCs. **Box 1** highlights the important barriers to overcome to improve the detection and management of TB disease among children.

UPDATES IN PEDIATRIC TUBERCULOSIS CASE DETECTION AND DIAGNOSIS

Diagnosis of pediatric TB may be made based on bacteriologic testing, clinical criteria, or a combination of supportive evidence provided by biomarkers and radiological imaging. Despite advances in each of these, diagnosis of pediatric TB remains difficult in clinical settings.

Clinical Diagnosis

Clinical judgment remains valuable in the diagnosis of pediatric TB. A detailed history of contact with a known TB case (mostly an adult household) is highly suggestive of active TB in a sick child. Healthy children in this situation should be evaluated for LTBI.

Initial signs and symptoms of pulmonary and extrapulmonary TB are nonspecific in younger (<2–3 years) children. However, childhood TB is highly responsive to antituberculous treatment especially if detected early. Early detection in younger children requires a meticulous history taking for failure to thrive, irritability, reduced playfulness, poor appetite, vomiting, and abdominal pain. Sleep disturbances may also be observed.[22,23]

Box 1
Barriers to childhood tuberculosis control and elimination in high-burden settings

Health system barriers
- Incomplete health care access to marginalized populations
- Inability of health system infrastructure to support integrated care
- Lack of programmatic linkages
- Lack of political commitment to new strategies (eg, lack of commitment to LTBI treatment)
- Lack of prioritization of children and pregnant women
- Disproportionate financing (lack of funds to support programs)
- Systematic corruption
- High turnover (low retention) of trained health care personnel in programs

Case finding barriers
- Difficult diagnosis, difficult sampling in children
- Insufficiently sensitive diagnostic tests
- Inadequate physician training in clinical diagnosis
- Unavailable diagnostic tools (lack of availability or scale-up)
- Underreporting (incomplete data)
- Overdiagnosis

Socioeconomic barriers
- Poverty
- Lack of trust in medical care
- Poor health literacy
- Social stigma

Presence of chronic cough alone in children increases the odds of being diagnosed with TB (odds ratio, 13.8; 95% confidence interval [CI], 2–83).[24] A wide confidence interval, however, indicates a high level of heterogeneity within the pediatric population, stemming from differences in underlying health, age, and weight; these differences may be more relevant within pediatric populations in HBCs. A combination of persistent cough, weight loss, and listlessness has a positive predictive value of greater than 80% in children with pulmonary TB.[23] However, positive predictive values of various combinations of symptoms may vary significantly in undernourished or HIV-infected children, due to masking of symptoms in young, malnourished, or immune-deficient children.

Studies of clinical diagnostic criteria in HBCs are therefore required, especially using clinical diagnostic criteria proposed for pulmonary TB in children.[25] Owing to the lower standalone specificity of clinical signs and symptoms and risk of overdiagnosis even in HBCs, bacteriologic confirmation should be sought.

Bacteriologic Confirmation with Conventional and Advanced Tools

HBCs rely heavily on smear microscopic diagnosis of TB, because laboratory capacity for culture and molecular testing is limited.[1] However, smear microscopy for the diagnosis of pediatric TB is insensitive. Culture of *Mycobacterium tuberculosis* provides results after a minimum of 10 days (2–4 weeks), which is not ideal for urgent situations in which TB is considered. Clinical diagnosis therefore takes precedence over a negative smear and culture result, particularly in situations requiring urgent treatments such as TB meningitis or disseminated TB in infants or HIV-infected children, especially where alternative rapid diagnostic tools are not available. Rapid molecular diagnosis is recommended by WHO using prequalified diagnostic tools.[26]

Global Fund-supported disbursement of rapid molecular diagnostics has been initiated in some HBCs, but is not available at large scale and remains underutilized.[27]

Xper Ultra assay is an automated, integrated, cartridge-based molecular assay to identify TB as well as rifampicin resistance directly from sputum. The development of such assay with its high sensitivity is ideal for pediatric populations, wherein lower bacillary load prevents good performance of microscopic smear and culture. Of note, such rapid tests have been shown to perform well with extrapulmonary specimens, except urine and pleural fluid.[26]

A major obstacle that prevents uptake of microbiological diagnostic tools even when available is the difficulty of obtaining appropriate samples from children. Younger children often do not produce sputum and thus require gastric lavage after overnight fasting in a hospital setting, or where available, bronchoscopy to obtain respiratory samples. Recently, stool has been evaluated as an alternative specimen for TB diagnosis.[26] Use of noninvasive stool specimens for the diagnosis of pulmonary TB in children is valuable, and the scale-up of stool-based Xpert Ultra assay can increase case detection rates in HBCs. Bacteriologic confirmation of extrapulmonary TB without coexisting pulmonary disease often requires invasive sampling techniques such as lumbar puncture, needle aspirations, needle biopsies, or surgical biopsies. Such sampling may, however, be made less invasive in selected cases by interventional radiology.

Histopathological diagnosis

Histopathological diagnosis demonstrating caseation and granulomas in biopsy specimens often proves valuable especially in situations with coexisting tumor pathology, or where a diagnosis is questionable, for instance, in low-prevalence settings. In HBCs, histopathological diagnosis is less often used because of the unavailability and inadequacy of pathology and laboratory medicine services.[28] Efforts to improve the pathology and laboratory medicine services in LMICs will improve clinical care beyond improving TB case detections, by preventing overdiagnosis and misdiagnoses in children with illnesses that mimic TB.[29]

Biomarkers

Accurate biomarker-supported diagnosis has 2 potential advantages over bacteriologic diagnosis in children. First, biomarkers are usually evaluated and performed in relatively easy-to-access specimens as opposed to invasive procedures required for obtaining samples for culture. Second, biomarkers provide supportive evidence of TB in children with a high likelihood of the disease but negative bacteriologic tests. Furthermore, biomarkers can potentially allow disease monitoring and prognostication.

Urine lipoarabinomannan lateral flow point-of-care test has a sensitivity of 43% (95% CI, 23%–66%) and specificity of 80% (95% CI, 69%–88%) as an add-on test for detection of TB in children living with HIV.[30] WHO recommends use of this test among HIV-positive children with CD4 counts less than 100/mm^3 in outpatient settings, in combination with clinical diagnosis.[30] Use in HBCs with high HIV prevalence can enhance case detections; however, only 13 of 30 HBCs have adopted this test in their diagnostic algorithms,[1] highlighting policy and implementation gaps.

Candidate biomarkers under development and evaluation include microRNAs, interleukins, and cytokines. Complex methodological issues prevent wider usage, and a recent systematic review also highlighted the need for further studies in diagnostic evaluations to avoid overestimates of accuracy.[31]

Biosignatures comprising several integrated biomarkers may have higher overall accuracy than single biomarkers. Immune cytokine profiles, proteins (proteomic), metabolic end products (metabolomic), and messenger as well as microRNA (transcriptomic) biosignatures[32] hold promise as a point-of-care biomarker of active TB disease with high accuracy regardless of HIV status.[33]

Radiological Diagnosis

Plain radiography and ultrasonography are both low cost and widely available in HBCs. The limitations are low sensitivity in pulmonary and extrapulmonary TB in children and the impact of operator variability for ultrasonography.[34,35] Advances in digital-assisted interpretation can overcome operator and reader subjectivity but cannot account for inherently lower sensitivity. To be able to uncover small lesions of extrapulmonary TB and lymphadenopathy in children and facilitate diagnostic or therapeutic drainage, computed tomography or MRI may be required. Given that such facilities are not widely available in HBCs, facilitated referral of children identified through clinical diagnosis or scoring (see later) as being high risk for TB can enhance case detection and management.

Diagnostic Markers of Latent Tuberculosis Infection in Children

Immune response to *M tuberculosis* antigens is considered a diagnostic surrogate for TB. Currently available tests (tuberculin skin test and interferon gamma assays) are methodologically complex and highly variable in children younger than 4 years.[36] Testing, however, is not a prerequisite before preventive treatment can be given to household contacts of patients with infectious TB. However, in a few instances, diagnosis of LTBI holds value in children, viz, in refugees or internationally displaced children from high-burden settings, in children with immunodeficiencies with uncertain contact history, and in children who will receive immunosuppressive or myeloablative therapies in high-burden settings and with uncertain contact histories. Moreover, evidence of LTBI serves as a criterion in clinical scoring systems for active TB in children. The test result does not have standalone value as a diagnostic element but adds to the certainty of diagnosis when used in combination with other suggestive criteria.

Clinical Scoring and Nonscoring Diagnostic Systems

Challenges surrounding the difficulty of using a single ideal diagnostic tool for the detection of TB in children necessitate the development of composite scoring systems or unscored diagnostic systems. Several scoring systems have been in use in clinical settings for decades; a systematic review in 2012 found that validity of scoring systems is not systematically evaluated.[37] The relatively recent Brazilian Ministry of Health scoring system has undergone rigorous evaluation and has been shown to have 48.3% (95% CI, 35.2%–61.6%) sensitivity and 76.5% (95% CI, 62.5%–87.2%) specificity in HIV-infected children.[38] Nonscoring systems such as the Marais criteria have greater sensitivity of 84.4% (95% CI, 73.1%–92.2%) but lower specificity of 29.8% (95% CI, 18.4%–43.4%) in the absence of microbiological diagnosis and has previously been shown to have high sensitivity in HIV-uninfected children.[37]

However, both the Marais system and the Brazilian Ministry of Health score were developed for the diagnosis of pulmonary TB. Older scoring systems such as the Kenneth Jones and Keith Edwards criteria also focus on extrapulmonary TB and therefore remain in wide usage for difficult clinical situations to rule in extrapulmonary TB. Moreover, these latter scoring systems also have improved specificity, allowing their use as rule-out scoring systems.[39] **Table 1** summarizes the various diagnostic tests and strategies for the detection of TB in children.

Programmatic Challenges and Implementation Gaps

Gaps in bacteriologic confirmation of pediatric TB and MDR TB are the limited laboratory and diagnostic capacity in HBCs.[1] Multiple factors prevent routine bacteriologic confirmation of TB in children, viz, paucibacillary disease, difficult sampling of clinical specimens, and unavailability of diagnostic tools (see **Box 1**). Lack of investment in diagnostic tools by programs leads to limited rollout of rapid and ultrasensitive molecular diagnostic tools.[1] Moreover, human resource, biomedical support, and connectivity are major obstacles in implementation of recommended diagnostic algorithms.[28] Moreover, physician training in algorithms and interpretation of laboratory and imaging tools is limited.[40] Such gaps, obstacles, and training must be addressed in the fight against pediatric TB globally.

UPDATES IN TREATMENT IN HIGH-BURDEN COUNTRIES

Treatment of Drug-Susceptible Tuberculosis in Children

TB disease in children has traditionally been treated with the agents used to treat adult disease. First-line regimens for drug-susceptible TB across the world still contain isoniazid, rifampin, ethambutol, and pyrazinamide. Dosages have recently been increased by WHO[41,42] with 2 months of rifampicin (R) (10–20 mg/kg, maximum [max] dose 600 mg/d), pyrazinamide (Z) (30–40 mg/kg), isoniazid (H) (10–15 mg/kg, max dose 300 mg/d), and sometimes ethambutol (E) (15–25 mg/kg, in areas of high HIV or isoniazid resistance prevalence) followed by 4 months of rifampicin and isoniazid at the aforementioned doses.[43,44] There are still remaining concerns over suboptimal plasma concentrations especially in resource-constrained settings where therapeutic drug monitoring is nonexistent.[45] WHO recommends the fixed drug combinations over separate formulations for children based on evidence from trials in adults.[46] A revised isoniazid range of 7 to 15 mg/kg/d was advised to national programs as adequate even in children younger than 2 years or fast acetylators (subgroups at risk of suboptimal serum drug concentrations) based on the impossibility of meeting recommended isoniazid range (10–15 mg/kg/d) with the existing fixed drug combination for children (H50R75Z150) without exceeding the therapeutic dose range of pyrazinamide.[42,44,47,48]

In rifamycin group (rifampicin, rifabutin, and rifapentine), despite revision in rifampicin dosage (15 mg/kg/d), there is an increasing focus on higher doses (30–35 mg/kg) with early reports of acceptable tolerance and higher serum levels.[49] For children with HIV-TB coinfection, rifabutin at the dose of 5 mg/kg (children) and 150 to 300 mg/d (adults) has been recommended based on lesser HIV-TB drug interactions and side effects.[50]

A 4-month fluoroquinolone-based regimen (2 months of isoniazid [H], rifampicin [R], prothionamide [pt], pyrazinamide [Z], and moxifloxacin [Mfx] [2HRptZMfx] followed by 2 months of HRptMfx) has been compared with 6-month standard regimens (2HRZE/4HR) in adults and have been found to have higher relapse rates.[51–53] Only recently in 2021, two 4-month regimens (first regimen, 2 months of isoniazid [H], rifapentine [RPT], pyrazinamide [Z], and ethambutol [E] followed by 9 weeks of RPT and H, and second regimen, 2 months of HRPTZMfx followed by 9 weeks of HRPTMfx) were compared with standard 6-month rifampicin-based regimen (2HRZE/4HR) and showed noninferiority to the standard of care for drug-susceptible TB in adults[54]; however, this has not translated into guidelines yet.

Drug-Susceptible Pulmonary Tuberculosis

A new possible alternative to the classic 6-month rifampicin-based regimen (2HRZE/4HR) is a 4-month rifapentine-based regimen[41] composed of rifapentine, isoniazid,

Table 1
Clinical application and limitations of various diagnostic tools for detection of TB in children with reference to needs of high-burden settings

Diagnostic Element	Settings Where Applicable[a]	Clinical Utility	Limitations
Clinical diagnosis			
History, symptoms, and signs	All	Can be applied in all settings, indispensable in informing physicians' "clinical judgment" *History of exposure* essential for both active infection and screening for latent infection	Do not perform well as standalone criteria; sensitivity and PPV vary with underlying conditions in children and are low in HIV-infected children Potential for overdiagnosis due to low specificity
Scoring/diagnostic systems	All; some scoring systems perform better in referral settings	Increase certainty of diagnosis and sensitivity by using multiple composite criteria Useful in both HIV-infected and uninfected children Systems with better performance are BMOH (clinical manifestations, radiograph, contact history, nutritional status, tuberculin skin test) and Marais criteria (in addition to BMOH, includes other risk factors, viz, HIV, extrapulmonary signs and symptoms, and microbiological evaluation)	Higher sensitivity than clinical signs and symptoms alone Issue of overdiagnosis may remain when bacteriologic diagnosis not used Need to train health care workers in use and interpretation Systems with high sensitivity for PTB do not perform well for children with EPTB
In vitro diagnosis			
Smear and culture	Need small laboratory for direct smear and advanced biosafety level for concentrated smear and culture	When positive have high PPV for TB in children in HBCs Culture allows further susceptibility testing and whole-genome sequencing where	Direct smear is highly insensitive Concentrated smear and culture limited by need for laboratories with advanced biosafety levels; culture results are not rapid

(*continued on next page*)

Table 1
(continued)

Diagnostic Element	Settings Where Applicable[a]	Clinical Utility	Limitations
		advanced service linkages available, to delineate molecular epidemiology	Positive smear may be found in NTM infections, especially in low-burden settings
Rapid molecular diagnosis with capability to detect rifampin resistance	All (new point-of-care platforms expected to be available in 2021)	1–2 h to results in most settings allows use in all settings in which equipment can be placed New tests with sensitivity comparable to concentrated culture are recommended for use in children Allow rapid detection of rifampin resistance and exclude NTM infection	Require connectivity for rapid result communication if not placed in clinic settings Biomedical maintenance is required, which may be unavailable in HBCs
Biomarkers of active infection	Inpatient and outpatient settings serving HIV-infected children, all levels; point-of-care, no need for laboratory	Available for use as point-of-care lateral flow devices Allow culture-independent testing in easy-to-access specimens (urine) in children with HIV where bacteriologic confirmation may not be possible	Not recommended for use in HIV-uninfected children Performance limited in children without symptoms or in children with CD4 counts greater than $200/mm^3$
Biomarkers of latent infection	Laboratory setting, referral centers	Allow diagnosis of "infection" as surrogate for exposure as part of some diagnostic systems	Do not diagnose active TB in children IGRAs limited by methodological issues and interlaboratory variability of results
Radiological diagnosis			

Radiography and ultrasonography	Secondary care and with annexed services in some primary care settings	Wider availability and acceptability as diagnostic tools May allow diagnostic and therapeutic aspiration in EPTB	Interobserver agreement and interpretation issues Have limited sensitivity and specificity with potential for overdiagnosis when used without bacteriologic confirmation
Advanced: CT, MRI, or fluoroscopic imaging	Referral centers	Advanced-level diagnostic tools for use in referral centers, allow detection as well as diagnostic and therapeutic drainage in EPTB	Limited availability and expertise in HBCs

Abbreviations: BMOH, Brazilian Ministry of Health; CT, computed tomography; EPTB, extrapulmonary tuberculosis; NTM, nontuberculous mycobacteria; PPV, positive predictive value; PTB, pulmonary tuberculosis.

[a] Primary and/or secondary versus referral center or laboratory versus point of care.

pyrazinamide, and moxifloxacin.[54,55] The noninferiority trial enrolled participants aged 12 years and older with newly diagnosed pulmonary TB confirmed by a WHO-recommended diagnostic test and who were susceptible to isoniazid, rifampicin, and fluoroquinolones. Preliminary results from the multicenter SHINE trial comparing a 4-month rifampicin-based regimen (2HRZE/2HR) with the standard 6-month regimen (2HRZE/4HR) in participants aged less than 16 years (median age 3.5 years) has shown noninferiority in treatment failure and relapse rates[56]; this may eventually influence future recommendations on duration of treatment of nonsevere TB in children.[57]

Drug-Susceptible Extrapulmonary Tuberculosis

Recommended regimens for extrapulmonary TB by WHO guidance to national programs are in **Table 2**. Classic regimens are 6 months long except for meningeal and osteoarticular TB, which should be 12 months. Adjuvant corticosteroid therapy with dexamethasone or prednisolone is recommended for meningeal and pericardial TB.

Dosing Frequency for Treatment of Tuberculosis Disease in Children

Directly Observed Treatment, Short Course (DOTS) strategy has largely targeted adults leading to less evidence on intermittent dosing in children.[58–60] There is no change in the recommendation of daily dosing for children with TB disease.[61] Data on trials comparing intermittent with daily dosing are insufficient to support intermittent regimens over daily treatment in children with TB.[43,62] However, recognizing practical limitations, WHO guidance to national programs is flexible in stating that thrice weekly dosing can be considered in continuation phase for new patients with pulmonary TB provided they do not have HIV and they are directly observed.

Treatment of Latent Tuberculosis Infection in Children

Chances of progression of latent disease to active inflates from 10% in healthy adults to as high as 50% in children younger than 5 years.[63,64] Risk of TB is particularly high in children younger than 3 years of age. Children older 2 years of age can be treated for LTBI with once-weekly isoniazid-rifapentine (3HP) for 3 months (see **Table 2**). Higher weight-adjusted doses may be required for efficacy in treating children with LTBI.[65]

Four months of rifampicin (4R) or 3 months of daily isoniazid plus rifampicin (3HR) is now preferred over 6 to 9 months of isoniazid (6H/9H) monotherapy.[66,67] Even though these regimens are equally acceptable, patients may be more likely to complete shorter treatment regimens. **Table 2** shows LTBI regimens recommended for children.

Treatment of Drug-Resistant Tuberculosis in Children

Oxazolidinones (cycloserine and linezolid) are core drugs in drug-resistant TB regimens. There are scarce data available about the use in children for drug-resistant TB, but data from adults point toward utility.[68]

Imipenem-cilastatin and meropenem are enlisted in WHO Group C for treatment of drug-resistant TB.[69]

New Drugs for Drug-Resistant Tuberculosis

Initially WHO recommended bedaquiline as part of second-line therapy in patients older than 18 years. Now it can be used conditionally in treatment of patients with MDR and RR TB aged 3 years or more. Delamanid (nitroimidazole) has been studied more extensively than pretomanid. WHO recommends delamanid for 6 months of intensive phase in patients with MDR TB and XDR TB with high baseline risk for poor outcomes.[70] Delamanid has been associated with increased sputum culture

Table 2
Recommended regimens for children with tuberculosis infection and DS disease in international settings modified from WHO guidelines[41,42,64]

Drug	Recommended Regimen/DT Strength (mg)	Number of Tablets by Weight Band Once Daily: Less Than 2 kg	2–2.9 kg	3–3.9 kg	4–7.9 kg	8–11.9 kg	12–15.9 kg	16–24.9 kg	Strength of Adult Tablet (mg)	Number of Tablets by Weight Band: 25–39.9 kg	40–54.9 kg	>55 kg
TB treatment regimens for children (low HIV prevalence [and HIV-negative children] and low-isoniazid-resistance settings)												
Smear-negative pulmonary TB Intrathoracic lymph node TB Tuberculous peripheral lymphadenitis	*2HRZ/4HR* (50/75/150)/(50/75)	0.25/0.25	0.5/0.5	0.75/0.75	1/1	2/2	3/3	4/4	*2HRZE/4HR* (75/150/400/245)/(75/150)	2/2	3/3	4/4
Extensive pulmonary disease Smear-positive pulmonary TB Severe forms of extrapulmonary TB (other than tuberculous meningitis/osteoarticular TB)	*2HRZ + E/4HR* (50/75/150) + 100/(50/75)			0.75 + 0.75/0.75	1 + 1/1	2 + 2/2	3 + 3/3	4 + 4/4	*2HRZE/4HR* (75/150/400/245)/(75/150)	2/2	3/3	4/4
TB treatment regimens for children (high HIV prevalence, high isoniazid resistance, or both)												
Smear-positive TB Smear-positive PTB ± extensive parenchymal disease All forms of EPTB except	**2HRZ + E/4HR** (50/75/150) + 100/(50/75)	0.25/0.25	0.5/0.5	0.75 + 0.75/0.75	1 + 1/1	2 + 2/2	3 + 3/3	4 + 4/4	**2HRZE/4HR** (75/150/400/245)/(75/150)	2/2	3/3	4/4

(continued on next page)

Table 2
(continued)

Drug	Recommended Regimen/DT Strength (mg)	Number of Tablets by Weight Band Once Daily: Less Than 2 kg	2–2.9 kg	3–3.9 kg	4–7.9 kg	8–11.9 kg	12–15.9 kg	16–24.9 kg	Strength of Adult Tablet (mg)	Number of Tablets by Weight Band: 25–39.9 kg	40–54.9 kg	>55 kg
meningeal/ osteoarticular TB												
All regions												
Meningeal/ osteoarticular TB	**2HRZ + E/10HR** (50/75/150) + 100/(50/75)	0.25/0.25	0.5/0.5	0.75 t+ 0.75 t/0.75 t	1 + 1/1	2 + 2/2	3 + 3/3	4 + 4/4	**2HRZE/10HR** (75/150/400/ 245)/(75/150)	2/2	3/3	4/4
TB prophylaxis regimens for children (LTBI)												
				<5 kg	**5.1–9.9 kg**	**10–13.9 kg**	**14–19.9 kg**	**20–24.9 kg**		**25–34.9 kg**	**40–54.9 kg**	**>55 kg**
B6	50 mg			-	0.5 EOD	0.5 EOD	1 OD	1 OD	50	1 OD	1 OD	1 OD
6H	100 mg			0.5	1	1.5	2	2.5	100 mg	3		
				<5 kg	**5.1–9.9 kg**	**10–14 kg**	**14.1–20 kg**	**20.1–25 kg**		**25.1–32 kg**	**32.1–50 kg**	**>50 kg**
3RH	75/50			0.75	1	2	3	4	150/75	2	3	4
3HP	Isoniazid (100 mg) +rifapentene (150 mg)					(25 mg/kg rounded) + (300 mg) 2 tab per wk for 12 wk	(25 mg/kg rounded) + (450 mg) 3 tablets per wk for 12 wk	(25 mg/kg rounded) + (450 mg) 3 tab per wk for 12 wk	Isoniazid (100 mg) +rifapentene (150 mg)	(15 mg/kg rounded) + (600 mg) 4 tab per wk for 12 wk	(15 mg/kg rounded) + (750 mg) 5 tab per wk for 12 wk	(15 mg/kg rounded) + (900 mg) 6 tab per wk for 12 wk

Abbreviations: B6, vitamin B6 (PYRIDOXINE); 3HP, once-weekly isoniazid-rifapentine for 3 months; 6H, 6 months of isoniazid; DS, drug susceptibility to first line anti-TB therapy; DT, dispersible tablet; EPTB, extrapulmonary tuberculosis; PTB, pulmonary tuberculosis; 3RH, 3 months of rifampicin isoniazid as prophylaxis; EOD, every other day or 3 days a week; OD, once daily.

Note: Treatment regimens for MDR TB are not shown in this table and can be accessed through WHO treatment guidelines for MDR TB.[73,79,80] conversion and lower mortality in patients with drug-resistant TB.[71] This drug can now be used conditionally in treatment of patients with MDR and RR TB aged 3 years or more. Pretomanid has also shown encouraging bactericidal activity in murine models.[72] In 2016, WHO recommended use of delamanid in children and adolescents with MDR TB (resistance to fluoroquinolones or second-line injectables or both). In children, this drug is a useful adjunct during the initial intensive phase (6 months) in longer (18–24 months) rather than shorter MDR TB regimens.[73] A shorter (9–12 months) regimen has recently been approved for patients with uncomplicated MDR TB (Bangladeshi regimen) containing 4 to 6 months of intensive phase (kanamycin, moxifloxacin, prothionamide, clofazimine, high-dose isoniazid, pyrazinamide, and ethambutol) and 5 months of continuation phase (moxifloxacin, clofazimine, pyrazinamide, and ethambutol).[74]

Recommendations on Treatment and Care for Isoniazid-Resistant Tuberculosis

WHO treatment guidelines for children with confirmed isoniazid-resistant TB are extrapolated from adult data. Only 2% of patients with isoniazid-resistant TB in WHO Individual Patient Data review were children. Recommended treatment includes rifampicin, ethambutol, pyrazinamide, and levofloxacin for 6 months ((H)REZ-Lfx).[42,75,76] Adding streptomycin and other injectable agents is not recommended. Customization is required if additional resistance (especially to pyrazinamide) is suspected or confirmed. Surveillance of isoniazid resistance mutations (katG or inhA) and host acetylator status at country or regional levels can be useful in guiding national treatment policy.[12]

Recommendations on Treatment and Care for Multidrug/Rifampicin-Resistant Tuberculosis

Longer MDR TB regimens with effective agents are associated with higher cure and lower mortality rates in adults and children.[77] Recommendations on composition of longer regimens (18–20 months with 15–17 months after culture conversion) include a minimum of 3 group A agents (levofloxacin/moxifloxacin, bedaquiline, linezolid) and one group B agent (clofazimine, cycloserine/terizidone) to ensure that the regimen contains at least 4 effective agents. If the regimen cannot be composed with agents from groups A and B alone, group C agents (ethambutol, delamanid, pyrazinamide, imipenem-cilastatin, meropenem, amikacin [streptomycin], ethionamide/prothionamide, *p*-aminosalicylic acid) are added to complete it.

Longer regimens containing aminoglycosides should have an intensive phase of 6 to 7 months (amikacin/kanamycin, levofloxacin, ethambutol, pyrazinamide, ethionamide, and cycloserine) and 18 months of continuation phase with levofloxacin, ethambutol, ethionamide and cycloserine.[78] Bedaquiline can be used in younger children (6–17 years) based on available pharmacokinetic data.[79] Delamanid can now be used conditionally in treatment of patients with MDR/RR TB aged 3 years or more on longer regimens.[80]

There is interest in shorter-duration regimens for MDR TB. Clinical effectiveness of shorter regimens (9–12 months) under programmatic and trial conditions has been reported.[81–85] However, the diligent monitoring of treatment response required for shorter regimens (ie, monthly sputum smear and culture during therapy) is resource intensive and difficult to implement in most HBCs, making this option potentially unsafe.

Need for Supportive Surgery

Since the advent of antituberculous drugs, surgery has receded to a less important but, nevertheless, viable treatment option.[86] Pulmonary resection combined with antituberculous drugs has shown success and reduced all-cause mortality in 88% to 92% of adult MDR TB cases.[87–89] Even with these encouraging outcomes, surgery remains controversial, at least in children. It has potential utility in complications such as massive hemoptysis, bronchiectasis, bronchopleural fistula, and aspergilloma and, mostly, in treatment failures.[89]

Adverse Effects of First-Line Agents

Even though children have a more sensitive therapeutic index,[90–92] side effects to common first-line drugs including isoniazid (neuropathy and hepatotoxicity), rifampicin (drug interactions, hepatotoxicity), pyrazinamide (hepatotoxicity, nongouty arthralgia and gout-induced arthritis), and ethambutol (optic neuritis) have been rarely reported.

Isoniazid-associated hepatitis is rare in children. Slow acetylators experience more toxicity than intermediate or fast acetylators.[93] There is limited evidence of hepatic adverse events when rifampicin is administered alone in children; however, it has potential for interactions with other drugs with hepatic metabolism.[94] Pyrazinamide-related hepatotoxicity is dose and duration dependent in adults,[95] and it has been rarely reported in children.[96] Nongouty polyarthralgia and gout-induced arthritis seen in adults has not been reported in children. Ocular toxicity with ethambutol is dose and duration dependent and is difficult to detect in younger children who cannot self-report changes in vision.[97]

Adverse Effects of Second-Line Agents

Second-line regimens have higher adverse event frequency with toxicity occurring in up to 40%.[98] Aminoglycoside association with nephrotoxicity and ototoxicity needs further study in TB regimens.[91,99] Traditional restriction of long-term fluoroquinolone use in children due to fear of arthropathy has not been substantiated by evidence. Nevertheless, side effects in children on prolonged fluoroquinolones need to be monitored. Monitoring for QT interval prolongation in children on bedaquiline and delamanid is also essential.

VULNERABLE POPULATIONS

Human Immunodeficiency Virus and Tuberculosis

HIV-infected children are at high risk of acquiring and developing TB after exposure. These children require immediate preventive therapy after exclusion of active disease, irrespective of age and immune status. Although preventive therapy should be provided at each TB exposure, continuous isoniazid prophylaxis is not recommended.

For all patients with HIV and drug-susceptible TB, antiretrovirals should be started regardless of their CD4 cell count; however, TB treatment should be initiated first, followed by antiretrovirals as soon as possible within the first 8 weeks of TB treatment. Those with severe immune suppression should receive antiretrovirals within the first 2 weeks of TB treatment initiation.

Tuberculosis and Migrant/Refugee Children

TB in migrants may vary based on incidence of TB in the countries of origin (17 new cases per 100,000 population in the Syrian Arab Republic to 338 per 100,000 in Nigeria). In high-income countries with stringent entry screening, it can be contained and appropriately addressed.[100] In LMICs with less-stringent criteria on entry and limited resources for detection and treatment of displaced and refugee populations, there is imminent risk of outbreaks.[101]

Primary Immune Deficiency and Tuberculosis

Natural immunity to TB relies on functional interleukin-12/23-interferon-gamma axis in macrophages.[102] In contrast to children with severe primary immune deficiency disorders who present with various infections, children with interleukin-12/23-interferon-gamma pathway errors (Mendelian susceptibility to the mycobacterial disease phenotype) are particularly susceptible to mycobacterial infections and nontyphoidal *Salmonella* infections. Although these children usually present with BCG-induced disease and nontuberculous *Mycobacterium* infections, they are exceedingly vulnerable to the more virulent TB especially in high-prevalence countries.[103–105]

Newborns and Tuberculosis

Worldwide the burden of TB in pregnant women is the greatest in Africa and Southeast Asia. Most of these countries also have poor implementation of Integrated Management of Pregnancy and Childbirth and even poorer linkage to existing TB programs.[106] Valuable opportunities are therefore lost to screen pregnant women for TB to prevent vertical transmission in utero and/or droplet transmission after giving birth. Very little is known about the burden of congenital TB in HBCs. Even China with relatively higher case finding and notification rates in pregnant women and a better health system reports very high mortality in sporadic cases.[107] Most HBCs also have concurrent high neonatal mortality and poor antenatal and newborn health service utilization rates thereby discouraging early identification of congenital TB and screening of newborns and infants whose mothers or household contacts have TB. Low preventive therapy coverage in infants is an important surrogate for TB program performance in 2 high-risk populations, namely, pregnant women and infants.

PREVENTING AND CONTROLLING THE EPIDEMIC

Preventive Therapy

Contact investigation is not routinely implemented in most HBCs. Case finding is passive at best with very little community engagement or empowerment of first-line health professionals[108]; this leads indirectly to poor coverage rates of preventive treatment to children. In 2017, preventive therapy was not accessed by more than 75% of 1.3 million eligible household contacts younger than 5 years of age. There is a need to address persistent policy-practice gaps in screening children for TB exposure and early implementation of preventive therapy[109] with focus on health system strengthening[91] and health literacy.

BCG Vaccination

In HBCs, all healthy newborns should be vaccinated with a single dose of BCG vaccine.[110,111] This vaccination is also safe in healthy preterm infants born at 32 to 36 weeks of gestation.[112,113] However, safety data in very preterm infants less than 32 weeks' gestation is lacking.

Vaccine efficacy and effectiveness against TB has been extensively studied. BCG vaccination has the potential to prevent primary infection (19% less infection in BCG-vaccinated children than unvaccinated children). Among those vaccinated as neonates, protection against pulmonary TB was 59% (risk ratio, 0.41; 95% CI, 0.29–0.58).[114] In studies in which BCG was given in childhood and with stringent tuberculin skin test screening, protection against pulmonary TB was 74% (risk ratio, 0.26; 95% CI, 0.18–0.37). BCG efficacy and effectiveness in reducing meningeal and miliary TB is 85% (risk ratio, 0.15; 95% CI, 0.08–0.31). The combined strategy of vaccination with BCG early in life during neonatal period and stringent tuberculin skin testing is associated with the highest protection against severe TB disease.

Patient-Centered Care and Prevention

Most progress in care and support of children with TB has been the inclusion of children and adolescents in clinical practice guidelines, the development of training and reference materials on childhood TB, the collection of better age- and sex-disaggregated data from programs, and the availability of pediatric drug formulations.

Poor integration of national TB program with other services accessed by women and children such as reproductive health, HIV, nutrition and immunization results in missed opportunities for identification of TB exposure, infection, and disease in women and children.[115] Achieving continuum of care requires a high level of multisectoral collaboration and political commitment, which is lacking in most HBCs. Interventions such as transportation vouchers, convenient clinic hours and location, reminder systems for missed appointments, social support schemes (housing, food stamps, stipends), and outreach workers to implement adherence have all shown positive impact[116] on detection and notification rates.[117,118]

New Developments

Research and innovation is essential for meeting the Sustainable Development Goals and End TB Strategy targets set for 2030.[1] Priorities include progress in exposure and infection prevention (new vaccines, better tests for LTBI, clinical trials evaluating short-course preventive therapy for children exposed to drug-susceptible and drug-resistant TB), diagnosis (collection of pediatric specimens and monitoring of drug resistance in children in HBCs), and treatment (pharmacokinetic and pharmacodynamic studies of antituberculous drugs in children; optimal regimens for children, pregnant women, and HIV-infected children; and complications of disease and therapy in children).[119]

The diagnostic pipeline seems robust so far in terms of the number of tests, products, or methods in development. Examples include several cartridge-based technologies for the detection of drug resistance, next-generation sequencing assays for detecting drug-resistant TB directly from sputum specimens, and newer skin tests and interferon-gamma release assays.

The crusade to control TB by permeating and implementing known and tested knowledge and interventions at all levels (community, patients, health care providers, laboratory personnel, policy makers, governance) is an ongoing step toward universal health especially in HBCs and in keeping with the Global Strategy for TB Research and Innovation adopted by WHO member states through a World Health Assembly Resolution in August 2020.

CLINICS CARE POINTS

- When biopsying tissue for histopathological diagnosis of suspected exptrapulmonary TB (EPTB) in LMICs, it should be ensured that tissue (lymph node, bone marrow, skin lesions refractory to standard treatment, lumps/masses) is sent for Xpert and/or AFB culture to avoid missing nontuberculous mycobacterial infections, fungal infection, and lymphoma (TB mimics).
- TB should be part of most chronic presentations by default because it can have atypical presentations in endemic HBCs such as isolated psoas abscess (without vertebral involvement), dactylitis, and ossicular osteomyelitis (chronically draining ear).
- Establishing radiological resolution at end of therapy may be helpful even in children with good clinical response if they have disseminated disease because it may unmask treatment

failure and lead to considering risk factors such as fast acetylator status or immune deficiency.

- Signs of clinical improvement should be observed (appetite, weight gain, defervescence, work of breathing [pulmonary TB]) and improvement in presenting signs and symptoms (EPTB) as intensive phase progresses because lack of improvement by end of intensive phase should lead to suspicion of alternate diagnosis (including MDR TB).
- Patients should only get their anti-tuberculous therapy (ATT) from certified sources like National TB Programs (over-the-counter counterfeit medicine is a potential risk in countries with poor health systems monitoring and evaluation).
- Preparing parents for drug-related effects like reddish urine, nausea after early morning medication, and repetition of dosage if vomiting within half hour of intake will keep them committed to adherence.

DISCLOSURE

The authors have nothing to disclose.

REFERENCES

1. Organization WH. Global tuberculosis report 2020. Geneva (Switzerland): WHO; 2020. p. 2020.
2. Campbell JR, Bastos ML. No time to waste: preventing tuberculosis in children. Lancet 2020;395(10228):924–6.
3. Kim J, Keshavjee S, Atun R. Health systems performance in managing tuberculosis: analysis of tuberculosis care cascades among high-burden and non-high-burden countries. J Glob Health 2019;9(1):010423.
4. Osman M, Karat AS, Khan M, et al. Health system determinants of tuberculosis mortality in South Africa: a causal loop model. BMC Health Serv Res 2021; 21(1):1–11.
5. Wingfield T, Karmadwala F, MacPherson P, et al. Challenges and opportunities to end tuberculosis in the COVID-19 era. Lancet Respir Med 2021;9(6):556–8.
6. Dodd PJ, Sismanidis C, Seddon JA. Global burden of drug-resistant tuberculosis in children: a mathematical modelling study. Lancet Infect Dis 2016; 16(10):1193–201.
7. Jenkins HE, Tolman AW, Yuen CM, et al. Incidence of multidrug-resistant tuberculosis disease in children: systematic review and global estimates. The Lancet 2014;383(9928):1572–9.
8. Harausz EP, Garcia-Prats AJ, Law S, et al. Treatment and outcomes in children with multidrug-resistant tuberculosis: a systematic review and individual patient data meta-analysis. PLoS Med 2018;15(7):e1002591.
9. Smith SE, Pratt R, Trieu L, et al. Epidemiology of pediatric multidrug-resistant tuberculosis in the United States, 1993–2014. Clin Infect Dis 2017;65(9): 1437–43.
10. Chiang SS, Khan FA, Milstein MB, et al. Treatment outcomes of childhood tuberculous meningitis: a systematic review and meta-analysis. Lancet Infect Dis 2014;14(10):947–57.
11. Suarez I, Fuenger SM, Jung N, et al. Severe disseminated tuberculosis in HIV-negative refugees. Lancet Infect Dis 2019;19(10):e352–9.
12. Wang J-Y, Hsueh P-R, Wang S-K, et al. Disseminated tuberculosis: a 10-year experience in a medical center. Medicine 2007;86(1):39–46.

13. Snow K, Bekker A, Huang G, et al. Tuberculosis in pregnant women and neonates: A meta-review of current evidence. Paediatr Respir Rev 2020;36:27–32.
14. Dodd PJ, Yuen CM, Sismanidis C, et al. The global burden of tuberculosis mortality in children: a mathematical modelling study. Lancet Glob Health 2017;5(9): e898–906.
15. HIV estimates with uncertainty bounds 1990-2019. Available at: https://www.unaids.org/en/resources/documents/2020/HIV_estimates_with_uncertainty_bounds_1990-present. Accessed May 14, 2021.
16. UNAIDS. Global HIV & AIDS statistics — Fact sheet. 2021. Available at: https://www.unaids.org/en/resources/fact-sheet. Accessed May 14, 2021.
17. HIV and Children: fact sheet. 2016. Available at: https://www.unaids.org/sites/default/files/media_asset/FactSheet_Children_en.pdf. Accessed May 14, 2021.
18. Chiang C-Y, Bam TS. Should tobacco control intervention be implemented into tuberculosis control program? In: Taylor & Francis; 2018.
19. Abdelmoez B, Abd-El-Nasser A, Baheeg MG, et al. Prevalence of tuberculosis among children who had type 1 diabetes and were admitted to Elminia University Hospital. Pediatrics 2008;121(Suppl 2):S151.
20. Jakaza TN, Nyoni C. Emerging dynamics of substance abuse among street children in Zimbabwe. A case of Harare Central Business District. Afr J Soc Work 2018;8(2):63–70.
21. Martyn LA. Health knowledge, attitudes, and practices among street children in LMICs. Doctoral dissertation: Duke University; 2016.
22. Thwaites G, Fisher M, Hemingway C, et al. British Infection Society. British Infection Society guidelines for the diagnosis and treatment of tuberculosis of the central nervous system in adults and children. J Infect 2009;59(3):167–87.
23. Chiappini E, Vecchio AL, Garazzino S, et al. Recommendations for the diagnosis of pediatric tuberculosis. Eur J Clin Microbiol Infect Dis 2016;35(1):1–18.
24. Wong KS, Huang Y, Lai S, et al. Validity of symptoms and radiographic features in predicting positive AFB smears in adolescents with tuberculosis. Int J Tuberc Lung Dis 2010;14(2):155–9.
25. Graham SM, Cuevas LE, Jean-Philippe P, et al. Clinical case definitions for classification of intrathoracic tuberculosis in children: an update. Clin Infect Dis 2015;61(suppl_3):S179–87.
26. Organization WH. Molecular assays intended as initial tests for the diagnosis of pulmonary and extrapulmonary TB and rifampicin resistance in adults and children: rapid communication. 2020.
27. Cazabon D, Pande T, Kik S, et al. Market penetration of Xpert MTB/RIF in high tuberculosis burden countries: a trend analysis from 2014-2016. Gates Open Res 2018;2:35.
28. Sayed S, Cherniak W, Lawler M, et al. Improving pathology and laboratory medicine in low-income and middle-income countries: roadmap to solutions. Lancet 2018;391(10133):1939–52.
29. Shakoor S, Mir F, Hasan R. Common alternative diagnoses among a pediatric hospital-based cohort evaluated for tuberculosis in Karachi, Pakistan: The need for facilitated referral in tuberculosis clinics. Int J Mycobacteriol 2019; 8(1):42.
30. Organization WH. Lateral flow urine lipoarabinomannan assay (LF-LAM) for the diagnosis of active tuberculosis in people living with HIV: policy update 2019. Geneva (Switzerland): World Health Organization; 2019. 9241550600.
31. Togun TO, MacLean E, Kampmann B, et al. Biomarkers for diagnosis of childhood tuberculosis: A systematic review. PLoS One 2018;13(9):e0204029.

32. Maertzdorf J, Kaufmann SH, Weiner J. Toward a unified biosignature for tuberculosis. Cold Spring Harb Perspect Med 2015;5(1):a018531.
33. Goussard P, Walzl G. Biosignatures: The answer to Tuberculosis diagnosis in children? EBioMedicine 2020;60:102977.
34. Jain SK, Andronikou S, Goussard P, et al. Advanced imaging tools for childhood tuberculosis: potential applications and research needs. Lancet Infect Dis 2020; 20(11):e289–97.
35. Cruz AT, Starke JR. Clinical manifestations of tuberculosis in children. Paediatr Respir Rev 2007;8(2):107–17.
36. Bergamini BM, Losi M, Vaienti F, et al. Performance of commercial blood tests for the diagnosis of latent tuberculosis infection in children and adolescents. Pediatrics 2009;123(3):e419–24.
37. Pearce EC, Woodward JF, Nyandiko WM, et al. A systematic review of clinical diagnostic systems used in the diagnosis of tuberculosis in children. AIDS Res Treat 2012;2012:401896.
38. David SG, Lovero KL, Maria de Fátima B, et al. A comparison of tuberculosis diagnostic systems in a retrospective cohort of HIV-infected children in Rio de Janeiro, Brazil. Int J Infect Dis 2017;59:150–5.
39. Holm M, Wejse C. New optimism to the use of clinical scoring systems for the diagnosis of child tuberculosis–even among HIV co-infected. Int J Infect Dis 2017;59:148–9.
40. Das J, Holla A, Das V, et al. In urban and rural India, a standardized patient study showed low levels of provider training and huge quality gaps. Health Aff (Millwood) 2012;31(12):2774–84.
41. Organization WH. Guidelines for treatment of drug-susceptible tuberculosis and patient care. 2017.
42. Organization WH. Guidance for national tuberculosis programmes on the management of tuberculosis in children. Geneva (Switzerland): World Health Organization; 2014. 9241548746.
43. Mukherjee A, Velpandian T, Singla M, et al. Pharmacokinetics of isoniazid, rifampicin, pyrazinamide and ethambutol in HIV-infected Indian children. Int J Tuberc Lung Dis 2016;20(5):666–72.
44. Aruldhas BW, Hoglund RM, Ranjalkar J, et al. Optimization of dosing regimens of isoniazid and rifampicin in children with tuberculosis in India. Br J Clin Pharmacol 2019;85(3):644–54.
45. Hiruy H, Rogers Z, Mbowane C, et al. Subtherapeutic concentrations of first-line anti-TB drugs in South African children treated according to current guidelines: the PHATISA study. J Antimicrob Chemother 2015;70(4):1115–23.
46. Albanna AS, Smith BM, Cowan D, et al. Fixed-dose combination antituberculosis therapy: a systematic review and meta-analysis. Eur Respir J 2013;42(3): 721–32.
47. Thee S, Seddon J, Donald P, et al. Pharmacokinetics of isoniazid, rifampin, and pyrazinamide in children younger than two years of age with tuberculosis: evidence for implementation of revised World Health Organization recommendations. Antimicrob Agents Chemother 2011;55(12):5560–7.
48. McIlleron H, Willemse M, Werely CJ, et al. Isoniazid plasma concentrations in a cohort of South African children with tuberculosis: implications for international pediatric dosing guidelines. Clin Infect Dis 2009;48(11):1547–53.
49. Seijger C, Hoefsloot W, Bergsma-de Guchteneire I, et al. High-dose rifampicin in tuberculosis: Experiences from a Dutch tuberculosis centre. PLoS One 2019; 14(3):e0213718.

50. Moultrie H, McIlleron H, Sawry S, et al. Pharmacokinetics and safety of rifabutin in young HIV-infected children receiving rifabutin and lopinavir/ritonavir. J Antimicrob Chemother 2015;70(2):543–9.
51. Gillespie SH, Crook AM, McHugh TD, et al. Four-month moxifloxacin-based regimens for drug-sensitive tuberculosis. N Engl J Med 2014;371(17):1577–87.
52. Jindani A, Harrison TS, Nunn AJ, et al. High-dose rifapentine with moxifloxacin for pulmonary tuberculosis. N Engl J Med 2014;371:1599–608.
53. Jawahar MS, Banurekha VV, Paramasivan CN, et al. Randomized clinical trial of thrice-weekly 4-month moxifloxacin or gatifloxacin containing regimens in the treatment of new sputum positive pulmonary tuberculosis patients. PLoS One 2013;8(7):e67030.
54. Dorman SE, Nahid P, Kurbatova EV, et al. Four-Month Rifapentine Regimens with or without Moxifloxacin for Tuberculosis. N Engl J Med 2021;384(18):1705–18.
55. Organization WH. Treatment of drug-susceptible tuberculosis: rapid communication. 2021.
56. Chabala C, Turkova A, Thomason MJ, et al. Shorter treatment for minimal tuberculosis (TB) in children (SHINE): a study protocol for a randomised controlled trial. Trials 2018;19(1):1–12.
57. Organization WH. SHINE trial on shorter treatment for children with minimal TB. 2020. Available at: https://www.who.int/news/item/26-10-2020-shine-trial-on-shorter-treatment-for-children-with-minimal-tb. Accessed October 26, 2020.
58. Starke JR. Improving tuberculosis care for children in high-burden settings. Pediatrics 2014;134(4):655–7.
59. Jaganath D, Mupere E. Childhood tuberculosis and malnutrition. J Infect Dis 2012;206(12):1809–15.
60. Marais BJ, Gie RP, Schaaf HS, et al. Childhood pulmonary tuberculosis: old wisdom and new challenges. Am J Respir Crit Care Med 2006;173(10):1078–90.
61. Ramachandran G, Hemanth Kumar A, Bhavani P, et al. Age, nutritional status and INH acetylator status affect pharmacokinetics of anti-tuberculosis drugs in children. Int J Tuberc Lung Dis 2013;17(6):800–6.
62. Ranjalkar J, Mathew SK, Verghese VP, et al. Isoniazid and rifampicin concentrations in children with tuberculosis with either a daily or intermittent regimen: implications for the revised RNTCP 2012 doses in India. Int J Antimicrob Agents 2018;51(5):663–9.
63. Borisov AS, Morris SB, Njie GJ, et al. Update of recommendations for use of once-weekly isoniazid-rifapentine regimen to treat latent Mycobacterium tuberculosis infection. Morb Mortal Wkly Rep 2018;67(25):723.
64. Organization WH. Guidelines on the management of latent tuberculosis infection. Geneva (Switzerland): World Health Organization; 2015.
65. Weiner M, Savic RM, Kenzie WRM, et al. Rifapentine pharmacokinetics and tolerability in children and adults treated once weekly with rifapentine and isoniazid for latent tuberculosis infection. J Pediatr Infect Dis Soc 2014;3(2):132–45.
66. Ferebee S. Controlled chemoprophylaxis trials in tuberculosis. Adv Tuberc Res 1969;17:28–106.
67. Hsu KH. Isoniazid in the prevention and treatment of tuberculosis: a 20-year study of the effectiveness in children. JAMA 1974;229(5):528–33.
68. Lee M, Lee J, Carroll MW, et al. Linezolid for treatment of chronic extensively drug-resistant tuberculosis. N Engl J Med 2012;367(16):1508–18.
69. Gonzalo X, Drobniewski F. Is there a place for β-lactams in the treatment of multidrug-resistant/extensively drug-resistant tuberculosis? Synergy between

meropenem and amoxicillin/clavulanate. J Antimicrob Chemother 2013;68(2): 366–9.

70. Organization WH. The use of delamanid in the treatment of multidrug-resistant tuberculosis: interim policy guidance. Geneva (Switzerland): World Health Organization; 2014.
71. Gupta R, Gao M, Cirule A, et al. Delamanid for extensively drug-resistant tuberculosis. N Engl J Med 2015;373(3):291–2.
72. Diacon AH, Dawson R, Hanekom M, et al. Early bactericidal activity and pharmacokinetics of PA-824 in smear-positive tuberculosis patients. Antimicrob Agents Chemother 2010;54(8):3402–7.
73. Organization WH. The use of delamanid in the treatment of multidrug-resistant tuberculosis in children and adolescents: interim policy guidance. 2016.
74. Sotgiu G, Tiberi S, Centis R, et al. Applicability of the shorter 'Bangladesh regimen' in high multidrug-resistant tuberculosis settings. Int J Infect Dis 2017;56:190–3.
75. Fregonese F, Ahuja SD, Akkerman OW, et al. Comparison of different treatments for isoniazid-resistant tuberculosis: an individual patient data meta-analysis. Lancet Respir Med 2018;6(4):265–75.
76. Organization WH. WHO treatment guidelines for isoniazid-resistant tuberculosis: supplement to the WHO treatment guidelines for drug-resistant tuberculosis. Geneva (Switzerland): World Health Organization; 2018. 9241550074.
77. Seddon JA, Hesseling AC, Godfrey-Faussett P, et al. High treatment success in children treated for multidrug-resistant tuberculosis: an observational cohort study. Thorax 2014;69(5):458–64.
78. Khurana AK, Dhingra B. What is new in management of pediatric tuberculosis? Indian Pediatr 2019;56(3):213–20.
79. Organization WH. WHO best-practice statement on the off-label use of bedaquiline and delamanid for the treatment of multidrug-resistant tuberculosis. World Health Organization; 2017.
80. Organization WH. WHO consolidated guidelines on tuberculosis: module 4: treatment: drug-resistant tuberculosis treatment. World Health Organization; 2020.
81. Nunn AJ, Rusen I, Van Deun A, et al. Evaluation of a standardized treatment regimen of anti-tuberculosis drugs for patients with multi-drug-resistant tuberculosis (STREAM): study protocol for a randomized controlled trial. Trials 2014; 15(1):1–10.
82. Van Deun A, Maug AKJ, Salim MAH, et al. Short, highly effective, and inexpensive standardized treatment of multidrug-resistant tuberculosis. Am J Respir Crit Care Med 2010;182(5):684–92.
83. Piubello A, Harouna SH, Souleymane M, et al. High cure rate with standardised short-course multidrug-resistant tuberculosis treatment in Niger: no relapses. Int J Tuberc Lung Dis 2014;18(10):1188–94.
84. Trébucq A, Schwoebel V, Kashongwe Z, et al. Treatment outcome with a short multidrug-resistant tuberculosis regimen in nine African countries. Int J Tuberc Lung Dis 2018;22(1):17–25.
85. Organization WH. Position statement on the continued use of the shorter MDR-TB regimen following an expedited review of the STREAM Stage 1 preliminary results. 2018.
86. Dara M, Zaleskis R, Acosta C, et al. The role of surgery in the treatment of pulmonary TB and multidrug-and extensively drug-resistant TB. 2014.

87. Marrone M, Venkataramanan V, Goodman M, et al. Surgical interventions for drug-resistant tuberculosis: a systematic review and meta-analysis. Int J Tuberc Lung Dis 2013;17(1):6–16.
88. Pontali E, Matteelli A, D'Ambrosio L, et al. Rediscovering high technology from the past: thoracic surgery is back on track for multidrug-resistant tuberculosis. Expert Rev Anti-infect Ther 2012;10(10):1109–15.
89. Man MA, Nicolau D. Surgical treatment to increase the success rate of multidrug-resistant tuberculosis. Eur J Cardiothorac Surg 2012;42(1):e9–12.
90. Frydenberg AR, Graham SM. Toxicity of first-line drugs for treatment of tuberculosis in children. Trop Med Int Health 2009;14(11):1329–37.
91. Seddon JA, Furin JJ, Gale M, et al. Caring for children with drug-resistant tuberculosis: practice-based recommendations. Am J Respir Crit Care Med 2012; 186(10):953–64.
92. Organization WH, Initiative ST. Treatment of tuberculosis: guidelines. Geneva (Switzerland): World Health Organization; 2010.
93. Golka K, Selinski S. NAT2 Genotype and isoniazid medication in children. EBioMedicine 2016;11:11–2.
94. Hoagland D, Zhao Y, E Lee R. Advances in drug discovery and development for pediatric tuberculosis. Mini Rev Med Chem 2016;16(6):481–97.
95. Pasipanodya JG, Gumbo T. Clinical and toxicodynamic evidence that high-dose pyrazinamide is not more hepatotoxic than the low doses currently used. Antimicrob Agents Chemother 2010;54(7):2847–54.
96. Corrigan D, Paton J. Hepatic enzyme abnormalities in children on triple therapy for tuberculosis. Pediatr Pulmonol 1999;27(1):37–42.
97. Donald PR, Schaaf HS. Old and new drugs for the treatment of tuberculosis in children. Paediatr Respir Rev 2007;8(2):134–41.
98. Ettehad D, Schaaf HS, Seddon JA, et al. Treatment outcomes for children with multidrug-resistant tuberculosis: a systematic review and meta-analysis. Lancet Infect Dis 2012;12(6):449–56.
99. Seddon JA, Hesseling AC, Marais BJ, et al. Paediatric use of second-line anti-tuberculosis agents: a review. Tuberculosis 2012;92(1):9–17.
100. Taylor EM, Painter J, Posey DL, et al. Latent tuberculosis infection among immigrant and refugee children arriving in the United States: 2010. J Immigr Minor Health 2016;18(5):966–70.
101. Legesse T, Admenur G, Gebregzabher S, et al. Tuberculosis (TB) in the refugee camps in Ethiopia: trends of case notification, profile, and treatment outcomes, 2014 to 2017. BMC Infect Dis 2021;21(1):1–12.
102. Lee W-I, Huang J-L, Yeh K-W, et al. Immune defects in active mycobacterial diseases in patients with primary immunodeficiency diseases (PIDs). J Formos Med Assoc 2011;110(12):750–8.
103. Altare F, Ensser A, Breiman A, et al. Interleukin-12 receptor β1 deficiency in a patient with abdominal tuberculosis. J Infect Dis 2001;184(2):231–6.
104. Caragol I, Raspall M, Fieschi C, et al. Clinical tuberculosis in 2 of 3 siblings with interleukin-12 receptor β1 deficiency. Clin Infect Dis 2003;37(2):302–6.
105. Özbek N, Fieschi C, Yilmaz BT, et al. Interleukin-12 receptor β1 chain deficiency in a child with disseminated tuberculosis. Clin Infect Dis 2005;40(6):e55–8.
106. Sugarman J, Colvin C, Moran AC, et al. Tuberculosis in pregnancy: an estimate of the global burden of disease. Lancet Glob Health 2014;2(12):e710–6.
107. Li C, Liu L, Tao Y. Diagnosis and treatment of congenital tuberculosis: a systematic review of 92 cases. Orphanet J Rare Dis 2019;14(1):1–7.

108. Organization WH. Roadmap towards ending TB in children and adolescents. 2018.
109. Safdar N, Hinderaker SG, Baloch NA, et al. Are children with tuberculosis in Pakistan managed according to National programme policy guidelines? A study from 3 districts in Punjab. BMC Res Notes 2010;3(1):1–7.
110. Organization WH. BCG Evidence to Recommendation Framework 2017.
111. Organization WH. BCG vaccine: WHO position paper, February 2018–recommendations. Vaccine 2018;36(24):3408–10.
112. Saroha M, Faridi M, Batra P, et al. Immunogenicity and safety of early vs delayed BCG vaccination in moderately preterm (31–33 weeks) infants. Hum Vaccines Immunother 2015;11(12):2864–71.
113. Dawodu A. Tuberculin conversion following BCG vaccination in preterm infants. Acta Pædiatrica 1985;74(4):564–7.
114. Li J, Zhao A, Tang J, et al. Tuberculosis vaccine development: from classic to clinical candidates. Eur J Clin Microbiol Infect Dis 2020;39(8):1405–25.
115. Mandalakas AM, Starke JR. Current concepts of childhood tuberculosis. Paper presented at: Seminars in pediatric infectious diseases. Geneva: World Health Organization, March 2-4, 2021.
116. Nahid P, Dorman SE, Alipanah N, et al. Official American thoracic society/centers for disease control and prevention/infectious diseases society of America clinical practice guidelines: treatment of drug-susceptible tuberculosis. Clin Infect Dis 2016;63(7):e147–95.
117. Liu Q, Abba K, Alejandria MM, et al. Reminder systems to improve patient adherence to tuberculosis clinic appointments for diagnosis and treatment. Cochrane Database Syst Rev 2014;(11):CD006594.
118. Lutge EE, Wiysonge CS, Knight SE, et al. Material incentives and enablers in the management of tuberculosis. Cochrane Database Syst Rev 2012;1:CD007952.
119. Organization WH. WHO consultation on the translation of tuberculosis research into global policy guidelines: 2-4 March 2021: meeting report. Geneva: World Health Organization, March 2-4, 2021.

Pediatric Malaria

Global and North American Perspectives

Ella M.E. Forgie, BSc, MA[a], Hannah M. Brooks, MSc[b], Michelle Barton, MD, MSc[c], Michael T. Hawkes, MD, PhD[d,e,f,g,*]

KEYWORDS

- Malaria • Children • North America • Artesunate • Artemether-lumefantrine

KEY POINTS

- Malaria is a common cause of child mortality globally. Roughly 2400 imported cases are diagnosed each year in the United States and Canada.
- Frontline clinicians need to recognize that malaria is a potential diagnosis in any febrile child with recent travel or residence in a malaria-endemic zone.
- Severe malaria is more common in children less than 5 years of age, and it generally presents as cerebral malaria, severe malarial anemia, respiratory distress, and/or acute renal failure.
- Uncomplicated malaria is generally treated with artemisinin combination therapy and severe malaria is generally treated with parenteral artesunate.
- Artemisinin resistance, mutant parasites that escape detection by rapid diagnostic tests, and insecticide-resistant mosquitoes complicate the treatment, diagnosis, and prevention of malaria globally.

[a] Department of Anthropology, University of Alberta, Tory Building, 11211 Saskatchewan Drive, Edmonton, Alberta T6G 2H4, Canada; [b] Faculty of Nursing, University of Alberta, 5-143 Edmonton Clinic Health Academy, 11405 87 Avenue Northwest, Edmonton, Alberta T6G 1C9, Canada; [c] Department of Paediatrics, Division of Pediatric Infectious Diseases, Schulich School of Medicine, Western University, Children's Health Research Institute, Lawson Health Research Institute, London Health Sciences Centre, 800 Commissioners Road East, London, Ontario N6A 5W9, Canada; [d] Department of Pediatrics, Faculty of Medicine and Dentistry, University of Alberta, Edmonton Clinic Health Academy, 11405 87 Avenue Northwest, Edmonton, Alberta T6G 1C9, Canada; [e] Department of Medical Microbiology and Immunology, Faculty of Medicine and Dentistry, University of Alberta, Edmonton Clinic Health Academy, 11405 87 Avenue Northwest, Edmonton, Alberta T6G 1C9, Canada; [f] School of Public Health, University of Alberta, Edmonton Clinic Health Academy, 11405 87 Avenue Northwest, Edmonton, Alberta T6G 1C9, Canada; [g] Women and Children's Health Research Institute, Edmonton, Canada

* Corresponding author. Department of Pediatrics, Faculty of Medicine and Dentistry, University of Alberta, 3-588D, Edmonton Clinic Health Academy, 11405 87 Ave Northwest, Edmonton, Alberta T6G 1C9, Canada.
E-mail address: mthawkes@ualberta.ca
Twitter: michaelhawkesmd (M.T.H.)

Pediatr Clin N Am 69 (2022) 47–64
https://doi.org/10.1016/j.pcl.2021.08.008

INTRODUCTION

Malaria remains a major threat to child health globally. Clinicians in North America may encounter cases of imported malaria among children immigrating from or returning from travel to the tropics. Malaria is a medical emergency, requiring prompt recognition and treatment. Frontline clinicians need to recognize that malaria is a potential diagnosis in any febrile child with recent travel or residence in a malaria-endemic zone. Barriers to optimal outcomes may include delays in diagnosis and treatment owing to a lack of familiarity with a tropical disease that is uncommon in North America.

The present narrative review is aimed at general practitioners and pediatricians in the North American setting. Principles of epidemiology, diagnosis, treatment, and prevention are first reviewed from a global perspective, highlighting recent updates in malaria control. Specific considerations for the management of children with malaria in the United States and Canada are discussed, including the availability, pediatric dosing, and adverse effects of artemisinin derivatives (the first-line therapy for both uncomplicated and severe malaria).

ETIOLOGY

Most infections and deaths owing to malaria are caused by *Plasmodium falciparum*, the predominant parasite species in Africa. Other *Plasmodium* species that can cause malaria include *Plasmodium vivax*, *Plasmodium ovale* (of which there are 2 congenic species *P ovale wallekeri* and *P ovale curtisi*),[1] *Plasmodium malariae*, *Plasmodium knowlesi*, and *Plasmodium simium.*[2] These parasites are transmitted to humans through the bite of the female *Anopheles* mosquito, which acts as the disease vector.

The *P falciparum* life cycle requires successive infection of 2 hosts: humans and female *Anopheles* mosquitoes (**Fig. 1**). In the mosquito, the parasite undergoes its sporogenic cycle, whereby sporozoites are generated; sporozoites can then be released from the mosquito's saliva and injected into the human host as it takes its next blood meal. In humans, the parasite first replicates within the liver, then infects red blood cells and travels throughout the body. When in the blood stage, the parasite causes symptoms of malaria. Mosquitoes then ingest *P falciparum* gametocytes as they take a blood meal from an infected human.

EPIDEMIOLOGY

Malaria is a leading cause of child mortality worldwide, accounting for an estimated 429,000 deaths annually.[3] According to the World Health Organization (WHO), 106 countries remain at risk of malaria transmission.[4] Approximately 90% of malaria cases occur in sub-Saharan Africa, where children less than 5 years of age account for 68% of global malaria deaths.[3] It is estimated that 114 million individuals were infected with malaria in sub-Saharan Africa in 2015 alone.[3] Globally, there have been large decreases in the number of malaria cases and deaths over the past 2 decades and an increasing number of countries are moving toward malaria elimination. Children under the age of 5 years have yet to develop an effective adaptive immune response and are therefore particularly susceptible to infection and rapid disease progression.

Roughly 2400 cases of malaria are treated in the United States and Canada every year.[5,6] Nearly all of these cases are imported and more than 75% originate in Africa.[5,7,8] Other regions that contribute to imported malaria in North America include South and South-East Asia and the Caribbean.[9] *P falciparum* and *P vivax* are the most prevalent species identified in Canada and the United States, whereas *P ovale*,

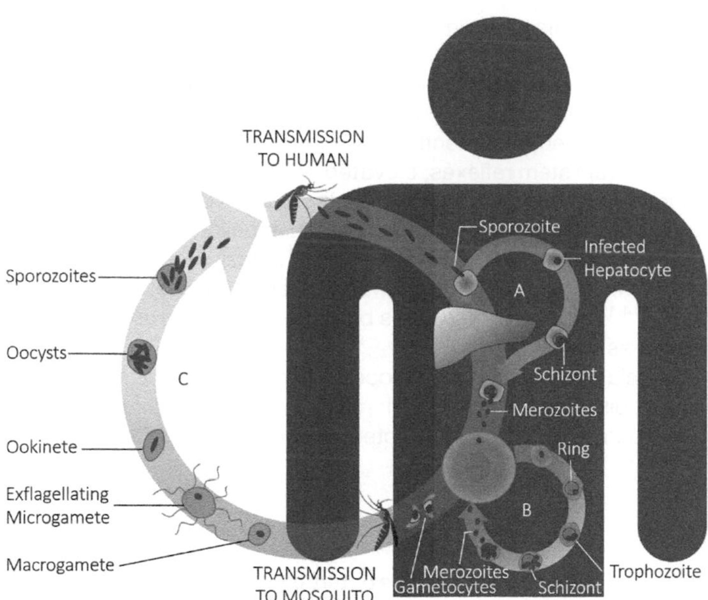

Fig. 1. Lifecycle of *P falciparum*.[63] During the course of its lifecycle, *P falciparum* must infect 2 hosts, the mosquito and the human, and go through various cycles including (A) the exo-erythrocytic cycle in the human liver, (B) the erythrocytic cycle in human red blood cells, and (C) the sporogenic cycle in mosquitoes.

P malariae, *P knowlesi*, and unknown *Plasmodium* spp. together account for only approximately 5% of cases.[5,10] The onset of illness differs by *Plasmodium* sp., but tends to occur within 1 month of departure from the endemic area.[5] Severe malaria is diagnosed in 5% to 15% of patients[5,11] and is more likely to occur in children less than 5 years of age and pregnant women.[5] In 2016 in the United States, 18% of cases of severe malaria occurred in children (<18 years old).[5] Similarly, over an 11-year period (2001–2012), 195 cases of severe malaria were reported to the Canadian Malaria Network, of which approximately 20% were children (<18 years old), and 11% were less than 5 years of age.[12]

CLINICAL MANIFESTATIONS

Symptoms and severity are affected by age and immune status as well as level of parasitemia. Nonimmune individuals such as individuals who are born in nonendemic countries or immigrants who have been living outside of endemic home countries periods longer than 6 months are at higher risk of severe disease than semi-immune individuals. Symptoms of uncomplicated malaria infection are nonspecific and include headache, fatigue, and myalgia, followed by fever, chills, sweats, and malaise. The disease may progress to severe malaria, which usually manifests with 1 or more of the following syndromes: cerebral malaria (coma and convulsions), severe anemia, respiratory distress, or acute renal failure.[13]

Most cases of severe malaria are caused by *P falciparum* infection. The criteria for severe malaria are based on clinical or laboratory parameters: impaired consciousness, prostration, convulsions, respiratory distress, acute pulmonary edema, circulatory collapse, clinical jaundice, abnormal bleeding, acute kidney injury, hemoglobinuria, severe anemia, hypoglycemia, lactic acidosis, or hyperparasitemia.

Hyperparasitemia is defined using percentage of infected red blood cells: 2% or more in children less than 5 years; 5% or more in children 5 years of age or older who are nonimmune; and 10% or more in children 5 years of age or older who are semi-immune (eg, residing in a malaria-endemic area).[12]

Severe malaria presents differently in children and adults.[14] For example, convulsions, abnormal brain stem reflexes, elevated cerebrospinal fluid pressure, neurologic deficits, neurologic sequelae, severe anemia, retinal vessel color changes, papilledema, and ring hemorrhages are more common in children. Conversely, coma, jaundice, and fatal outcomes are more common in adults. Renal failure, which may be associated with hemoglobinuria ("blackwater fever"), is a classic complication of adult severe malaria.[14,15] More recently, it has become recognized as a common complication in children, as well.[15]

Congenital malaria is a rare form that occurs in newborns who acquire malaria transplacentally or at birth from a mother with malaria. Congenital infection is more likely to be symptomatic in infants born to infected mothers who are from countries with low endemicity.

DIAGNOSIS

A potential diagnosis of malaria should be entertained in travelers returning from malaria-endemic destinations who have a fever. To avoid missing the diagnosis, frontline practitioners should always ask for a travel history in any patient with fever and should always order a thin and thick blood smear (or other appropriate diagnostic test) in all febrile children with recent (particularly <30 days) travel to a malaria-endemic area.

A prompt diagnosis is essential for early intervention in children with malaria to prevent the development and/or progression of severe malaria. Owing to the nonspecific clinical features of both uncomplicated and severe malaria, clinical diagnosis is often challenging, and bacterial and viral causes of fever should also be considered. The current WHO guidelines recommend that all suspected cases of malaria have a parasitologic test to confirm diagnosis.[13] The use of parasitologic tests ensures that only confirmed cases receive treatment, avoiding adverse drug effects and limiting drug exposure, which may drive resistance. In the WHO Africa Region, diagnostic testing has increased dramatically from 36% of suspected cases being tested in 2005 to 65% in 2014,[4] likely owing to an increase in availability of malaria rapid diagnostic tests (mRDTs). The main 3 diagnostic modalities currently in use are microscopy of peripheral blood smears, mRDTs, and polymerase chain reaction (PCR).

Microscopy

Microscopy is an accurate and inexpensive means of diagnosing malaria that allows for species determination and estimation of parasite density through light microscopic visualization of Giemsa-stained peripheral thin and thick blood smears.[16,17] A diagnosis of malaria should not be excluded on the basis of a single negative smear; instead, if the initial is negative, smears should be repeated at 12- and 24-hour intervals until there are 3 negative smears. Globally, microscopy is considered the gold standard for a malaria diagnosis.[17] However, microscopic detection relies on a continuous electrical supply to the detection facility and trained malaria microscopists, both of which may be limited in endemic areas.[16,17] Moreover, false-negative tests may occur at low parasite density using microscopy. Mixed species infection may also be difficult to detect. In North America, where malaria cases are relatively rare, maintenance of the necessary skills and competence for timely and accurate microscopic detection is challenging.

Malaria Rapid Diagnostic Tests

Malaria RDTs are monoclonal antibody tests used to detect *Plasmodium*-specific antigens in blood samples, such as *P falciparum* histidine-rich protein-2 (HRP-2), pan-plasmodium parasite lactate dehydrogenase, and pan-plasmodium aldolase.[16,17] They are accurate and cost effective, and unlike microscopy, mRDTs are easy to use even by untrained personnel. The sensitivity of mRDTs may be compromised by inadequate handling and storage before use.[16] Recently, deletion of the *Pfhrp2/3* genes has been detected in some *P falciparum* strains, which encodes HRP-2, the target of the most widely used mRDTs globally.[18] This deletion may lead to false-negative mRDTs,[17] which could have important implications in malaria-endemic areas for missed diagnoses. In North America, the use of mRDTs is often followed up with microscopy before a definitive diagnosis is given.[12,19]

Polymerase Chain Reaction

PCR is the most sensitive and specific diagnostic modality for malaria.[16,17] It allows for species determination even at low levels of parasite density (1–5 parasites/μL of blood) compared with microscopy and mRDTs (50–100 parasites/μL of blood).[16,20–22] PCR is a very useful tool for the detection of mutations associated with drug resistance. Many PCR methods can be used to detect malaria, including conventional, nested, real-time, droplet digital, and isothermal PCR.[16,17] Despite the many advantages associated with PCR detection, the accompanying costs are often prohibitive in many endemic regions.[17] Even in North America, access to PCR testing is limited, and it is used less frequently than other diagnostic methods.[12]

TREATMENT

The guidelines for the treatment of malaria are available from the WHO,[9] US Centers for Disease Control and Prevention (CDC)[23] and the Committee to Advise on Travel Medicine and Tropical.[12] Treatment depends on the disease severity (uncomplicated vs severe), the infecting species (*P falciparum*, *P vivax*, or other species), likelihood of resistance (generally based on the geographic area where the malaria was acquired), as well as other patient factors (eg, the ability to tolerate the oral medication). In addition, for travelers who acquire malaria despite chemoprophylaxis, the treatment regimen should generally not include the medication used for prevention. Treatment principles are summarized elsewhere in this article; however, consultation with a pediatric infectious diseases specialist is recommended for the management of malaria in children.

Uncomplicated Malaria caused by P falciparum

The WHO guidelines for treatment of uncomplicated malaria recommend oral artemisinin combination therapy (ACT; eg, artemether–lumefantrine, artesunate–amodiaquine, artesunate–mefloquine, dihydroartemisinin–piperaquine, ad artesunate–sulfadoxine-pyrimethamine).[9] Monotherapy with artemisinin derivatives may select for drug resistance and is discouraged.

In the United States, the preferred treatment is artemether–lumefantrine. Artemether–lumefantrine is prescribed as a 3-day oral treatment course, administered twice daily, with dosage based on weight. Where artemether–lumefantrine is not available, other effective options include (1) atovaquone–proguanil; (2) quinine plus clindamycin or doxycycline; or (3) mefloquine.[24] In Canada, treatment differs from international standards because of a lack of availability of ACT.[12,24] The recommended treatment is atovaquone–proguanil.[12] Chloroquine may be used for *P falciparum* infection known to be acquired in geographic areas where chloroquine resistance has not been detected.

For pediatric malaria, weight-based dosing of artemether–lumefantrine and atovaquone–proguanil is available for children with a body weight of 5 kg or more. When used in combination with quinine, clindamycin may be preferred over doxycycline in children less than 8 years of age. However, the American Academy of Pediatrics now recommends that doxycycline can be safely administered for short durations ($\leq$21 days) regardless of age.

Medications and dosing for uncomplicated malaria are provided in **Table 1**.

Uncomplicated Malaria caused by P vivax and Other Species

The WHO guidelines recommend oral chloroquine for the treatment of chloroquine-sensitive *P vivax*.[9] Primaquine, which targets the hypnozoite stage of *P vivax*, must be prescribed in addition to chloroquine as a radical cure.[9] If the illness originates in a chloroquine-resistant region (ie, Papua New Guinea[25]) or if species determination is unavailable or inconclusive, treatment should follow the WHO guidelines for the treatment of uncomplicated *P falciparum*.[9]

Other *Plasmodium* species (*P ovale* and *P malariae*) should be treated with chloroquine.[9,26] *P ovale* also has a hypnozoite stage and requires primaquine for radical cure.

Medications and dosing for uncomplicated malaria are provided in **Table 1**.

Severe Malaria

The current WHO guidelines recommend parenteral artesunate for the treatment of severe malaria.[27] In several large, randomized, controlled trials in Asia and Africa among children and adults, a head-to-head comparison of quinine and artesunate demonstrated improved survival with artesunate.[28–30] Furthermore, severe adverse effects of quinine including hypoglycemia and cardiac arrhythmias are not associated with artesunate treatment. Artesunate use in clinical practice is expanding in Africa and Asia, replacing quinine as the mainstay of severe malaria treatment.[31]

In North America, intravenous artesunate was approved for clinical use by the US Food and Drug Administration in May 2020. Previously, the US CDC distributed artesunate under an investigational new drug protocol, a process that will continue until stocking of the drug in pharmacies and hospitals is complete.[24] Previously used for the treatment of severe malaria in the United States, quinidine gluconate was discontinued by the manufacturer, and the last remaining stocks expired in March 2019. In Canada, artesunate is available 24 hours per day through the Canadian Malaria Network and Health Canada's Special Access Program.[32] Dosing of intravenous artesunate is provided in **Table 2**. Once the patient is able to tolerate oral medications, the treatment can be switched to either oral artemether–lumefantrine or atovaquone–proguanil. The oral follow-on therapy is a full treatment course for uncomplicated malaria (see **Table 1**).

Postartesunate Delayed Hemolysis

Parenteral artesunate has an excellent safety profile, with lower incidence of hypoglycemia, new seizures, and development of coma during treatment than quinine.[30,33] Nonetheless, a recently described adverse event among patients receiving artesunate is postartesunate delayed hemolysis (PADH), which occurs well after parasite clearance and resolution of clinical symptoms[34,35] and involves a distinct mechanism of hemolytic anemia.[36] PADH was first recognized among nonimmune travelers with severe malaria treated with intravenous artesunate.[37] This adverse event was not reported in

Table 1
Drug regimens for the treatment of uncomplicated malaria

Drug	Dose	Side-effects	Comments
P falciparum – Chloroquine resistant[a]			
Artemether-lumefantrine	*<5 kg:* Not recommended *5 kg to < 15 kg:* 1 tablet (20 mg/120 mg) as a single dose, then 1 tablet again after 8 h, then 1 tablet every 12 h × 2 d *15 kg to < 25 kg:* 2 tablets (40 mg/240 mg) as a single dose, then 2 tablets again after 8 h, then 2 tablets every 12 h × 2 d *25 kg to < 35 kg:* 3 tablets (60 mg/360 mg) as a single dose, then 3 tablets again after 8 h, then 3 tablets every 12 h × 2 d *≥35 kg:* 4 adult tablets (80 mg/480 mg) as a single dose, then 4 tabs again after 8 h, then 4 tabs every 12 h × 2 d	Cough, pain, vomiting, anemia, headache, and diarrhea	Take with food. Repeat dose if patient vomits within 30 min. If resistance suspected (eg, infection acquired in Greater Mekong subregion), monitor parasitemia and consider extending therapy until parasite clearance.
Atovaquone-proguanil Two tablet strengths are available: Adult tablet: 250 mg/100 mg Pediatric tablet: 62.5 mg/25 mg	*<5 kg:* Not recommended *5–8 kg:* 2 pediatric tablets in a single dose daily × 3 d *9–10 kg:* 3 pediatric tablets in a single dose daily × 3 d *11–20 kg:* 1 adult tablet in a single dose daily × 3 d *21–30 kg:* 2 adult tablets in a single dose daily × 3 d *31–40 kg:* 3 adult tablets in a single dose daily × 3 d *>40 kg:* 4 adult tablets in a single dose daily × 3 d	Maculopapular rash, nausea, diarrhea, and headache	Take with food. Repeat dose if patient vomits within 30 min.

(*continued on next page*)

Table 1
(*continued*)

Drug	Dose	Side-effects	Comments
P falciparum – chloroquine sensitive[b]			
Chloroquine phosphate	10 mg/kg of base orally; then 5 mg/kg of base at 6, 24, and 48 h. Total: 25 mg/kg base Adult (maximum) dose: 600 mg of base orally, then 300 mg of base in 6 h, then 300 mg of base daily × 2 d. Total: 1500 mg of base	Use with caution in patients with epilepsy. QT prolongation. Pruritus, nausea, vomiting, diarrhea, retinitis pigmentosa, blurred vision, insomnia.	According to WHO guidelines, an ACT may be used for all species of malaria.
P vivax[c]			
Chloroquine phosphate[d]	*Pediatric:* 10 mg/kg of base orally; then 5 mg/kg of base at 6, 24, and 48 h. Total: 25 mg/kg base (never exceed adult dose) *Adult (maximum) dose:* 600 mg of base orally, then 300 mg of base in 6 h, then 300 mg of base daily × 2 d. Total: 1500 mg of base	Use with caution in patients with epilepsy. QT prolongation. Pruritus, nausea, vomiting, diarrhea, retinitis pigmentosa, blurred vision, insomnia.	According to WHO guidelines, an ACT may be used for all species of malaria.
AND Primaquine phosphate[d]	*Pediatric:* 0.5 mg/kg of base orally once daily × 14 d. *Adult (maximum) dose:* 30 mg of base (2 tablets) orally once daily × 14 d. Total dose of primaquine in patients ≥70 kg should be adjusted to a total dose of 6 mg/kg, given in daily doses of 30 mg/d times the number of days to complete the total dose.	Hemolysis in people with glucose-6-phosphate dehydrogenase deficiency, nausea, dizziness, vomiting	

P ovale, P malariae, and P knowlesi			
Chloroquine phosphate[d]	*Pediatric:* 10 mg/kg of base orally; then 5 mg/kg of base at 6, 24, and 48 h. Total: 25 mg/kg base (never exceed adult dose) *Adult (maximum) dose:* 600 mg of base orally, then 300 mg of base in 6 h, then 300 mg of base daily × 2 d. Total: 1500 mg of base	Use with caution in patients with epilepsy. QT prolongation. Pruritus, nausea, vomiting, diarrhea, retinitis pigmentosa, blurred vision, insomnia.	According to WHO guidelines, an ACT may be used for all species of malaria.
For *P ovale* only, add: primaquine phosphate[d]	*Pediatric:* 0.5 mg/kg of base orally once daily × 14 d. *Adult (maximum) dose:* 30 mg of base (2 tablets) orally once daily × 14 d. Total dose of primaquine in patients ≥70 kg should be adjusted to a total dose of 6 mg/kg, given in daily doses of 30 mg/d × number of days to complete the total dose.	Hemolysis in people with glucose-6-phosphate dehydrogenase deficiency, nausea, dizziness, vomiting	Must check for glucose-6-phosphate dehydrogenase deficiency before prescribing

[a] *P falciparum* can be acquired in most areas of the world.
[b] *P falciparum* is known to be acquired in the Caribbean or Central America north of the Panama Canal.
[c] In some areas (eg, Papua New Guinea), chloroquine-resistant *P vivax* has been detected.
[d] The dose is sometimes given in mg of salt and sometimes in mg of base, which leads to frequent confusion. Dosing in the table is in mg of base.

Table 2
Drug regimen for the treatment of severe *P falciparum* malaria

Drug	Dose	Side-effects	Comments
Artesunate	2.4 mg/kg IV at 0, 12, and 24 h, then every 24 h until able to tolerate oral regimen[a]	Rash, dizziness, nausea, diarrhea, anorexia	Artesunate for Injection (Amivas) is now commercially available in the US through major distributors (https://ivartesunate.com) or through the CDC (tel: 770–488–7788; 770–488–7100 after hours) In Canada, artesunate is available through the Canadian Malaria Network.
Followed by complete oral course of antimalarials for uncomplicated malaria	See **Table 1** for dosing of Artemether-lumefantrine or Atovaquone-proguanil	See **Table 1**	See **Table 1**

[a] The WHO guidelines recommend a higher dose of 3.0 mg/kg for children under 20 kg, based on pharmacokinetic considerations.

randomized controlled trials, which monitored hemoglobin levels during acute infection but not beyond hospital admission.[30]

The incidence of PADH is estimated to be 15% among adult travelers with malaria treated with artesunate.[38] The severity of anemia is variable, with 73% of patients requiring a blood transfusion in 1 systematic review.[39] The incidence among children with severe malaria in endemic areas has been estimated at 7%; however, the hemoglobin reduction is modest (<10 g/L) in almost all patients.[40] If a more stringent definition of PADH is applied (requiring laboratory evidence of hemolysis), the incidence rate estimate may be lower.[41] No fatal outcome of PADH has been reported in the literature to date.

The mechanism of PADH is novel. Artesunate rapidly kills intra-erythrocytic parasites, which are removed from erythrocytes by the spleen, leaving behind once-infected erythrocytes. These once-infected erythrocytes remain in circulation with a pitted appearance and a decreased lifespan of 7 to 21 days,[42,43] which correlates with the timing of PADH. There is a higher incidence of PADH among patients with high parasite burden. Thus, PADH seems to be a consequence of rapid parasite killing by artesunate, resulting in a synchronized population of short-lived pitted erythrocytes.

Pediatric Pharmacokinetics and Dosing of Artesunate

Regarding the pediatric dosing of artesunate, some differences between treatment guidelines by the US CDC and the WHO are worth noting. The pharmacokinetics of artesunate differ in children compared with adults, leading to lower exposure to the active metabolite dihydroartemisinin in children.[44,45] These considerations led to revised dosing recommendations in the WHO[9] and the Committee to Advise on Travel

Medicine and Tropical[12] malaria treatment guidelines: children weighing less than 20 kg should receive 3.0 mg/kg/dose of artesunate, rather than the dose in larger children or adults of 2.4 mg/kg/dose. However, the product monograph for artesunate for injection lists the same dose (2.4 mg/kg/dose) for infants and children, regardless of weight.

Emerging Artemisinin Resistance

Malaria control efforts are increasingly threatened by antimalarial drug resistance. *P falciparum* resistance to current first-line ACT drugs has been detected in multiple Asian countries in the Greater Mekong subregion.[3] Cambodia has seen the greatest prevalence of drug resistance, with high rates of treatment failure for ACTs.[3] Resistance is manifested initially by a phenotype of delayed parasite clearance.[46] Genetic determinants of resistance include mutations in the propeller domain of the *Pfkelch13* gene.[47–50] Resistance to ACT partner drugs (eg, mefloquine and piperaquine) has also been detected, and high rates to ACT failure have now been reported from Cambodia, Thailand, and Vietnam.[46] In African countries, data (2010–2018) from the WHO showed that the clinical efficacy of ACT for uncomplicated malaria was 98.0%, 98.5%, and 99.3% for artemether–lumefantrine, artesunate–amodiaquine, and dihydroartemisinin–piperaquine, respectively. The high efficacy remained constant over the period of study.[9] Partial resistance to artemisinin derivatives has been recently reported in Rwanda with *Pfkelch13* mutations in more than 13% of cases, associated with delayed parasite clearance.[51]

In North America, guidelines for the treatment of malaria continue to recommend the use of artemisinin derivatives for uncomplicated and severe malaria.[12,24] There are a few case reports of travelers returning from Africa with malaria and not responding as expected to treatment. However, molecular markers or blood levels of the partner medicines could not confirm resistance.[9] Clinicians should remain alert for possible delayed clearance and should monitor parasite density throughout treatment, particularly in travelers retuning from Southeast Asia. In cases of delayed response to artemisinin-based therapies in travelers from this region, it may be necessary to extend the duration of therapy for several days until the parasitemia clears.

PREVENTION

In malaria-endemic regions, vector control is the main mode of malaria prevention and is achieved primarily using insecticide-treated bed nets (ITNs) or indoor residual spraying (IRS). Case management of infected individuals, which includes prompt diagnosis and treatment of infections, is another component of malaria control and the prevention of onward transmission. In some areas, chemoprevention using a variety of strategies (eg, mass drug administration, seasonal malaria chemoprophylaxis, or intermittent preventative treatment) has been used. A new vaccine against malaria is being pilot tested in 3 countries as a possible addition to the armamentarium of prevention strategies. For North American travelers to endemic areas, advice for vector avoidance and chemoprophylaxis are the principal methods for malaria prevention during the well-defined period of exposure.

Insecticide-treated Bed Nets

ITNs act as both a physical and chemical barrier to *Anopheles* mosquitoes.[12] A systematic review on the efficacy of ITNs found that the incidence of uncomplicated malaria was halved in regions with ITNs compared with regions with no nets.[52]

Long-lasting insecticide nets treated with pyrethroids are the standard recommended by the WHO.[9] Unfortunately, gaps in coverage are widespread. An estimated 269 million individuals continue to live in malaria-endemic regions of sub-Saharan Africa without ITNs.[4] Reasons for low coverage are complex, compounded by low domestic government spending on health care in malaria-endemic countries.

Indoor Residual Spraying

IRS using insecticide applied to the inner walls of homes is another effective way to decrease *Anopheles* mosquito bites.[9] Several chemical classes of insecticides are available (eg, pyrethroids, organophosphates, carbamates, and organochlorines), each with a good safety and efficacy profile.[9] However, insecticide resistance of mosquitoes has increased, decreasing the effectiveness of both ITNs and IRS. Of the malaria-endemic countries with monitoring data, 82% reported resistance to at least 1 insecticide, and 68% reported resistance to 2 or more insecticide classes.[3] The WHO recommends combining 2 or more insecticides with different modes of action when spraying to mediate resistance.[9] Other barriers to IRS implementation include cost and community acceptability.

Chemoprevention of Malaria in Endemic Areas

In malaria-endemic areas, several strategies have been tested for malaria prophylaxis and preventive treatment using antimalarial medications. Mass drug administration rapidly decreases the burden of malaria in the target population in the short term, but the long-term impact, barriers to community uptake, and potential contribution to drug resistance require further study.[53] Sulfadoxine–pyrimethamine may be used for intermittent preventative therapy in pregnancy and in infancy.[46] In 2015, however, only 31% of pregnant women in 36 African countries received 3 or more doses of intermittent preventative therapy in pregnancy.[3] Seasonal malaria chemoprevention (eg, using sulfadoxine–pyrimethamine and amodiaquine) in preschool children has been applied in the Sahel region of Africa (ie, geographic region between the Sahara desert and the savanna).[46]

Vaccine

The leading malaria vaccine candidate is known as RTS,S/AS01 vaccine (Mosquirix). This vaccine targets the *P falciparum* circumsporozoite protein.[54] Recombinant circumsporozoite protein epitopes (represented by the letters “R” and “T”) are fused to the hepatitis B surface antigen and expressed together with free hepatitis B surface antigen (represented by the letter “S”).[54] The resulting proteins (RTS,S) self-assemble into virus-like particles.[55] RTS,S is formulated with an adjuvant system (AS01).[55] The RTS,S/AS01 vaccine is the first malaria vaccine shown to provide partial protection against malaria in young children.[56] Phase III trials of the RTS,S/AS01 conducted at 11 centers in sub-Saharan Africa enrolled at total of 15,459 participants in 2 age groups (infants aged 6–12 weeks and children aged 5–17 months).[56] The vaccine efficacy against clinical malaria was 20% in infants and 35% in children over 32 months of follow-up.[56] In a 7-year follow-up study, vaccine efficacy waned over time.[57] In particular, negative efficacy (higher clinical infection rates in the vaccine group relative to the placebo group) were seen during the fifth year among children in areas with high malaria exposure.[57] Given its modest vaccine efficacy, the WHO considers RTS,S/AS01 as a potential complementary tool in combatting the global malaria burden.[58] In a coordinated evaluation of malaria vaccine introduction, pilot implementation of the vaccine in 3 countries (Ghana, Kenya, and Malawi) began in 2019.[59] Of note, the vaccine remains experimental and is not available to North American travelers to malaria-endemic regions.

Malaria Prevention in Travelers

Travelers to the tropics from North America should be counseled on the risk of acquiring malaria, which varies widely according to travel destination (eg, greatest risk in sub-Saharan Africa). In addition to geographic considerations, a high-risk demographic group for malaria acquisition is the traveler visiting friends and relatives. Visiting friends and relatives include children of immigrants returning to home countries for family visits, who may have higher levels of exposure (eg, rural areas), a lower perception of risk, and lower levels of immunity relative to children living in the endemic area.

All travelers should be counseled on mosquito precautions. Physical barriers include long-sleeved shirts, full-length pants, and other full-coverage garments, especially at dusk, when *Anopheles* mosquitoes are most likely to feed.[12] Insect repellents may be used, with the following considerations for efficacy and safety in children. Topical repellents that contain 10% to 30% DEET or 20% icaridin are effective against *Anopheles* bites when applied properly.[12] Safe and protective concentrations of DEET vary by age: children aged 6 months to 2 years should use 10% DEET no more than once daily; children aged 2 to 12 should use 10% DEET no more than thrice daily; and adults and children greater than 12 years of age should use 30% DEET every 6 hours.[60] The 20% icaridin is safe and effective for all ages except children less than 6 months of age. Mosquito nets should be used in place of topical repellents for children less than 6 months of age.

Antimalarial drugs are highly effective at preventing severe malaria, but they require strict adherence to the dosing regimen.[12] All antimalarial drug regimens should begin before departure to assess tolerability. For individuals traveling to *P falciparum* chloroquine-resistant zones (most of the world), atovaquone–proguanil, doxycycline, or mefloquine all provide adequate protection. Atovaquone–proguanil regimens should begin 1 to 2 days before departure and end 1 week after leaving the malaria-endemic region. Atovaquone–proguanil is available in pediatric and adult tablets, with dosing based on weight, but is not licensed for children weighing less than 5 kg. Doxycycline is also a daily medication, but should be taken for 4 weeks after departure of the malaria-endemic region because it is not active against liver stages of the parasite. Doxycycline is associated with photosensitivity, vaginal candidiasis, rare cases of esophageal erosion, and should not be used for malaria chemoprophylaxis in children less than 8 years of age.[61] Mefloquine is dosed once weekly, but should not be prescribed to individuals traveling to chloroquine- and mefloquine-resistant regions.[12] Additionally, prescribing physicians must warn patients about potential for mefloquine to cause or aggravate neuropsychiatric illness.[62] Children seem to have a lower incidence of neuropsychiatric side effects, although this may be related to lower reporting of symptoms. Primaquine taken once daily is an alternative to atovaquone–proguanil, doxycycline, or mefloquine, but it cannot be taken by children with glucose-6-phosphate dehydrogenase deficiency.[12] Primaquine may also be taken as terminal prophylaxis by individuals traveling to *P vivax* or *P ovale* endemic regions. For individuals traveling only to chloroquine-sensitive regions (eg, Caribbean and Central America north of the Panama Canal), chloroquine or hydroxychloroquine can be considered, beginning 1 week before departure, and ending 4 weeks after return from the malaria-endemic region. Medications and dosing from chemoprophylaxis in travelers is given in **Table 3**.

Table 3
Chemoprophylaxis regimens for the prevention of malaria in North American travelers

Drug	Dose	Side Effects	Comments
Atovaquone-proguanil Two tablet strengths are available: Adult tablet: 250 mg/100 mg Pediatric tablet: 62.5 mg/25 mg	Take *daily* beginning 1–2 d before, during, and for *7 d* after travel in endemic area at the following dose: *<5 kg:* Not recommended *5–8 kg:* 1/2 pediatric tablet daily *9–10 kg:* 3/4 pediatric tablet daily *11–20 kg:* 1 pediatric tablet daily *21–30 kg:* 2 pediatric tablets daily *31–40 kg:* 3 pediatric tablets daily *>40 kg:* 1 adult tablet daily	Maculopapular rash, nausea, diarrhea, and headache	Take with food.
Doxycycline	Take *daily* beginning 1–2 d before, during, and for *4 wk* after travel in an endemic area at the following dose: 2.2 mg/kg once daily up to 100 mg/d	Nausea, vomiting, diarrhea, sun sensitization, odynophagia, headache, vaginal candidiasis	Avoid in children <8 y of age.[a]
Mefloquine	Take *weekly* beginning 2 wk before, during, and for *4 wk* after travel in endemic area at the following dose: *<9 kg:* 5 mg/kg weekly *10–19 kg:* ¼ adult tablet weekly *20–30 kg:* ½ adult tablet weekly *31–45 kg:* ¾ adult tablet weekly *>45 kg:* 1 tablet weekly	Not recommended if cardiac conduction abnormalities, seizures, or psychiatric disorders. QT interval prolongation. Neuropsychiatric adverse reactions.	FDA "black box" warning states that neuropsychiatric and vestibular adverse reactions may persist indefinitely, even after discontinuation of drug.

[a] Although the American Academy of Pediatrics now recommends that doxycycline can be safely administered for a short duration (≤21 d) regardless of patient age, prophylaxis will require prolonged duration of dosing.

SUMMARY

Recent progress and setbacks in malaria control in the tropics are analogous to an escalating arms race of human versus parasite and vector. Potent artemisinin derivatives for the treatment of severe malaria have been accompanied by an increase in *Pfkelch13*-mutant *P falciparum* and artemisinin resistance. Rapid diagnostic tests to replace the microscope have been met with *Pfhrp2/3* stealth mutations that avoid parasite detection. ITNs are challenged by insecticide-resistant *Anopheles* mosquitoes. Even the newest tool in the armamentarium, the RTS,S circumsporozoite vaccine, has proven only modestly effective against such an antigenically variable parasite. It seems that the battle against malaria is far from over and that combined strategies on multiple fronts will be needed, together with sustained international commitment. Meanwhile, physicians need to remain vigilant for malaria among febrile returning travelers or new immigrants from the tropics. Owing to its nonspecific clinical presentation, the diagnosis may be missed. Children with severe malaria in nonendemic regions frequently have a history of multiple emergency department visits before an accurate diagnosis is made. Nonetheless, if promptly recognized, diagnosed, and treated, pediatric outcomes can be excellent.

CLINICS CARE POINTS

- Ask for a travel history in every febrile child.
- In case of recent (particularly <30 days) travel to a malaria-endemic area, urgently obtain thin and thick blood smears for malaria microscopy and/or a sensitive rapid molecular test (eg, PCR). To confidently exclude malaria, smears should be repeated at 12 and 24 hours until there are 3 negative smears.
- In case of a positive smear, consult a pediatric infectious disease specialist. Initiate treatment without delay for uncomplicated or severe malaria, according to clinical presentation.
- Guidelines are available for treatment according to *Plasmodium* species and severity. Expert consultation is recommended.
- Chemoprophylaxis should be prescribed for all travelers to malaria endemic areas for the entire duration of the exposure.

DISCLOSURE

The authors have nothing to disclose.

REFERENCES

1. Sutherland C, Tanomsing N, Nolder D, et al. Two nonrecombining sympatric forms of the human malaria parasite Plasmodium ovale occur globally. J Infect Dis 2010;201(10):1544–50.
2. Brasil P, Zalis MG, de Pina-Costa A, et al. Outbreak of human malaria caused by Plasmodium simium in the Atlantic Forest in Rio de Janeiro: a molecular epidemiological investigation. Lancet Glob Health 2017;5(10):e1038–46.
3. WHO. World malaria report 2016. Geneva: World Health Organization; 2016:186.
4. WHO. In: Organization WH, editor. World malaria report 2015. Switzerland: WHO Press; 2015. p. 280.
5. Mace KE, Arguin PM, Lucchi NW, et al. Malaria surveillance — United States, 2016. Surveill Summ 2019;68(5):1–35.
6. Boggild AK, McCarthy AE, Libman MD, et al. Underestimate of annual malaria imports to Canada. Lancet Infect Dis 2017;17(2):141–2.
7. Davies HD, Keystone J, Lester M, et al. Congenital malaria in infants of asymptomatic women. CMAJ 1992;146(10):1755–6.
8. Slinger R, Giulivi A, Bodie-Collins M, et al. Transfusion-transmissed malaria in Canada. CMAJ 2001;164(3):377–9.
9. World Health Organization. WHO Guidelines for malaria. Geneva: World Health Organization; 2021.

10. McCarthy AE, Morgan C, Prematunge C, et al. Severe malaria in Canada, 2001-2013. Malar J 2015;14:151.
11. Boggild AK, Geduld J, Libman M, et al. Malaria in travellers returning or migrating to Canada: surveillance report from CanTravNet surveillance data 2004-2014. CMAJ Open 2016;4(3):E352–8.
12. Committee to Advise on Tropical Medicine and Travel (CATMAT). Canadian recommendations for the prevention and treatment of malaria. Public Health Agency of Canada; 2020. Available at: https://www.canada.ca/en/public-health/services/catmat/canadian-recommendations-prevention-treatment-malaria.html. Accessed June 8, 2021.
13. WHO. Guidelines for the treatment of malaria. 2nd edition. Geneva: World Health Organization; 2010. Available at: http://www.who.int/malaria/publications/en/Malaria.
14. Hawkes M, Elphinstone RE, Conroy AL, et al. Contrasting pediatric and adult cerebral malaria. Virulence 2013;4(6):543–55.
15. Conroy AL, Hawkes M, Elphinstone RE, et al. Acute kidney injury is common in pediatric severe malaria and is associated with increased mortality. Open Forum Infect Dis 2016;3(2):ofw046.
16. Hawkes M, Kain KC. Advances in malaria diagnosis. Expert Rev Anti Infect Ther 2007;5(3):485–95.
17. Makanjuola RO, Taylor-Robinson AW. Improving accuracy of malaria diagnosis in underserved rural and remote endemic areas of sub-Saharan Africa: a call to develop multiplexing rapid diagnostic tests. Scientifica 2020;2020:3901409.
18. Golassa L, Messele A, Amambua-Ngwa A, et al. High prevalence and extended deletions in *Plasmodium falciparum hrp2/3* genomic loci in Ethiopia. PLoS One 2020;15(11):e0241807.
19. Centers for Disease Control and Prevention. Malaria diagnostic tests. 2020. Available at: https://www.cdc.gov/malaria/diagnosis_treatment/diagnostic_tools.html. Accessed June 7, 2021.
20. Snounou G, Viriyakosol S, Jarra W, et al. Identification of the four human malaria parasite species in field samples by the polymerase chain reaction and detection of a high prevalence of mixed infections. Mol Biochem Parasitol 1993;58(2):283–92.
21. Snounou G, Viriyakosol S, Zhu X. High sensitivity of detection of human malaria parasites by the use of nested polymerase chain reaction. Mol Biochem Parasitol 1993;61(2):315–20.
22. Oliveira D, Shi Y, Oloo A. Field evaluation of a polymerase chain reaction-based nonisotopic liquid hybridization assay for malaria diagnosis. J Infect Dis 1996;173(5):1284–7.
23. Center for Disease Control and Prevention (CDC). Treatment of malaria: guidelines for clinicians (United States). Part 3: alternatives for pregnant women and treatment of severe malaria. Atlanta, GA: Center for Disease Control and Prevention (CDC); 2013.
24. Centers for Disease Control and Prevention. Treatment of malaria: guidelines for clinicians (United States). 2020. Available at: https://www.cdc.gov/malaria/resources/pdf/Malaria_Treatment_Guidelines.pdf. Accessed June 6, 2021.
25. Schuurkamp GJ, Spicer PE, Kereu RK, et al. Chloroquine-resistant Plasmodium vivax in Papua New Guinea. Trans R Soc Trop Med Hyg 1992;86(2):121–2.
26. Maguire JD, Sumawinata IW, Masbar S, et al. Chloroquine-resistant Plasmodium malariae in south Sumatra, Indonesia. Lancet 2002;360:58–60.

27. WHO. Guidelines for the treatment of malaria. Third Edition 2015. Available at: http://www.who.int/malaria/publications/atoz/9789241549127/en/.
28. Dondorp AM, Nosten F, Yi P, et al. Artemisinin resistance in Plasmodium falciparum malaria. N Engl J Med 2009;361(5):455–67.
29. Sinclair D, Donegan S, Isba R, et al. Artesunate versus quinine for treating severe malaria. Cochrane Database Syst Rev 2012;2012(6):CD005967.
30. Dondorp AM, Fanello CI, Hendriksen ICE, et al. Artesunate versus quinine in the treatment of severe falciparum malaria in African children (AQUAMAT): an open-label, randomised trial. Lancet 2010;376(9753):1647–57.
31. Noubiap JJ. Shifting from quinine to artesunate as first-line treatment of severe malaria in children and adults: saving more lives. J Infect Public Health 2014; 7(5):407–12.
32. Boggild A, Brophy J, Charlebois P, et al. Summary of recommendations for the diagnosis and treatment of malaria by the Committee to Advise on Tropical Medicine and Travel (CATMAT). Can Commun Dis Rep 2014;40–7.
33. Dondorp A, Nosten F, Stepniewska K, et al. South East Asian Quinine Artesunate Malaria Trial g. Artesunate versus quinine for treatment of severe falciparum malaria: a randomised trial. Lancet 2005;366(9487):717–25.
34. Zoller T, Junghanss T, Kapaun A, et al. Intravenous artesunate for severe malaria in travelers, Europe. Emerg Infect Dis 2011;17(5):771–7.
35. Kreeftmeijer-Vegter AR, van Genderen PJ, Visser LG, et al. Treatment outcome of intravenous artesunate in patients with severe malaria in the Netherlands and Belgium. Malar J 2012;11:102.
36. Jaureguiberry S, Ndour PA, Roussel C, et al. Postartesunate delayed hemolysis is a predictable event related to the lifesaving effect of artemisinins. Blood 2014; 124(2):167–75.
37. Rolling T, Schmiedel S, Wichmann D, et al. Post-treatment haemolysis in severe imported malaria after intravenous artesunate: case report of three patients with hyperparasitaemia. Malar J 2012;11:169.
38. Roussel C, Caumes E, Thellier M, et al. Artesunate to treat severe malaria in travellers: review of efficacy and safety and practical implications. J Trav Med 2017; 24(2):1–9.
39. Rehman K, Lotsch F, Kremsner PG, et al. Haemolysis associated with the treatment of malaria with artemisinin derivatives: a systematic review of current evidence. Int J Infect Dis 2014;29:268–73.
40. Rolling T, Agbenyega T, Issifou S, et al. Delayed hemolysis after treatment with parenteral artesunate in African children with severe malaria–a double-center prospective study. J Infect Dis 2014;209(12):1921–8.
41. Arguin P. Case definition: postartemisinin delayed hemolysis. Blood 2014;124(2): 157–8.
42. Newton PN, Chotivanich K, Chierakul W, et al. A comparison of the in vivo kinetics of Plasmodium falciparum ring-infected erythrocyte surface antigen-positive and -negative erythrocytes. Blood 2001;98(2):450–7.
43. Chotivanich K, Udomsangpetch R, Dondorp A, et al. The mechanisms of parasite clearance after antimalarial treatment of Plasmodium falciparum malaria. J Infect Dis 2000;182(2):629–33.
44. Hendriksen I, Mtove G, Kent A, et al. Population pharmacokinetics of intramuscular artesunate in African children with severe malaria: implications for a practical dosing regimen. Clin Pharmacol Ther 2013;93:443–50.

45. Zaloumis S, Tarning J, Krishna S, et al. Population pharmacokinetics of intravenous artesunate: a pooled analysis of individual data from patients with severe malaria. CPT Pharmacometrics Syst Pharmacol 2014;3:e145.
46. Ashley EA, Phyo AP, Woodrow CJ. Malaria. Lancet 2018;391(10130):1608–21.
47. Ariey F, Witkowski B, Amaratunga C, et al. A molecular marker of artemisinin-resistant Plasmodium falciparum malaria. Nature 2014;505(7481):50–5.
48. Ashley EA, Dhorda M, Fairhurst RM, et al. Spread of artemisinin resistance in Plasmodium falciparum malaria. N Engl J Med 2014;371(5):411–23.
49. Mok S, Ashley EA, Ferreira PE, et al. Population transcriptomics of human malaria parasites reveals the mechanism of artemisinin resistance. Science 2015; 347(6220):431–5.
50. Takala-Harrison S, Jacob CG, Arze C, et al. Independent emergence of artemisinin resistance mutations among plasmodium falciparum in Southeast Asia. J Infect Dis 2015;211(5):670–9.
51. Uwinmana A, Umulisa N, Venkatesan M, et al. Association of *Plasmodium falciparum kelch13* R561H genotypes with delayed parasite clearance in Rwanda: an open-label, single-arm, multicentre, therapeutic efficacy study. Lancet Infect Dis 2021;21(8):1120–8.
52. Lengeler C. Insecticide-treated bed nets and curtains for preventing malaria. Cochrane Database Syst Rev 2004;2:CD000363.
53. Poirot E, Skarbinski J, Sinclair D, et al. Mass drug administration for malaria. Cochrane Database Syst Rev 2013;12:CD008846.
54. Gordon DM, McGovern TW, Krzych U, et al. Safety, immunogenicity, and efficacy of a recombinantly produced Plasmodium falciparum circumsporozoite protein-hepatitis B surface antigen subunit vaccine. J Infect Dis 1995;171(6):1576–85.
55. Hoffman SL, Vekemans J, Richie TL, et al. The march toward malaria vaccines. Vaccine 2015;33(Suppl 4):D13–23.
56. Rts SCTP. Efficacy and safety of RTS,S/AS01 malaria vaccine with or without a booster dose in infants and children in Africa: final results of a phase 3, individually randomised, controlled trial. Lancet 2015;386(9988):31–45.
57. Olotu A, Fegan G, Wambua J, et al. Seven-year efficacy of RTS,S/AS01 malaria vaccine among young African children. N Engl J Med 2016;374(26):2519–29.
58. WHO. World Health Organization. Malaria vaccine implementation Programme (MVIP). Available at: http://www.who.int/immunization/diseases/malaria/malaria_vaccine_implementation_programme/about/en/. Accessed June 4, 2021.
59. Baral R, Levin A, Odero C, et al. Costs of continuing RTS,S/ASO1E malaria vaccination in the three malaria vaccine pilot implementation countries. PLoS One 2021;16(1):e0244995.
60. Government of Canada. Personal insect repellents 2021. Available at: https://www.canada.ca/en/health-canada/services/about-pesticides/insect-repellents.html#a2. Accessed June 8, 2021.
61. Centers for Disease Control and Prevention. Choosing a drug to prevent malaria 2018. Available at: https://www.cdc.gov/malaria/travelers/drugs.html. Accessed June 8, 2021.
62. McCarthy S. Malaria prevention, mefloquine neurotoxicity, neuropsychiatric illness, and risk-benefit analysis in the Australian defence force. J Parasitol Res 2015;2015:287651.
63. Brooks HM. Anti-malarial strategies among vulnerable populations: exploring bed net underutilization among internally displaced persons and novel adjunctive therapies for cerebral malaria. Edmonton, Canada: University of Alberta; 2017.

Salmonellosis Including Enteric Fever

Farah Naz Qamar, MBBS, FCPS, MSC, FRCP[a,*], Wajid Hussain, MBBS, FCPS[b], Sonia Qureshi, MBBS, FCPS ,MSC[b]

KEYWORDS

- Salmonellosis • Enteric fever • XDR Typhoid

KEY POINTS

- *There are more than 2500 serotypes (serovars) of Salmonella; but less than 100 serotypes are known to cause infections in humans.*
- *Nontyphoidal Salmonellosis (NTS) is one of the leading causes of foodborne disease globally.*
- *Enteric fever is a potentially life-threatening acute febrile illness.*
- *S. enterica serovar Typhi (S. typhi), is a gram-negative, facultative anaerobic bacillus, belonging to the family Enterobacteriaceae, transmitted via feco-oral route.*
- *Typhoid vaccination, clean drinking water, and careful attention to hygiene are essential preventive control measures against enteric fever.*

INTRODUCTION

Salmonellosis is one of the significant causes of food-borne disease worldwide and a major public health concern. It is caused by the genus Salmonella, named after Daniel E. Salmon, who first isolated the bacteria in 1884. Salmonella is a gram-negative, motile, nonsporulating, facultative anaerobic bacillus, belongs to the family *Enterobacteriaceae*.[1] *S. enterica* serovar typhi (*S. typhi*) and *S. enterica* serovar paratyphi (*S. paratyphi* A B C) cause enteric fever, whereas nontyphoidal *Salmonella* serotypes (NTS) cause diarrhea.

Taxonomy

According to the recent nomenclature, the genus *Salmonella* is broadly categorized into 2 species, *S. enterica* and *Salmonella bongori*. *S. enterica* is further divided into 6 different subspecies *S. enterica* subspecies enterica, *S. enterica* subspecies salamae, *S. enterica* subspecies arizonae, *S. enterica* subspecies arizona, *S. enterica*

[a] Department of Paediatrics & Child Health, The Aga Khan University Hospital, Stadium Road, P.O Box 3500, Karachi 74800, Pakistan; [b] Department of Paediatrics & Child Health, The Aga Khan University Hospital, Stadium Road, P.O Box 3500, Karachi 74800, Pakistan
* Corresponding author.
E-mail address: farah.qamar@aku.edu

Pediatr Clin N Am 69 (2022) 65–77
https://doi.org/10.1016/j.pcl.2021.09.007 pediatric.theclinics.com
0031-3955/22/

subspecies houtenae, and *S. enterica* subspecies indica. More than 2500 different serotypes or serovars of *S. enterica* have been identified to date but less than 100 serotypes are known to cause infections in humans.[2]

Salmonella can survive for several months in water.[3] *S. enterica* serotype Dublin and *S. enterica* serotype Choleraesuis are host-specific and reside in animal species such as cattle and pigs, respectively. These particular serotypes often cause invasive and life-threatening diseases in human.[4] Fecal-oral route remains an important mode of transmission of salmonellosis in humans in low and middle-income countries (LMICs). *Salmonella* spp. live in the intestines of humans and animals. Most people are infected with *Salmonella* through direct contact with an infected person or indirect contact by means of contaminated water or food.[5]

Epidemiology

Salmonellosis accounts for 93.8 million food-borne illnesses and 155,000 deaths per year.[1]The reported annual incidence of salmonellosis was 14.9 cases per 100,000 population in the United States.[5]

Salmonellosis is the second most common reported zoonosis in Europe, after campylobacteriosis, with *S. enterica* serotype enteritidis being the most commonly reported serotype.[6] This bacterium remains one of the major causes of food-borne outbreaks.[7] Diarrheal disease caused by Salmonella ranged from 0.44 to 0.99 episodes per person-year, such an incidence would translate into an order of 2.8 billion cases of diarrheal illness each year world wide.[8] Salmonella was responsible for 95.1 million cases of enterocolitis and 50,771 deaths in 2017.[9] In 2017, an estimated 535,000 cases of invasive NTS disease occurred globally affecting the children younger than 5 years with a total death of 77,500. The incidence of invasive NTS in East Asia was estimated to be 1.2 cases per 100,000.[9]

Enteric fever is more common in children[10] and is prevalent in areas that are overcrowded and have poor sanitation practices. Globally, 14·3 million cases of typhoid and paratyphoid fevers occurred in 2017, a 44·6% decline from 25·9 million in 1990.[9] Incidence of enteric fever is highest in Southeast Asia[10] Up to 100 enteric fever cases, per 100,000 person-years have been reported from south-central Asia, Southeast Asia, and southern Africa. See **Table 1**.[11]

Pathophysiology

Several factors influence the pathophysiology of salmonellosis such as the infecting species, infectious dose, and the gastric PH. In general, about 10^6 bacterial cells are needed to cause infection. Low gastric acidity among individuals who use antacids can decrease the infective dose to 10^3 cells. In the small intestine, Salmonella induces an influx of macrophages (typhoidal strains) or neutrophils (nontyphoidal strains). After access to the small intestine, *S. typhi* penetrates the epithelium, via the M-cells, a specialized epithelial cell or direct penetration then enters the lymphoid tissue and disseminates through the lymphatic or hematogenous route, whereas nontyphoidal Salmonella generally precipitates a localized response.

Nontyphoidal Salmonellosis

NTS is one of the leading causes of foodborne disease globally. Most frequently isolated serotypes are *S. enteritidis*, *S. Newport*, and *S. typhimurium*. NTS is most commonly associated with ingestion of poultry, eggs, milk products, fresh produce, meats, as well as contact with pets, such as reptiles and other animals.

Risk factors for the disease include watering of crops from drains or other contaminated water sources, living in close proximity to a farm and other domestic animals,

Table 1
Differences between typhoidal and nontyphoidal Salmonella associated with human disease

	Typhoidal Salmonella	Nontyphoidal Salmonella
Serovars	Typhi, Paratyphi A B C	Ubiquitous serovars Typhimurium and Enteritidis, but ~1500 other serovars of *S.enterica* ssp. are known
Epidemiology	Endemic in developing countries especially Southeast Asia, Africa, and South America	Most common in Southeast Asia and Africa
Host	Human	Pets, poultry, pigs, cattles
Incubation period	7–21 d	6–24 h
Disease course	Symptoms (3 d to 3 wk). 2%–5% of infected individuals become long-term (≥1 y) carriers.	Brief duration of symptoms (<10 d). Long-term carriage is rare
Long-term carriage	Chronic carrier	Rare
Reservoir	Human to human transmission	poultry, beef, pork, eggs, milk, seafood, and fresh produce
Clinical manifestations	Systemic disease (fever, abdominal pain, rash, nausea, anorexia, hepatosplenomegaly, diarrhea or constipation, headache, dry cough)	Self-limiting gastroenteritis in immunocompetent individuals (diarrhea, vomiting, abdominal cramps). In immunocompromised patients (inherited deficiency of the IL-12/IL-23 system, young infants, elderly, and those with HIV), the disease is associated with invasive extraintestinal infections.
Immune response	Minimal intestinal inflammation, leukopenia, Th1 response	Robust intestinal inflammation, neutrophil recruitment, Th1 response
Vaccination	(i) Live attenuated oral vaccine (Ty21a), (ii) Vi polysaccharide capsule-based vaccine. (iii) Typhoid conjugate vaccine Typbar TCV® (Bharat Biotech)	Monovalent and bivalent vaccines for *S. typhimurium* and *S. enteritidis* are under development

using animal feces as manure in subsistence farming along with unhygienic practices of slaughtering of animals and meat processing.

5% of individuals with documented NTS gastroenteritis develop bacteremia and invasive disease (iNTS), such as those with underlying immunocompromised conditions like human immunodeficiency virus (HIV), malaria, sickle cell disease, young infants, elderly, and malnourished children. NTS species, such as *Salmonella choleraesuis* and *Salmonella Heidelberg* have higher predilection for invasive disease.[12]

Clinical features

NTS present with gastroenteritis, bacteremia, or invasive systemic disease. Salmonella gastroenteritis typically manifests within 8 to 72 hours following exposure to contaminated food or water. Clinical features include diarrhea, nausea, vomiting, fever, and abdominal cramps along with other constitutional symptoms. Severity of diarrhea, the duration of illness, and weight loss correlate with the ingested dose of bacteria.[13] Salmonellosis may present as dysentery in children.[14] In addition to diarrheal disease, nontyphoidal Salmonella infections can invade normally sterile sites, resulting in bacteremia. Invasive NTS (iNTS) can present with systemic infection such as meningitis, septic arthritis, osteomyelitis, or visceral abscess.[15]

Diagnosis

On clinical ground, it is difficult to distinguish nontyphoidal gastroenteritis from other causes of acute infectious diarrhea such as *Rotavirus, Norovirus, E. coli, Shigella, Vibrio cholerae, Campylobacter, Clostridioides, Entamoeba, and Giardia*. Isolation of the pathogen in stool culture is diagnostic. Generally, 48 to 72 hours are required for the pathogen to grow on stool culture. Blood culture and additional tests such as lumbar puncture are indicated depending on the presence of complications in patients with suspected invasive disease.

Management

Nontyphoidal salmonellosis is a self-limiting disease, fever generally resolves within 48 to 72 hours, whereas diarrhea may last for 4 to 10 days. Appropriate hydration remains the mainstay of management. Antimicrobial therapy is limited to patients presenting with severe disease, invasive nontyphoidal salmonellosis with systemic symptoms, and immunocompromised hosts including young infants. Hospitalization and antibiotics (typically third-generation cephalosporins [ceftriaxone or cefotaxime]) are indicated for all individuals with NTS extraintestinal disease.[16] Fluoroquinolones may be used safely in children over short courses,[17] especially if other agents such as trimethoprim-sulfamethoxazole, azithromycin, and a third-generation cephalosporin are not readily available. Optimal duration of antibiotic therapy is variable, and most trials have documented the use of antibiotics for 3 to 14 days, majority recommending for 5 days.[18] Local antibiotic resistance patterns must be taken into account when choosing empiric therapy.

Prognosis

Most cases of NTS are mild to moderate whereas invasive nontyphoidal Salmonella is associated with a case fatality of 20% to 25%.[19] Delayed diagnosis and treatment of invasive nontyphoidal Salmonella with inappropriate antibiotics lead to mortality, particularly in developing countries. Multidrug-resistant and even extensively drug-resistant Salmonella serotypes further compound the high fatality from invasive nontyphoidal Salmonella disease. The rising trend in mortality from invasive nontyphoidal Salmonella in the presence of risk factors such as HIV infection, malnutrition, and malaria, has prompted investigations into the burden of this disease.

Prevention

Monovalent and bivalent vaccines for *S. typhimurium* and *S. enteritidis* are under development.[20] Nontyphoidal Salmonella disease has clearly defined risk factors and is preventable through relatively simple measures involving safe water, sanitation, and personal hygiene.

Typhoidal and Paratyphoidal Salmonellosis (enteric fever)

Enteric fever is a potentially life-threatening infection, with an estimated 21 million illnesses globally and ~ 200,000 deaths annually, in LMICs.[21] Inadequate sanitation and hygiene, poor food, water, and disposal of human excreta are the major contributors to the disease. The infection is transmitted via fecal-oral route, when an individual ingests food or water that is contaminated with infected human feces.[22] *S. enterica* serotype Typhi causes disease only in humans; it has no known animal reservoir. In the preantibiotic era, mortality rates were 15% or greater, whereas, in the postantibiotic era, the average mortality rate from enteric fever is estimated to be less than 1%.[23]

In the early 1970s, the emergence of *S. typhi* strains with resistance to first-line antibiotics (ampicillin, trimethoprim/sulfamethoxazole, and chloramphenicol) was detected and these strains were considered MDR *S. typhi* strains. Soon in the 1990s, resistance to fluoroquinolones was reported.[24]In 2016, a highly resistant strain of *Salmonella typhi*, known as extensively drug resistant (XDR) was identified in an outbreak from Sindh Province of Pakistan, with resistance to ampicillin, trimethoprim/sulfamethoxazole, chloramphenicol, ciprofloxacin, and third-generation cephalosporins.[25] The resistance is mediated by both plasmid-borne and chromosome-borne resistance genes[26] see **Table 2**. By the end of 2018, more than 5000 cases of XDR *S. typhi* strain were reported, with imported cases in the United Kingdom and the United States.[27]

Clinical features

After the ingestion of the causative microorganism through contaminated food or water, symptoms appear around 7 to 14 days. The clinical presentation of enteric fever is nonspecific and varies from a mild illness with low-grade fever, malaise, and dry cough to a severe illness with abdominal discomfort, altered mental status, and multiple complications. In the endemic setting, patients typically present with a high-grade fever for more than 3 days with no clear focus of infection. Along with fever patients may have anorexia, nausea, vomiting, abdominal pain, loose stools, dry cough, headache, myalgia, lethargy, and convulsions. Complications of enteric fever occur in 10% to 15% of patients. Common complications are intestinal (usually ileal) perforation, encephalopathy, hepatitis, cystitis, pyelonephritis, myocarditis, endocarditis, shock, and meningitis. Intestinal perforation is a serious complication and causes a high mortality.[28] Complications due to XDR strains are similar but are expected at a much higher rate because of delays in appropriate antibiotic treatment.

Diagnosis

Microbiological and serologic laboratory methods are used to diagnose enteric fever. However, each one has its own limitation. Isolation of *S. typhi* and *S. paratyphi* on blood culture is considered the gold standard for diagnosis; it is limited by its sensitivity of 40% to 80%.[29] Despite its limitations, blood culture is the only diagnostic method that permits identification for drug resistance. Laboratory documentation of

Table 2
Summary table of antibiotic resistance in Salmonella typhi and the genes encoding the resistance

Resistant Strains	Definition	Genetic Mutation
Multidrug-resistant(MDR) Salmonella strains	Isolates fully resistant to amoxicillin, trimethoprim/ sulfamethoxazole and chloramphenicol	blaTEM-1 dfrA7, sul1, sul2 catA1
Quinolone-resistant Salmonella strains	Isolates fully resistant to fluoroquinolones (ciprofloxacin)	qnrS
Extensively drug-resistant (XDR) Salmonella Strains	Isolates fully resistant to amoxicillin, trimethoprim/ sulfamethoxazole, chloramphenicol, fluoroquinolones, and cephalosporin	blaTEM-1 dfrA7, sul1, sul2 catA1 qnrS, blaCTX-M-15

the genus *Salmonella* is conducted by biochemical tests and the serologic type is established by serologic testing. *Salmonella* are nonlactose fermenters and grow well on several nonselective and selective agar media (Blood, MacConkey, *Salmonella shigella*, Xylose lysine deoxycholate Agars) as well as into enrichment broth such as selenite-F or tetrathionate. Further identification can be achieved using the API (analytical profile index) 20E system that permits the rapid testing of 10 to 20 different biochemical parameters concurrently. The probable biochemical identification of *Salmonella* can be confirmed by antigenic analysis of O and H antigens using polyvalent and specific antisera.[30]

In underdeveloped countries whereby culture facilities are limited, and several serologic methods have been used for the diagnosis of enteric fever for more than hundred years. The Widal test has been broadly used in endemic countries for over a century. It detects patient serum antibodies to *S. typhi* O and H antigens. However, it has limitations including poor specificity (other conditions can lead to increased antibody titers, including malaria) and a cutoff titer that fluctuates according to the endemicity of the disease.[31] Typhidot, an ELISA-based technique is another way for recognizing Salmonella. Typhidot was established for the identification of specific IgM and IgG antibodies. Another modified version of Typhidot, Typhidot-M, is a more specific indicator of acute illness and identifies anti-IgM to the similar protein.[31,32] There are many prototypes of these commercially available rapid diagnostic tests like TUBEX TF, Test-it Typhoid, and others for detecting enteric fever but lack the accuracy and fail to replace blood culture as the gold standard diagnostic test for enteric fever.[33] A major drawback of any rapid diagnostic method is the lack of isolating species and drug susceptibility testing. Therefore, rapid diagnostic tests are not recommended as part of the diagnostic workup because of their variable antibody response and because of the cross-reactivity of *S. typhi* (and *S. paratyphi* A) with other enteric bacteria.[34] Poor diagnostic tests complicate the management of enteric fever. Blood cultures should be sent instead in all cases of suspected enteric fever because the culture method regardless of its shortcomings is still beneficial for antibiotic sensitivity testing.

Advances in diagnostics. To overcome the limitations of the existing tests, new specific antigens and new diagnostic techniques have been used. Typhoid ELISA is a serologic technique that uses *S. typhi* lipopolysaccharide (LPS) and hemolysin E (HlyE) proteins to detect the total antibody response and has shown better sensitivity see **Table 3** when compared with Widal and Typhi Dot.[35,36] In addition to serologic methods, molecular techniques particularly polymerase chain reaction (PCR)-based assays have been developed over the last few decades. It is costly and its use is limited to the research laboratories. PCR precisely identifies *S. typhi* by amplifying the flagellin (fliC) gene locus and can also target virulence genes (tviA and tviB).[37]

To characterize *S. typhi,* genomes for antimicrobial resistance (AMR) and for the evolution of different lineages, whole-genome sequencing (WGS) is also under development. WGS has high sensitivity and specificity than serologic and bacteriologic methods and was studied in various typhoid endemic countries like Bangladesh, Nepal, and in a recent XDR enteric fever outbreak in Pakistan. XDR *S. typhi* has been reported in travelers from Pakistan to several countries (**Fig. 1**). WGS is useful for the identification of AMR phenotypes and to document the emergence, expansion, and spread of antimicrobial-resistant organisms.[38]

Management

Enteric fever is a systemic febrile illness requiring prompt antibiotic treatment. Various antimicrobials have been used for the treatment of enteric fever in the past see

Table 3
Various laboratory methods for diagnosing enteric fever

Method	Tests	Sensitivity/ Specificity	Limitations
Serologic methods			
Widal[39]	Detects agglutinating antibodies to LPS (O antigen) and flagella (H antigen)	74%/76%	Variable sensitivity/ specificity Need of paired sera Difficult to differentiate between acute and convalescent cases
Typhi Dot[31]	Detects specific IgM and IgG antibodies in contrast to a 50-kD *S. typhi* outer membrane protein	70%/80%	Cross-reactivity with infections with non-Salmonella organisms (Malaria, dengue, brucellosis, and so forth)
Typhi Dot- M[40]	Detects specific IgM antibodies in contrast to a 50-kD *S. typhi* outer membrane protein	91%/82%	Lack of isolating species and performing drug susceptibility testing
Tubex[33]	Detects antibody against *S. typhi* LPS	78%/87%	
Culture methods			Lack of quality microbiological laboratories in the endemic setting is challenging
Blood culture[29]	Isolation of species from blood	40%–80%	Isolation of a pathogen depends on the volume of blood collected, previous antibiotic use, and bacterial load
Bone marrow culture[41]	Isolation of species from bone marrow	More than 90%	Expensive and invasive technique
Stool, and bile or duodenal contents[29]	Isolation of species from stool,urine, or bile or duodenal contents	7%–50%	Need careful Interpretation because it may suggest acute infection or chronic carriage
Molecular methods			
PCR[37]	Identify *S. typhi* by amplifying the flagellin (fliC) gene locus	>90%/100%	Not commercially available and expensive

Table 4. In areas of increasing AMR in *S. typhi*, multidrug resistance (MDR) (resistant to chloramphenicol, ampicillin, and trimethoprim-sulfamethoxazole), resistance against fluoroquinolones, the first-line treatment of enteric fever is third-generation cephalosporins (eg, ceftriaxone, cefixime).[42] With the emergence of the XDR *S. typhi* clone, limited treatment options are available. The isolate is only susceptible to one oral drug, azithromycin, making treatment options for outpatient settings highly limited. Those who develop treatment failure or develop complications, treatment with injectable carbapenems is the only other treatment option. Antibiotic selection depends on the severity of illness, local resistance patterns, whether oral medications are feasible, the clinical setting, and available resources.

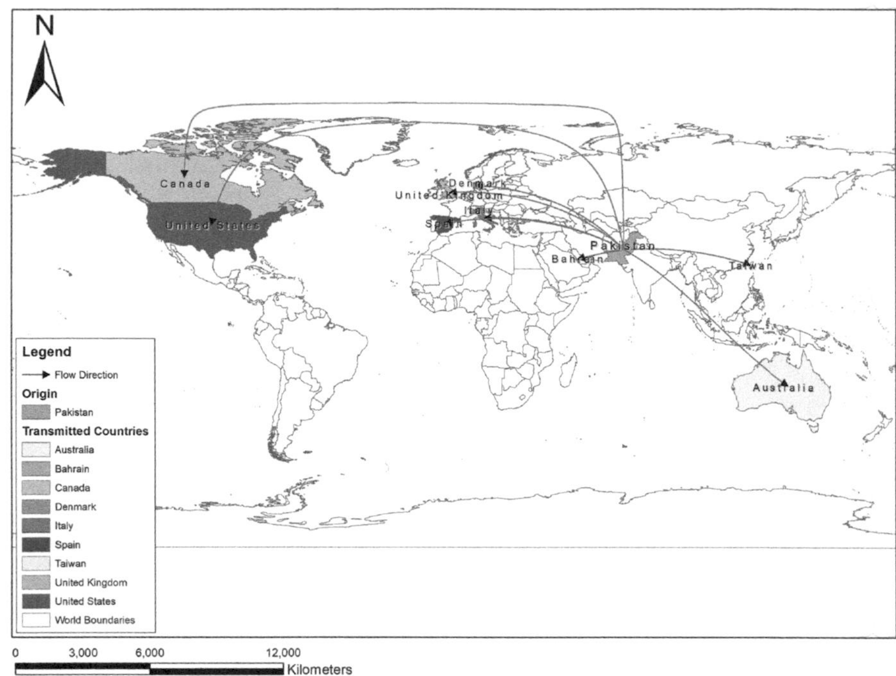

Fig. 1. Global spread of XDR- typhoid fever cases.

The current practice in most endemic countries is the initiation of therapy with a cephalosporin in patients with clinical suspicion of enteric fever.[43,44] This is ineffective if the infecting strain is XDR. A potential empiric strategy is the use of meropenem for the sick or hospitalized patient or a combination of ceftriaxone and azithromycin for the clinically stable particularly if there is a travel history from an XDR typhoid endemic country or there is poor response to oral cephalosporin (cefixime), with further rationalization once sensitivities become available.[45] Duration of treatment must be long enough (10–14 days) or $\geq$5 days after resolution of fever, whichever is longer.[46] For patients with complications like delirium, obtundation, stupor, coma, or shock, adjunctive therapy with dexamethasone (3 mg/kg followed by 1 mg/kg every 6 hours for a total of 48 hours) is recommended. Reports from other countries have also recognized successful recovery with meropenem in cases of extensively drug-resistant *S. typhi*.[45]

Azithromycin has been shown to be effective against uncomplicated enteric fever caused by MDR *S. typhi* that remain susceptible to azithromycin, with a cure rate of greater than 90%. Good clinical outcomes have also been observed with the use of carbapenems.[47] Nonetheless, there are significant cost implications as these drugs are expensive and require administration in the hospital. There is extensive data, particularly for gram-negative MDR organisms, favoring combination treatments. For enteric fever, it has been observed that those who are treated with single agent have an increased time to defervescence in comparison to those treated with combination regimens.[48] However, there are no randomized control trials on the clinical efficacy of combination therapy with meropenem with azithromycin for the treatment of XDR enteric fever. Large randomized control trials are needed to identify the most effective treatment of XDR enteric fever.

Table 4
Antibiotic choices for the treatment of enteric fever in children

	Optimal Therapy		Alternative Therapy	
Susceptibility	**Choice of Antibiotic**	**Duration (days)**	**Choice of Antibiotic**	**Duration (days)**
Uncomplicated Typhoid Fever				
Fully sensitive	Chloramphenicol Or Amoxicillin	14–21 14	Fluoroquinolone, for example, ofloxacin or ciprofloxacin	5–7
Multidrug resistant	Fluoroquinolone or Cefixime	5–7 7–14	Azithromycin	7
Quinolone-resistant	Ceftriaxone	10–14	Cefixime Or Azithromycin	7–14 7
Extensively drug resistant (XDR)	Azithromycin	7–10	Meropenem	10–14
[a]*Complicated Typhoid Fever*				
Fully sensitive	Fluoroquinolone, for example, ofloxacin Or Chloramphenicol Or Ampicillin	10–14	Ceftriaxone Or Cefotaxime	10–14
Multidrug resistant	Fluoroquinolone	10–14	Ceftriaxone Or Cefotaxime	10–14 10–14
Quinolone -resistant	Ceftriaxone Or Cefotaxime	10–14	Azithromycin	7
Extensively drug resistant (XDR)	Meropenem	10–14	Azithromycin and Meropenem	7–10 10–14

[a] Additional treatment with dexamethasone (3 mg/kg for the initial dose, followed by 1 mg/kg every 6 h for 48 h) for patients with shock, obtundation, stupor, or coma, and with abdominal complications, for example, intestinal perforation.

Prevention and control

Vaccination, supply of clean and safe drinking water, and careful attention to cleanliness and hygiene during food preparation are essential preventive control measures to decrease Salmonella infections. Currently, commercially available enteric fever vaccines are the live oral vaccine Ty21a, licensed for children aged $\geq$6 years, the Vi polysaccharide vaccine (ViCPS or Vi) licensed for children aged $\geq$2 years, and the new conjugate vaccine TCV as a single-dose for infants and children aged greater than 6 month.[49] A parenteral heat-phenol-inactivated whole-cell vaccine first licensed in 1952 was associated with high rates of fever and systemic reactions and was discontinued in 2000.[20,50]

Typhoid vaccines provide a unique opportunity to reduce empirical use of antimicrobials in endemic countries and to reduce the global dissemination of AMR in many other bacterial pathogens apart from *S. typhi*. Primary vaccination with Vi polysaccharide consists of a single dose administered intramuscularly whereas live-attenuated Ty21a vaccine consists of one enteric-coated capsule taken on alternate days (day 0, 2, 4, and 6), for a total of 4 capsules. The oral vaccine is no longer available in LMIC. Booster doses of Vi polysaccharide vaccine are needed every 2 years, whereas the booster doses of live-attenuated Ty21a vaccine are every 5 years to maintain immunity.

After the outbreak of XDR enteric fever in Sindh Pakistan, the new conjugate vaccine (Typbar TCV) was introduced into the routine immunization program of Paksitan. Typbar TCV has an advantage of being administered at the age of 6 months has shown a protective efficacy of 87%.[51] The high immunogenicity of Typbar TCV makes it an ideal candidate in typhoid-endemic countries, especially for children aged less than 2 years.

CLINICS CARE POINTS

- Enteric fever should be suspected in a febrile patient living in, or traveling from, an endemic area, with a history of fever of more than 3 days.
- The gold standard for the diagnosis of enteric fever is blood culture serologic tests should not be used.
- Emergence of XDR typhoid has limited the therapeutic options for the treatment of typhoid.
- In addition to an effective vaccine, access to safe drinking water, hygiene, and improved sanitation is important for the prevention of salmonellosis.

DISCLOSURE

The authors have no conflict of interest, nothing to disclose.

REFERENCES

1. Rahman HS, Mahmoud BM, Othman HH, et al. A review of history, definition, classification, source, transmission, and pathogenesis of salmonella: a model for human infection. J Zankoy Sulaimani 2018;20(3–4):11–9.
2. Issenhuth-Jeanjean S, Roggentin P, Mikoleit M, et al. Supplement 2008–2010 (no. 48) to the white–Kauffmann–Le minor scheme. Res Microbiol 2014;165(7):526–30.
3. Salmonella (non-typhoidal)- World Health Organization. Secondary Salmonella (non-typhoidal)- World Health Organization 2018. Available at: https://www.who.int/news-room/fact-sheets/detail/salmonella-(non-typhoidal.
4. Luk-In S, Chatsuwan T, Pulsrikarn C, et al. High prevalence of ceftriaxone resistance among invasive Salmonella enterica serotype Choleraesuis isolates in Thailand: the emergence and increase of CTX-M-55 in ciprofloxacin-resistant S. Choleraesuis isolates. Int J Med Microbiol 2018;308(4):447–53.
5. Control CfD, Prevention. Preliminary FoodNet data on the incidence of infection with pathogens transmitted commonly through food–10 states, 2007. MMWR Morb Mortal Wkly Rep 2008;57(14):366–70.
6. Pijnacker R, Dallman TJ, Tijsma AS, et al. An international outbreak of Salmonella enterica serotype Enteritidis linked to eggs from Poland: a microbiological and epidemiological study. Lancet Infect Dis 2019;19(7):778–86.
7. Kalaba V, Golić B, Sladojević Ž, et al. Incidence of Salmonella Infantis in poultry meat and products and the resistance of isolates to antimicrobials. IOP Conference series: earth and environmental science. IOP Publishing; 2017.
8. Majowicz SE, Musto J, Scallan E, et al. The global burden of nontyphoidal Salmonella gastroenteritis. Clin Infect Dis 2010;50(6):882–9.
9. Stanaway JD, Reiner RC, Blacker BF, et al. The global burden of typhoid and paratyphoid fevers: a systematic analysis for the Global Burden of Disease Study 2017. Lancet Infect Dis 2019;19(4):369–81.

10. John J, Van Aart CJ, Grassly NC. The burden of typhoid and paratyphoid in India: systematic review and meta-analysis. PLoS Negl Trop Dis 2016;10(4):e0004616.
11. Radhakrishnan A, Als D, Mintz ED, et al. Introductory article on global burden and epidemiology of typhoid fever. Am J Trop Med Hyg 2018;99(3_Suppl):4–9.
12. Marks F, Von Kalckreuth V, Aaby P, et al. Incidence of invasive salmonella disease in sub-Saharan Africa: a multicentre population-based surveillance study. Lancet Glob Health 2017;5(3):e310–23.
13. Acheson D, Hohmann EL. Nontyphoidal salmonellosis. Clin Infect Dis 2001;32(2): 263–9.
14. Liu L-J, Yang Y-J, Kuo P-H, et al. Diagnostic value of bacterial stool cultures and viral antigen tests based on clinical manifestations of acute gastroenteritis in pediatric patients. Eur J Clin Microbiol Infect Dis 2005;24(8):559–61.
15. Cohen JI, Bartlett JA, Corey GR. Extra-intestinal manifestations of salmonella infections. Medicine 1987;66(5):349–88.
16. Worsena CR, Miller AS, King MA. Salmonella infections. Pediatr Rev 2019;40(10):543–545.
17. Grady R. Safety profile of quinolone antibiotics in the pediatric population. Pediatr Infect Dis J 2003;22(12):1128–32.
18. Onwuezobe IA, Oshun PO, Odigwe CC. Antimicrobials for treating symptomatic non-typhoidal Salmonella infection. Cochrane Database Syst Rev 2012;(11):CD001167.
19. Feasey NA, Dougan G, Kingsley RA, et al. Invasive non-typhoidal salmonella disease: an emerging and neglected tropical disease in Africa. Lancet 2012; 379(9835):2489–99.
20. Tennant SM, MacLennan CA, Simon R, et al. Nontyphoidal salmonella disease: current status of vaccine research and development. Vaccine 2016;34(26): 2907–10.
21. Crump JA, Luby SP, Mintz ED. The global burden of typhoid fever. Bull World Health Organ 2004;82:346–53.
22. Akullian A, Ng'eno E, Matheson AI, et al. Environmental transmission of typhoid fever in an urban slum. PLoS Negl Trop Dis 2015;9(12):e0004212.
23. Parry CM, Hien TT, Dougan G, et al. Typhoid fever. N Engl J Med 2002;347(22): 1770–82.
24. Andrews JR, Qamar FN, Charles RC, et al. Extensively drug-resistant typhoid—are conjugate vaccines arriving just in time? 2018;379(16):1493–5.
25. Yousafzai MT, Qamar FN, Shakoor S, et al. Ceftriaxone-resistant Salmonella Typhi outbreak in Hyderabad City of Sindh, Pakistan: high time for the introduction of typhoid conjugate vaccine. Clin Infect Dis 2019;68(Supplement_1):S16–21.
26. Klemm EJ, Shakoor S, Page AJ, et al. Emergence of an extensively drug-resistant Salmonella enterica serovar Typhi clone harboring a promiscuous plasmid encoding resistance to fluoroquinolones and third-generation cephalosporins. MBio 2018;9(1):e00105–18.
27. Akram J, Khan AS, Khan HA, et al. Extensively drug-resistant (XDR) typhoid: evolution, prevention, and its management. Biomed Res Int 2020;2020:6432580.
28. Rahman G, Abubakar A, Johnson AB, et al. Typhoid ileal perforation in Nigerian children: an analysis of 106 operative cases. Pediatr Surg Int 2001;17(8):628–30.
29. Parry CM, Ribeiro I, Walia K, et al. Multidrug resistant enteric fever in South Asia: unmet medical needs and opportunities. BMJ 2019;364:k5322.
30. Giannella RA. Salmonella. In: Baron SE, editor. Medical microbiology. 4th edition. Galveston (TX): University of Texas Medical Branch at Galveston; 1996. Chapter 21.

31. Siba V, Horwood PF, Vanuga K, et al. Evaluation of serological diagnostic tests for typhoid fever in Papua New Guinea using a composite reference standard. Clin Vaccin Immunol 2012;19(11):1833–7.
32. Olopoenia LA, King AL. Widal agglutination test– 100 years later: still plagued by controversy. Postgrad Med J 2000;76(892):80–4.
33. Wijedoru L, Mallett S, Parry CM. Rapid diagnostic tests for typhoid and paratyphoid (enteric) fever. Cochrane Database Syst Rev 2017;(5):CD008892.
34. World Health Organization. . Background document: the diagnosis, treatment and prevention of typhoid fever. Geneva: Secondary World Health Organization; 2003. Available at: http://www.who.int/iris/handle/10665/68122.
35. Fadeel MA, House BL, Wasfy MM, et al. Evaluation of a newly developed ELISA against Widal, TUBEX-TF and Typhidot for typhoid fever surveillance. New York: NAVAL MEDICAL research UNIT NO 3 FPO; 2011.
36. Kintz E, Heiss C, Black I, et al. Salmonella enterica Serovar Typhi Lipopolysaccharide O-antigen modification impact on serum resistance and antibody recognition. Infect Immun 2017;85(4):e01021.
37. Prabagaran SR, Kalaiselvi V, Chandramouleeswaran N, et al. Molecular diagnosis of Salmonella typhi and its virulence in suspected typhoid blood samples through nested multiplex PCR. J Microbiol Methods 2017;139:150–4.
38. Katiyar A, Sharma P, Dahiya S, et al. Genomic profiling of antimicrobial resistance genes in clinical isolates of Salmonella Typhi from patients infected with Typhoid fever in India. Scientific Rep 2020;10(1):8299.
39. Mengist H, Tilahun K. Diagnostic value of Widal test in the diagnosis of typhoid fever: a systematic review. J Med Microbiol Diagn 2017;6:248.
40. A Study on the evaluation of Typhidot M (IgM enzyme-linked immunosorbent assay) in the early diagnosis of enteric fever in children; 2018.
41. Gasem M, Dolmans W, Isbandrio B, et al. Culture of Salmonella typhi and Salmonella paratyphi from blood and bone marrow in suspected typhoid fever. Trop Geogr Med 1995;47(4):164–7.
42. Chatham Stephens K, Medalla F, Hughes M, et al. Emergence of extensively drug-resistant salmonella typhi infections among travelers to or from Pakistan—United States, 2016–2018. MMWR Morb Mortal Wkly Rep 2019;68(1):11.
43. Parry CM, Beeching NJ. Treatment of enteric fever. BMJ 2009;338:b1159.
44. Bhutta ZA. Current concepts in the diagnosis and treatment of typhoid fever. BMJ 2006;333(7558):78–82.
45. Wong W, Al Rawahi H, Patel S, et al. The first Canadian pediatric case of extensively drug-resistant Salmonella Typhi originating from an outbreak in Pakistan and its implication for empiric antimicrobial choices. IDCases 2019;15:e00492.
46. Khan EA. XDR Typhoid: the problem and its solution. J Ayub Med Coll Abbottabad 2019;31(2):139–40.
47. Kleine C-E, Schlabe S, Hischebeth GT, et al. Successful therapy of a multidrug-resistant extended-spectrum β-lactamase–producing and fluoroquinolone-resistant Salmonella enterica Subspecies enterica serovar typhi infection using combination therapy of meropenem and fosfomycin. Clin Infect Dis 2017;65(10):1754–6.
48. Izadpanah M, Khalili H. Antibiotic regimens for treatment of infections due to multidrug-resistant gram-negative pathogens: an evidence-based literature review. J Res Pharm Pract 2015;4(3):105.

49. Andrews JR, Qamar FN, Charles RC, et al. Extensively drug-resistant typhoid - are conjugate vaccines arriving just in time? N Engl J Med 2018;379(16):1493–5.
50. Wheaton AG, Cunningham TJ, Ford ES, et al. Employment and activity limitations among adults with chronic obstructive pulmonary disease–United States, 2013. MMWR Morb Mortal Wkly Rep 2015;64(11):289–95.
51. Vaccine WHOJ. Typhoid vaccines: WHO position paper, March 2018–Recommendations 2019;37(2):214–6.

Amebiasis and Amebic Liver Abscess in Children

Shipra Gupta, MD, FAAP[a,*], Layne Smith, PharmD[b], Adriana Diakiw, MD[a]

KEYWORDS

- Amebiasis • Children • Diarrhea • Colitis • Amebic liver abscess • Entamoeba

KEY POINTS

- Amebiasis causes a spectrum of intestinal illness ranging from diarrhea to colitis and dysentery as well as amebic liver abscess (ALA) which is associated with high mortality.
- Microscopic examination of stool does not differentiate between pathogenic and nonpathogenic entamoeba. More specific and sensitive tests such as antigen and molecular testing are preferred to decrease over diagnosis and treatment.
- Treatment with amebicidal drugs such as metronidazole/tinidazole and luminal cysticidal agents such as paromomycin for clinical disease is indicated.
- Asymptomatic carriers are treated with a luminal cysticidal agent to decrease the chances of invasive disease and transmission.
- Preventive measures include handwashing, preventing fecal contamination of water and food supply, and providing clean water and improving sanitation in endemic areas.

INTRODUCTION

Diarrheal illnesses continue to be a leading cause of death in children under 5 years of age in developing countries with about 1200 young children dying per day of diarrhea.[1,2] Annual mortality due to amebiasis has been estimated at 40,000–110,000 making it one of the deadliest parasitic infections.[3–5] *Entamoeba histolytica* infection in about 90% of cases results in asymptomatic infection. However, 10% of those infected can develop amebiasis which is a spectrum of illness from diarrhea to colitis and more severe amebic liver abscess (ALA) or cerebral amebiasis.[6] Amebic colitis is also a leading cause of infectious diarrhea in a traveler returning from endemic regions.[7] Transmission is fecal-oral with the ingestion of water or food contaminated with cysts as the most common method of transmission. Cysts are surrounded by a cell wall made of chitin which renders resistance to acid as well as chlorination performed routinely for water supplies. Low infectious dose, chlorine resistance, and

[a] West Virginia University School of Medicine, One Medical Center Drive, HSC 9214, Morgantown, WV 26506, USA; [b] West Virginia University School of Pharmacy, One Medical Center Drive, Morgantown, WV-26506, USA
* Corresponding author.
E-mail address: Shipra.gupta@hsc.wvu.edu

Pediatr Clin N Am 69 (2022) 79–97
https://doi.org/10.1016/j.pcl.2021.08.003
pediatric.theclinics.com

environmental stability make *E. histolytica* capable of outbreaks and are considered among the second highest priority biodefense pathogens per National Institute of Allergy and Infectious Diseases (NIAID).[8] ALA which is the most common extraintestinal amebiasis can present acutely with fever and right upper quadrant abdominal pain or a subacute presentation with weight loss, anemia, and hepatomegaly. Although rarely encountered in the developed world clinicians should have a high index of suspicion for amebiasis in recent immigrants and travelers returning from endemic regions as well as other high-risk groups.

EPIDEMIOLOGY

Disease burden

E. histolytica is ubiquitous but the major burden of amebiasis is endured by developing nations with poor sanitation and paucity of clean water supplies with high prevalence rates of up to 10% in these countries.[4,9,10] Developing countries in West and East Africa and Central and South America, particularly Mexico and regions in South and South East Asia especially India, Pakistan, and Bangladesh, have the highest infection rates.[4] Immigrants or travelers returning from endemic regions account for most cases in developed countries such as those in North America and Europe with prevalence estimated at 4% in the United States for *E. histolytica–E. dispar* complex.[11–13] Annually *E. histolytica* infects millions and is responsible for up to 100,000 deaths and ranks second in terms of mortality caused by protozoan parasites.[3,14]

E. histolytica is a nonflagellated protozoan parasite and attains its name for the pathologic feature of lysis in infected tissues. *E. histolytica* and *Entamoeba moshkovskii* are pathogenic with latter causing both asymptomatic infection and diarrhea in children.[15,16] These are morphologically similar to the nonpathogenic entamoeba species such as *E. dispar* and *Entamoeba bangladeshi* which cause asymptomatic colonization.[17]

Initial prevalence studies were based on the microscopic examination of stools for cysts in asymptomatic individuals. This testing was not sensitive and did not differentiate pathogenic and nonpathogenic species, therefore, the prevalence of amebiasis was overestimated as most asymptomatic individuals were colonized with *E. dispar*.[18–20] Isoenzyme electrophoresis was used to differentiate pathogenic and nonpathogenic strains or zymodemes.[21] Allason-Jones and colleagues used this method and found a 20% prevalence of *E. histolytica* in asymptomatic men who have sex with men (MSM) but only nonpathogenic zymodemes were isolated.[22] Advanced techniques using antigen detection and polymerase chain reaction (PCR) in the stool have been helpful in assessing the true prevalence and burden of infection and have confirmed that most of the previously identified infections were due to nonpathogenic entamoeba.[23–25] Using antigen testing in the stool of children presenting with diarrhea in Peru, the authors found that 26% of children were diagnosed with amebiasis based on stool microscopy but all were negative by antigen testing.[26]

Assessing the presence of antibodies to *E. histolytica* specific antigens has been used to study the prevalence of entamoeba infections.[27,28] Seroprevalence of 10% to 20% was reported in asymptomatic study participants in South Africa and Egypt.[29,30] A longitudinal seroprevalence study in preschool children (2–5 years) living in an urban slum in Bangladesh showed that 15% (170/1164) of screened children tested positive for antibodies.[31] Among those who completed the study 80% tested positive by antigen detection testing in stool and serum antibody was detected in 91% of the children at least once during the 4 year study period.[31] This study highlighted the high rates of infection with *E. histolytica* in children living in resource-limited settings. Haque and colleagues also noted that the presence of specific IgA antibodies in stool was associated with protection from amebiasis.[31]

Incidence and mortality of ALA vary across various endemic regions which are hypothesized due to the difference in *E. histolytica* infection rates and presence of invasive strains as well as host susceptibility. Blessmann and colleagues reported high incidence from central Vietnam, a highly endemic region for *E. histolytica* infections and estimated 21 cases of ALA per 100,000 population per year.[32] Higher incidence of amebic liver abscess in young adults and adults (20–50 years) and males (3–10 males per 1 female case) has been noted.[33,34] Despite the high seroprevalence rates of up to 50% in children especially in school-aged children by various studies, the incidence of ALA and other invasive diseases is low in children. [31,34–37] Acuna-Soto and colleagues reviewed publications from 1929 to 1997 and found that children comprised about 12% of liver abscess cases.[33]

Risk factors

Travelers visiting endemic areas for longer duration (>1 month) and immigrants from endemic regions are at increased risk of disease reported in developed nations.[7,38] Other recognized risk groups include people with underlying immunosuppression, AIDS, MSM, residents of group homes, or mental health facility.[13,39,40] High prevalence of 20% to 31.7% was reported in the late 1970s in MSM but further investigation by zymodeme analysis showed that nonpathogenic entamoeba was more prevalent.[22,41,42] However, sporadic cluster of cases of amebiasis in MSM from Barcelona, Spain underscored amebiasis as a reemerging pathogen of interest in this population.[43] Similar studies in patients with HIV infection showed that the prevalence of amebiasis had increased over time and receptive anal sex behavior was associated with higher seropositivity for *E. histolytica* antibodies.[44,45]

Transmission and life cycle

E. histolytica most commonly infects when a susceptible host ingests food or water contaminated with amebic cyst. Human to human transmission is rare in developed countries; however, household outbreaks have been reported with a history of household member returning from the endemic region.[46,47] *E. histolytica* can also be sexually transmitted by oral–anal sexual contact with both homosexual and heterosexual activity.[48]

E. histolytica has a less complex life cycle than other protozoan parasites and exists either as infectious cyst or trophozoite stage (**Fig. 1**). Humans are the natural host and reservoir of disease. Infectious cysts are almost spherical with an average diameter of 12 μm (5–20 μm) and 1 to 4 nuclei depending on the stage of maturation.[13,49] The cysts are surrounded by a refractile wall made of chitin and have a greenish tint in unstained preparation.[49] The cysts are capable of surviving in the environment weeks to months and are resistant to treatment with the chlorination of water supplies and acidic environment of the stomach. Once the cyst is ingested by the host it transforms into small or large bowel by losing the outer cyst and forming 8 trophozoites which measure 25 μm in diameter on average (10–60 μm) and have 1 nucleus.[13] The trophozoites of *E. histolytica* are morphologically indistinguishable from the nonpathogenic *E. dispar* but the presence of erythrocytes in the trophozoite is a unique feature of *E. histolytica* (**Fig 2**).[49]

Once in the intestine the trophozoites continue to multiply and can either colonize or invade the large bowel. Trophozoites have the potential to invade the bloodstream by entering through the portal venous system and invading other organs of the body. Trophozoites continue multiplication by binary fission and produce cysts. Cysts never cause tissue invasion. Both cysts and trophozoites are passed in the stool but

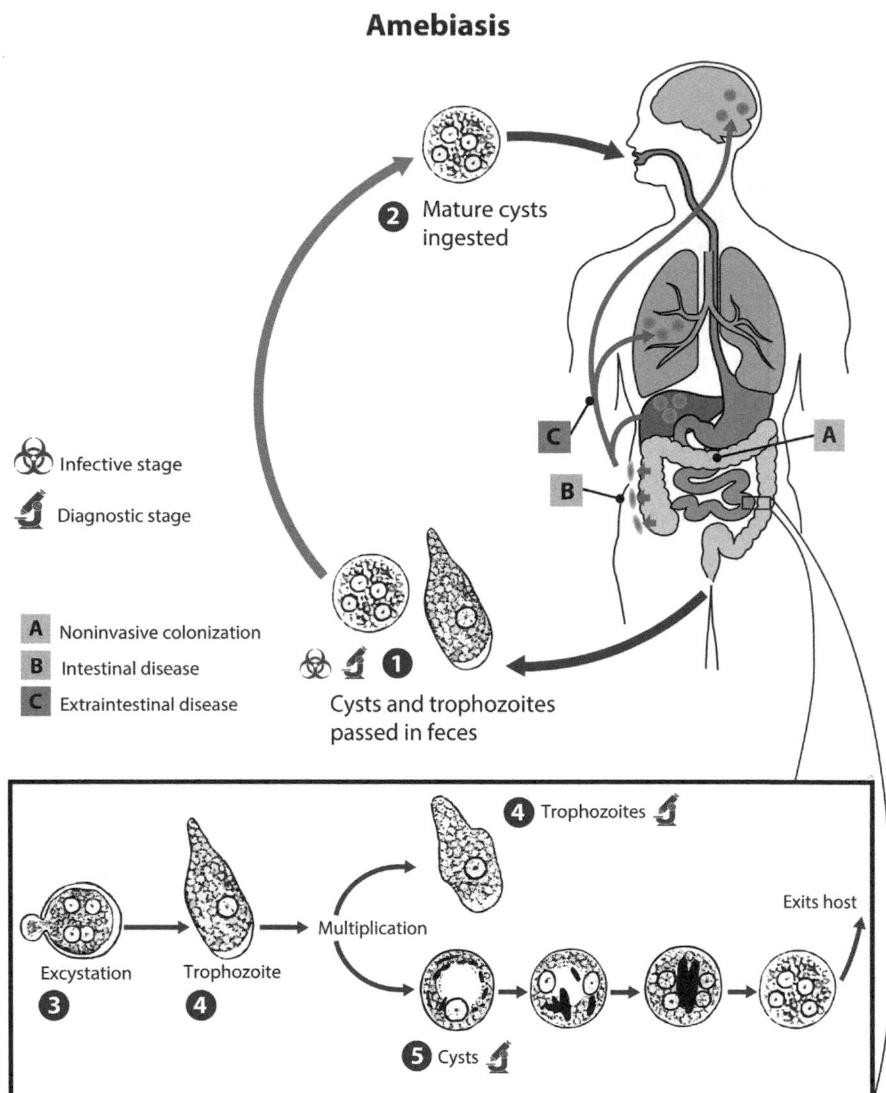

Fig. 1. Life cycle of *Entamoeba histolytica.*

1. Infected host passes both cysts and trophozoites in feces.
2. Susceptible host ingests mature cysts through fecally contaminated food, water, or hands.
3. Transformation occurs in the small intestine and quadrinucleate cyst loses its cyst wall and forms 8 trophozoites.
4. The trophozoites are released, which migrate to the large intestine.

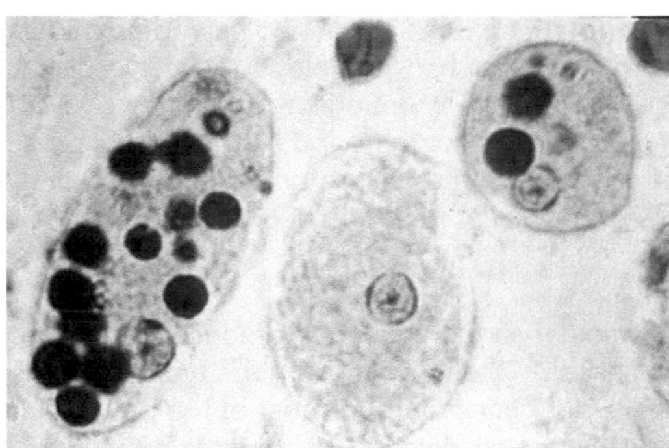

Fig. 2. Trophozoites of *E histolytica* with ingested erythrocytes stained with trichrome. The ingested erythrocytes appear as dark inclusions. (From - https://www.cdc.gov/dpdx/amebiasis/index.html URL https://www.cdc.gov/dpdx/amebiasis/index.html (image gallery))

trophozoites cannot survive in the external environment or the high acid content of stomach if ingested. On the other hand, cysts survive outside the host for prolonged periods awaiting a susceptible host.

CLINICAL FEATURES

Intestinal amebiasis

Noninvasive intestinal infection

Approximately 90% of *E. histolytica* infections are asymptomatic and self-limited.[34] Noninvasive infection, also referred to as asymptomatic intraluminal amebiasis, is characterized by the presence of Entamoeba trophozoites in the bowel and passage of Entamoeba cysts in the feces. The duration of cyst passage is highly variable. A longitudinal study of asymptomatic adult carriers in an endemic area of Vietnam found that the mean half-life of *E. histolytica* infection was approximately 13 months, and that untreated infections showed a regular exponential decline of about 3% per month.[50] A study of urban households in Brazil showed that 85% of colonized individuals cleared their infection within 30 to 45 days without treatment.[51]

Invasive intestinal amebiasis

Symptomatic amebiasis occurs when trophozoites breach the intestinal mucous layer and invade the underlying tissue. Asymptomatic colonization may progress to invasive disease at any time after initial infection. In a longitudinal study of asymptomatic

---

5. The trophozoites multiply by binary fission and produce cysts (5), and both stages are passed in the feces.In many cases, the trophozoites remain confined to the intestinal lumen (A: noninvasive infection) of individuals who are asymptomatic carriers, passing cysts in their stool.In some patients, the trophozoites invade the intestinal mucosa (B: intestinal disease), or, through the bloodstream, extraintestinal sites such as the liver, brain, and lungs (C: extraintestinal disease), with resultant pathologic manifestations. (From Centers for Disease Control and Prevention, National Center for Emerging and Zoonotic Infectious Diseases (NCEZID), Division of Foodborne, Waterborne, and Environmental Diseases (DFWED) and Global Health, Division of Parasitic Diseases and Malaria. https://www.cdc.gov/dpdx/amebiasis/index.html)

carriers in Durban, South Africa, 90% remained asymptomatic and resolved spontaneously within 1 year, whereas 10% developed invasive disease.[52] A prospective study in Bangladesh found that 3.1% of children with new *E. histolytica* infection progressed to dysentery over a 12-month period.[53] The clinical presentation of intestinal amebiasis is protean, manifesting across a broad spectrum of disease ranging from mild, watery diarrhea to fulminant necrotizing colitis.

Amebic colitis

Acute diarrhea and dysentery are the most common forms of intestinal amebiasis, accounting for 90% of cases.[54] Onset of symptoms is typically gradual, occurring over a period of 2 to 4 weeks after infestation in most of the patients; however, symptoms may also present acutely or be delayed for months after initial exposure. Patients are typically present with abdominal pain and diarrhea, sometimes accompanied by weight loss.[55] A study of the clinical characteristics of amebiasis cases in Ontario, Canada, found that the most common symptom was diarrhea, occurring in 70% of cases, followed by abdominal pain in 63% and abdominal bloating in 60%.[56]

Frequent loose, mucous, and small-volume stools are most characteristic of amebic colitis, but profuse watery diarrhea may also occur.[4] Due to the invasive nature of the disease, virtually all stool samples test positive for occult blood,[55] though grossly bloody stools are present in only about 7% to 8% of cases.[56,57] In some cases, amebic colitis may present as rectal bleeding without diarrhea, particularly in children.[58–60] Abdominal pain occurs in up to 80% of cases, and manifests on a spectrum of intensity ranging from mild discomfort to severe pain that may resemble acute abdomen.[61] Abdominal tenderness may be generalized or localized to the lower quadrants.[13,55] Vomiting may also be present; this symptom was reported in 63% of amebiasis cases in Ontario, Canada, and 62% of patients hospitalized for *E. histolytica* infection in Dhaka, Bangladesh.[56,57] Constitutional symptoms are frequently mild or absent. Fever is an uncommon finding, present in 6% to 25% of patients.[55,61] Anorexia and weight loss are frequently observed.[4,55,61]

The diagnosis of amebic colitis can be challenging due to the insidious onset of symptoms and wide variability in clinical presentation. However, certain findings, when present, may offer a clue to the diagnosis. In a retrospective study of patients diagnosed with *E. histolytica* infection at a tropical medicine clinic in Belgium, 40% of all infections were found to be asymptomatic. Of patients with symptomatic disease, many presented with nonspecific watery diarrhea; blood and mucus in the stools were not frequent findings, nor was cramping abdominal pain. However, despite the low prevalence of these symptoms, the presence of blood or mucus in the stools and crampy abdominal pain were found to be significant predictors of infection, with a specificity of 100%, 100%, and 90%, respectively.[62]

In most cases, symptoms of illness resolve within 1 month; approximately 20% of patients have a protracted course lasting more than 4 weeks.[61] Median disease duration in patients presenting to a Canadian travel clinic was 20 days.[56] A chronic form of nondysenteric amebiasis has been reported, consisting of abdominal pain, weight loss, and intermittent episodes of mucousy, nonbloody diarrhea, that may persist for months or years; however, these symptoms may, in fact, be attributable to irritable bowel disease rather than true *E. histolytica* infection, and the syndrome of chronic amebiasis, to the extent that it exists, is thought to be extremely rare.[63]

Acute fulminant amebic colitis and intestinal perforation

Fulminant or necrotizing colitis is a rare complication of intestinal amebiasis, occurring in about 0.5% of cases. Fulminant amebic colitis is characterized by transmural ulcerations that erode through the bowel wall, resulting in necrosis, and may involve all or part of the colon. In 75% of cases, necrotizing colitis progresses to intestinal perforation with subsequent bacterial peritonitis. Mucosal sloughing may also occur.[4] Symptoms of fulminant colitis are severe and rapidly progressive. Patients are ill-appearing, with fever, abdominal pain, and profuse bloody diarrhea.[13] Peritoneal signs, including abdominal distension and rebound tenderness, are present in most patients.[61] The mortality rate in fulminant amebic colitis ranges from 40% to 89%.[64–66] Risk factors for increased disease severity and mortality include young age, pregnancy, malnutrition, immunosuppression, and corticosteroid use, which is associated with the development of toxic megacolon.[67,68] Surgical intervention is indicated for acute abdomen, bowel perforation, toxic megacolon, massive colonic hemorrhage, and in cases that fail to improve with antiamebic therapy. Partial or total colectomy may be required for extensive disease.[64–66]

Ameboma

An ameboma, or amebic granuloma, is a mass of hyperplastic granulation tissue that forms in the cecum or ascending colon. Amebomas are thought to develop in response to inflammation from healing ulcers or amebic abscesses in the bowel wall. They are an uncommon manifestation of intestinal amebiasis, occurring in 0.5% to 1.5% of cases.[55,69] Symptoms of amebic dysentery are present in two-thirds of patients at the time of diagnosis. Patients may present with right lower quadrant pain or symptoms of bowel obstruction. A tender, palpable mass is usually present on the right side of abdomen. Barium enema reveals characteristic annular "apple core" lesions with narrowing of the intestinal lumen. Diagnosis requires colonoscopy with the biopsy of the mass. Intestinal strictures caused by granulation tissue in the colon occur in 0.8% of cases. Intestinal strictures range in size from a narrow band to several centimeters in length. Both amebomas and amebic strictures are highly responsive to medical therapy, often resolving within a few weeks of completing antiamebic therapy, and surgical intervention is rarely necessary.[55]

Amebic appendicitis

Acute amebic appendicitis is an unusual presentation that must be considered in patients with acute abdomen who have lived in or traveled to tropical or subtropical countries. Patients present with sudden onset of severe right lower quadrant or suprapubic abdominal pain, and rebound tenderness and guarding are invariably present on physical examination. In a systematic review of 174 cases, a history of travel from a low-risk country to a high/moderate-risk country was present in 64% of patients diagnosed with amebic appendicitis. Of note, the interval between travel and onset of clinical symptoms ranged from months to years, and only 3% of patients had a known diagnosis of amebiasis. Concurrent diarrhea was present in 14% of patients at presentation, and a history of diarrhea was reported in 7%, emphasizing the need for clinical suspicion of amebic appendicitis in patients who might be at risk. Amebic appendicitis was associated with a significantly higher risk of morbidity and mortality than bacterial appendicitis. The postoperative complication rate was 25.4% and the overall mortality rate was 3.2%.[70]

Extraintestinal amebiasis

Extraintestinal disease may occur simultaneously with symptoms of amebic colitis, but frequently manifests in the absence of any intestinal symptoms, and may develop months or years after the resolution of intestinal disease.[55]

Amebic liver abscess

ALA arises from hematogenous spread of trophozoites that penetrate the colonic mucosa and travel through the portal vein, seeding infection into the liver. It is the most common extraintestinal manifestation of amebiasis. Presentation in endemic areas may be acute, subacute, or insidious. Acute presentation is most common, with the onset of symptoms occurring within 2 to 4 weeks before diagnosis in 80% of patients.[71] Patients with acute presentation commonly present with fever and constant, dull right upper quadrant, or epigastric abdominal pain, which may radiate to the right shoulder. Nonproductive cough is present in some cases. Pleuritic chest pain may result from the involvement of the diaphragmatic surface of the liver. Because 80% of hepatic abscesses are located in the right lobe of the liver, pleuritic chest pain commonly occurs at the lower right chest; left-sided chest pain is less frequent, and indicates the presence of an abscess in the left hepatic lobe. Atelectasis, serous pleural effusion, and elevation of the right hemidiaphragm are found in 75% of patients.[61] Lung examination may reveal dullness or rales at the right base. Hepatic enlargement and point tenderness with palpation over the liver, subcostal, or intercostal spaces is a characteristic finding. Subacute presentation is less common, with the onset of symptoms occurring over a period of 2 to 12 weeks. Patients with subacute presentation present with weight loss, hepatomegaly, and anemia, and are less likely to have fever or abdominal pain.[71,72] Jaundice and peritoneal signs are uncommon. In nonendemic areas, presentation in returning travelers typically occurs within 8 to 20 weeks after leaving the endemic area, with an average interval of 12 weeks, but symptom onset may be delayed for months to years after travel or residency in an endemic area.[73,74]

Most patients with ALA have no history of antecedent colitis, and stool examination is often negative for cysts or trophozoites at the time of diagnosis. Gastrointestinal symptoms are present in 10% to 35% of cases, and may include nausea, vomiting, diarrhea, and cramping abdominal pain.[71,72] Than adults, children with ALA are more likely to present with high-grade fever, gastrointestinal symptoms, hepatomegaly, and cough or labored breathing.[75] ALA in children frequently presents with high-grade fever, right upper quadrant abdominal pain, and tender hepatomegaly.[76,77] By contrast, infants with ALA follow a disease course that resembles neonatal sepsis: they may be afebrile or hypothermic, and present with lethargy, irritability, abdominal distension, colitis, and respiratory distress.[78] Infants with ALA are more likely to present with hepatomegaly and symptoms of colitis, including diarrhea and bloody stools. Most cases of ALA in infants follow a fulminant course, with significantly higher rates of disease severity and mortality. In one case review of 18 infants with ALA in the United States, 92% of cases were fulminant, and the mortality rate was 47%.[79]

Most of the patients with ALA have leukocytosis ranging from 10,000 to 20,000/mm^3; higher leukocyte counts are associated with acute disease. Mild normochromic, normocytic anemia is common, and lower hemoglobin levels are associated with chronic disease. Elevated alkaline phosphatase is the most reliable biomarker for ALA occurring in 84% of cases. Alkaline phosphatase levels increase with prolonged duration of disease and may increase to twice normal level in chronic cases. Transaminase levels are elevated in acute cases and correlate with increased severity of disease.[72]

Diagnosis is established by serologic tests and imaging studies. Ultrasonography, computed tomography (CT) and magnetic resonance imaging (MRI) are all highly sensitive for detecting ALA. Occasionally, fine needle aspiration may be required to distinguish amebic from pyogenic abscesses.[13]

Rupture of hepatic abscess into the peritoneal cavity is a rare but serious complication. Patients present with sudden onset of severe abdominal pain and peritoneal signs including abdominal distension and rigidity, and progress rapidly to sepsis and shock.[71]

Pulmonary amebiasis

Pleuropulmonary amebiasis is the most common complication of ALA, and typically results from the erosion of the hepatic abscess through the diaphragm and rupture into the thoracic cavity, but may also arise via hematogenous or lymphatic spread from the liver, and hematogenous spread from the colon.[80] Risk factors include malnutrition and atrial septal defect with left-to-right shunt.[80] Manifestations of pleuropulmonary amebiasis include empyema, consolidation, pulmonary abscess, and hypobranchial fistula. The right lower lobe is most commonly involved, but any part of the lung may be affected. Patients present with fever, cough, respiratory distress, and right upper quadrant or pleuritic chest pain. Hemoptysis is frequently present. Cough may be productive of a characteristically thick, necrotic sputum that resembles the color of chocolate or anchovy paste. Chest radiograph may reveal infiltration or consolidation of the right lung base, pleural effusion, elevated hemidiaphragm, and hepatomegaly. Diagnosis is established by imaging studies and serologic testing. Thoracentesis with the aspiration of pus may be necessary to confirm the diagnosis. *E. histolytica* trophozoites are rarely present, but amebic antigen and PCR techniques can detect DNA in pus. Pulmonary amebiasis usually responds well to treatment with metronidazole.[80,81]

Pericardial amebiasis

Pericardial amebiasis is a rare complication that results from rupture of hepatic, pulmonary, or pleural abscess into the pericardium. Patients present with acute onset of severe chest pain, dyspnea, and signs of pericarditis, including tachycardia and pericardial friction rub, and may progress to cardiac tamponade and shock. Diagnosis is established by imaging (chest radiograph, ultrasound, CT scan, or echocardiogram) showing a pericardial effusion communicating with a liver abscess, and may be confirmed by pericardiocentesis. Urgent aspiration of pericardial fluid is needed in case of cardiac tamponade, and surgical drainage is occasionally necessary.[71,80]

Cerebral amebiasis

Cerebral amebiasis arises from hematogenous spread of Entamoeba trophozoites into the brain, and is an extremely rare complication of ALA. Symptoms may be insidious or sudden in onset and include mental status changes, focal neurologic signs, headache, vomiting, and seizure. Rapid progression to death occurs in half of patients without adequate treatment. CT scan and MRI are both highly accurate in establishing the presence of cerebral abscess. Biopsy and immunohistochemistry may be required to confirm the diagnosis. Treatment with metronidazole should be started immediately in suspected cases. Surgical drainage may be required.[82–85]

Cutaneous and genitourinary amebiasis

Cutaneous amebiasis arises when *E. histolytica* trophozoites from the bowel coming into contact with the skin and is usually found in the perineal, vulvar, and perianal areas. Infection of the diaper area is common in infants and children due to prolonged contact with infected stools. Rarely, infection may be transmitted by vaginal or anal intercourse, resulting in the ulceration of the vulva, cervix, or penis. Recto-vaginal fistulas have also been described. Cutaneous disease may be associated with intestinal symptoms, but also occurs in their absence. Children are more likely to present with symptoms of fever and amebic colitis.

Ulceration and necrosis of the skin may extend into the subcutaneous fat and muscle. Lesions can be intensely painful and tender to palpation, and typically appear as well-demarcated ulcers with central sloughing and a raised, hyperpigmented border that may appear purple to black in color. A halo of erythematous skin may surround the ulcer, and purulent exudate may be present. Microscopic evaluation of purulent exudate or a scraping from the edge of the ulcer reveals the presence of motile trophozoites. Diagnosis may also be confirmed by biopsy. Cutaneous disease responds well to treatment with amebicide. Early diagnosis and treatment are essential to prevent tissue destruction. Severe cases may require surgical debridement and skin grafting.

Differential diagnosis

The differential diagnosis of amebic colitis is extensive and includes bacterial infection with *Salmonella, Shigella,* enteroinvasive or enterohemorrhagic *Escherichia coli, Campylobacter,* and *Clostridioides difficile*. Viral gastroenteritis, intestinal tuberculosis, and infection with other parasites should also be excluded. Noninfectious causes such as inflammatory bowel disease, ischemic colitis, and diverticulitis may resemble amebic colitis. The differential diagnosis of ameboma includes intestinal neoplasm, lymphoma, bacterial abscess, tuberculosis, and intestinal stricture arising from other causes. The differential diagnosis of ALA includes pyogenic liver abscess, necrotic hepatoma, echinococcal cyst, and malignancy. Pleuropulmonary amebiasis may be misdiagnosed as bacterial pneumonia, bacterial lung abscess, or pulmonary tuberculosis.[80,86]

Diagnosis

Stool microscopy is the oldest tool used to make a diagnosis of amebiasis. However, due to morphologic similarities, it was hard to differentiate pathogenic and nonpathogenic entamoeba. Other tools such as antigen testing, molecular testing by PCR, and serology have improved the diagnosis of amebiasis leading to rapid diagnosis and detection as well as decreased overprescribing of antiamebic drugs. Diagnosis of amebiasis is made using a combination of diagnostic tools.[87] Serology testing offers noninvasive diagnosis of extraintestinal amebiasis as stool microscopy is often negative.

STOOL STUDIES

Stool microscopy

Identification of cysts and trophozoites in a fresh stool sample in either wet mount or stained preparation under a microscope has been the traditional method for diagnosis. At least 3 fresh stool samples increase the yield of identifying cysts and trophozoites as trophozoites are fragile once outside their host. The presence of erythrocytes in the cytoplasm of trophozoite is 100% specific and predictive of invasive amebiasis.[49,88]

However, in the absence of erythrophagocytosis, microscopy does not help differentiate between pathogenic and nonpathogenic entamoeba. Also, the differentiation of trophozoites from leukocytes as well as other intestinal protozoa requires training and experience. This method is used primarily in developing countries and is not recommended alone for diagnosis if other diagnostic modalities are available.[89]

Stool antigen detection

The introduction of enzyme-linked immunosorbent assay (ELISA) technique to detect *E. histolytica*-specific antigens in the stool advanced the understanding of epidemiology and clinical diagnosis of invasive disease. Commercially available antigen tests are readily available, simple to use with quick turnaround times. Antigen detection during acute illness in conjunction with stool microscopy can help make the distinction between pathogenic and nonpathogenic entamoeba.

Point-of-care testing using specific *E. histolytica* antigens have been developed which are useful in population screening and provide rapid results and are easy to use.[90,91] Although these tests are more sensitive and specific than microscopy in differentiating *E. histolytica/E. dispar*, the sensitivity of these point-of-care test was lower when compared with ELISA or PCR assays.[91,92]

PCR testing

Various PCR assays offer testing in stool as well as in tissues and abscess aspirate. The assays vary in DNA amplification techniques and allow the differentiation and detection of entamoeba species with great sensitivity and specificity. PCR testing is considered the gold standard and coupled with multiplex PCR can allow the detection of other enteric pathogens.[93] PCR testing is recommended by WHO for the diagnosis of amebiasis; however, the cost and technical expertise severely limit the widespread use of PCR testing in resource-limited settings.

Serology

Serum antibody

Detection of antibodies against *E. histolytica* has been a useful tool for defining seroprevalence in epidemiologic studies and diagnosing extraintestinal amebiasis especially because stool studies are often negative at the time of presentation. Ravdin and colleagues showed that antibodies to *E. histolytica* galactose-inhibitable adherence lectin were detectable by using the ELISA method in 99% of cases with ALA.[94] If the serum antibody test is negative in a patient with clinical presentation consistent with ALA, a follow-up specimen should be obtained 7 to 10 days later.

Rapid antibody testing developed by TechLab, Inc was compared with traditional ELISA test for antibody detection and showed comparable sensitivity and specificity providing bedside testing with minimal training and no equipment.[90] However, in endemic regions, asymptomatic individuals may remain seropositive for years following exposure to *E. histolytica* and a positive serologic test may be found in patients with similar presentations but different diagnoses like pyogenic liver abscess.

Serum antigen detection

Haque and colleagues showed that 96% of patients with ALA tested positive by the detection of serum antigen (Gal/GalNAc lectin) before the start of treatment but only 10% of patients who had received treatment tested positive for this antigen.[95] Also, 91% of patients with serum lecithin antigen positive became negative within 2 weeks of starting treatment; therefore, highlighting that these specific antigens can be used for diagnosis and for monitoring response to therapy.[95]

Imaging

Radiologic evidence of liver abscess can be detected as a cystic hypoechoic lesion in the liver by ultrasonography. CT scan or MRI can show a space-occupying lesion in the liver with the rim of inflammation. In conjunction with positive antibody test in serum and aforementioned imaging, such findings support the diagnosis of ALA.

Colonoscopy and biopsy

Most of the amebic ulcers develop in the cecum. A diagnostic colonoscopic biopsy may show characteristic flask shaped ulcers on histology. Trophozoites can also be identified in the tissue.

Treatment

Treatment is warranted in all *E. histolytica* infections, including asymptomatic carriers. Although many cases are asymptomatic, carriers are at risk of developing invasive disease and spreading the disease to others. For asymptomatic patients who excrete cysts, treatment with an intraluminal amebicide alone is recommended. Intraluminal amebicidal agents include paromomycin, iodoquinol/diiodohydroxyquinoline, and diloxanide furoate. These agents are generally given for a week-long duration. The recommended dose of paromomycin is 25 to 35 mg/kg/d orally divided 3 times daily.[96] Iodoquinol/diiodohydroxyquinoline and diloxanide furoate are currently unavailable in the United States.[97]

In patients with colitis or extraintestinal disease, including liver abscesses, a course of a nitroimidazole agent is recommended. Metronidazole and tinidazole are highly effective at eliminating invading trophozoites. Metronidazole may be given orally or intravenously, and recommended treatment duration is 7 to 10 days. The recommended dose of metronidazole for amebiasis is 35 to 50 mg/kg/d divided every 8 hours (maximum 750 mg/dose).[98] A 3-5-day course of tinidazole is also an appropriate regimen for intestinal or extraintestinal disease. Tinidazole is only available orally, and the recommended dose is 50 mg/kg/dose once daily (maximum 2000 mg/dose).[99] A systematic review of 41 trials including a total of 4999 participants found that compared with metronidazole, tinidazole may be more effective in reducing clinical failure and may be associated with fewer adverse events. However, most of these studies were completed more than 20 years ago, and only one trial used adequate methods of randomization and allocation concealment, was blinded, and analyzed all randomized patients.[100] Metronidazole and tinidazole are not effective in eradicating luminal cysts. Therefore, after the initial course of treatment with either metronidazole or tinidazole, an intraluminal amebicide aforementioned is recommended to ensure the luminal parasites are cleared and prevent relapse.[97,101]

In patients with liver abscess that are refractory to medical management, percutaneous or surgical aspiration and drainage may be required. This is generally recommended in patients who fail to respond to initial antiamebic therapy and patients at high risk for rupture. Patients at high risk for rupture include those with a large-diameter abscess (>5 cm) and those with an abscess in the left lobe of the liver, because the abscess may rupture into pericardium. If fulminant amoebic colitis develops, broad-spectrum antibacterial agents should be added due to the high risk of bacterial translocation.[101] Corticosteroids and antimotility drugs such as loperamide can worsen symptoms and the disease process. These medications should be avoided.[101]

After treatment is completed, a follow-up stool examination is recommended.

Prevention

Prevention in infected individuals

Hospitalized patient with amebiasis should be placed in a private room with standard precautions as nosocomial spread is rare. However, hand hygiene following defecation should be emphasized with the patient. Patients with diarrhea or incontinence can be placed in contact precautions until the resolution of diarrhea.[102] Health care workers should pay special attention to hand hygiene when handling soiled diapers or clothing.

Individuals diagnosed with amebiasis should avoid using public water venues, such as pools, spas, showers, recreation water parks, and so forth. Avoidance of these public areas should be continued till diarrhea has completely resolved and after the completion of luminal therapy.[97,101] Household members and other close contacts should be screened for symptoms and have stool examinations performed and be treated if results are positive for *E. histolytica.*[101]

PRIMARY PREVENTION

Public health measures

The spread of amebiasis is prevented by improving sanitation and preventing the contamination of water supplies and food with fecal material. Public health measures focusing on providing clean drinking water in endemic regions that have been adequately treated to prevent waterborne infections will help decrease the burden of amebiasis worldwide.

Personal measures

Hand hygiene is one of the most important measures in preventing the spread of amebiasis. Hands should be washed thoroughly with soap and water after defecation and before handling or preparing food. Amebic cysts can be eliminated by boiling water, addition of iodine, or water purification tablets or with the use of a portable water filter (<1 μm pore size).

Amebiasis can be transmitted sexually and proper use of condoms may aid in prevention, especially in high-risk population. Education about preventive measures for amebiasis and symptoms of illness should be provided to high-risk groups.

Vaccination

There are currently no vaccines approved for use in humans against *E. histolytica* disease. However, several recombinant antigens have been shown to provide protection in animal models. The most widely studied antigen is the Gal-lectin protein, which is localized on the surface of the ameba and aids in attachment to cell surfaces. Serine-rich *E. histolytica* protein (SREHP) and 29-kDa-reductase antigen have also been studied in animal models.[103] Thus far, vaccines against the Gal-lectin protein show the most promise, but clinical trials in humans are warranted to confirm the safety and efficacy in humans.

SUMMARY

Although rare in the developed world, amebiasis continues to be a leading cause of diarrhea and illness in underdeveloped nations with crowding, poor sanitation, and lack of clean water supply. Travelers or immigrants from endemic regions are at high risk of developing illness. A high index of suspicion for amebiasis should be maintained for other high-risk groups such as MSM, people with AIDS/HIV, immunocompromised hosts, residents of mental health facility, or group homes. Various diagnostic tools are available and when amebiasis is suspected the combination of tests should be sent to maximize the yield of testing. Treatment with amebicidal drugs such as metronidazole/tinidazole and luminal cysticidal agent such as paromomycin for clinical disease is indicated. However, asymptomatic disease treatment with luminal cysticidal agent decrease chances of invasive disease and transmission. Prevention of amebiasis focuses primarily on food and water safety, hand hygiene as well as the avoidance of exposure through sexual contact.98i

CLINICS CARE POINTS

- Immigrants or travelers returning from high endemic regions account for most of the cases of amebiasis in developed countries.
- High index of suspicion should be maintained for high-risk groups like men who have sex with men, people living with HIV/AIDS, residing in long-term health facilities, and so forth.
- Once a case is diagnosed, household members and close sexual contacts should be screened for symptoms and treated if testing is positive.
- An array of testing both stool and serology should be used for diagnosing amebiasis. Almost 100% of patients with ALA are seropositive and stool examination is usually negative for cysts or trophozoites.

DISCLOSURES

The authors have nothing to disclose.

REFERENCES

1. Collaborators GCoD. Global, regional, and national age-sex specific mortality for 264 causes of death, 1980-2016: a systematic analysis for the Global Burden of Disease Study 2016. Lancet 2017;390(10100):1151–210.
2. International Vaccine Access Center (IVAC), Johns Hopkins Bloomberg School of Public Health. *Pneumon*ia and diarrhea progress rep*ort 2020* 2020. Available at: https://www.jhsph.edu/ivac/resources/pdpr/.
3. Lozano R, Naghavi M, Foreman K, et al. Global and regional mortality from 235 causes of death for 20 age groups in 1990 and 2010: a systematic analysis for the Global Burden of Disease Study 2010. Lancet 2012;380(9859):2095–128.
4. Stanley SL Jr. Amoebiasis. Lancet 2003;361(9362):1025–34.
5. Walsh J. Prevalence of *Entamoeba histolytica* infection. In: Ravdin JI, editor. Amebiasis: human infection by *Entamoeba histolytic*a. New York: JohnWiley and Sons; 1988. p. 93–105.
6. Irusen EM, Jackson TF, Simjee AE. Asymptomatic intestinal colonization by pathogenic Entamoeba histolytica in amebic liver abscess: prevalence, response to therapy, and pathogenic potential. Clin Infect Dis 1992;14(4):889–93.
7. Hagmann SH, Han PV, Stauffer WM, et al. Travel-associated disease among US residents visiting US GeoSentinel clinics after return from international travel. Fam Pract 2014;31(6):678–87.
8. NIAID emerging infectious diseases/pathogens. Available at: https://www.niaid.nih.gov/research/emerging-infectious-diseases-pathogens.
9. Atabati H, Kassiri H, Shamloo E, et al. The association between the lack of safe drinking water and sanitation facilities with intestinal Entamoeba spp infection risk: a systematic review and meta-analysis. PLoS One 2020;15(11):e0237102.
10. Speich B, Croll D, Fürst T, et al. Effect of sanitation and water treatment on intestinal protozoa infection: a systematic review and meta-analysis. Lancet Infect Dis 2016;16(1):87–99.
11. CDC CfDCaP. Summary of notifiable diseases, United States 1994. MMWR Morb Mortal Wkly Rep 1994;43(53):1–80.
12. Herbinger KH, Fleischmann E, Weber C, et al. Epidemiological, clinical, and diagnostic data on intestinal infections with Entamoeba histolytica and Entamoeba dispar among returning travelers. Infection 2011;39(6):527–35.

13. Ravdin JI. Amebiasis. Clin Infect Dis 1995;20(6):1453–64 [quiz 1465–6].
14. Entamoeba taxonomy. Bull World Health Organ 1997;75(3):291–4.
15. Kyany'a C, Eyase F, Odundo E, et al. First report of. Trop Dis Trav Med Vaccin 2019;5:23.
16. Shimokawa C, Kabir M, Taniuchi M, et al. Entamoeba moshkovskii is associated with diarrhea in infants and causes diarrhea and colitis in mice. J Infect Dis 2012;206(5):744–51.
17. Royer TL, Gilchrist C, Kabir M, et al. Entamoeba bangladeshi nov. sp., Bangladesh. Emerg Infect Dis 2012;18(9):1543–5.
18. Diamond LS, Clark CG. A redescription of Entamoeba histolytica Schaudinn, 1903 (Emended Walker, 1911) separating it from Entamoeba dispar Brumpt, 1925. J Eukaryot Microbiol 1993;40(3):340–4.
19. Ali IK, Hossain MB, Roy S, et al. Entamoeba moshkovskii infections in children, Bangladesh. Emerg Infect Dis 2003;9(5):580–4.
20. Ximénez C, Morán P, Rojas L, et al. Reassessment of the epidemiology of amebiasis: state of the art. Infect Genet Evol 2009;9(6):1023–32.
21. Sargeaunt PG, Williams JE. Electrophoretic isoenzyme patterns of Entamoeba histolytica and Entamoeba coli. Trans R Soc Trop Med Hyg 1978;72(2):164–6.
22. Allason-Jones E, Mindel A, Sargeaunt P, et al. Entamoeba histolytica as a commensal intestinal parasite in homosexual men. N Engl J Med 1986;315(6): 353–6.
23. Guevara Á, Vicuña Y, Costales D, et al. Use of real-time polymerase chain reaction to differentiate between pathogenic. Am J Trop Med Hyg 2019;100(1):81–2.
24. Khairnar K, Parija SC. A novel nested multiplex polymerase chain reaction (PCR) assay for differential detection of Entamoeba histolytica, E. moshkovskii and E. dispar DNA in stool samples. BMC Microbiol 2007;7:47.
25. Heckendorn F, N'Goran EK, Felger I, et al. Species-specific field testing of Entamoeba spp. in an area of high endemicity. Trans R Soc Trop Med Hyg 2002;96(5):521–8.
26. Quispe-Rodríguez GH, Wankewicz AA, Luis Málaga Granda J, et al. *Entamoeba histolytica* identified by stool microscopy from children with acute diarrhoea in Peru is not *E. histolytica*. Trop Doct 2020;50(1):19–22.
27. Myung K, Burch D, Jackson TF, et al. Serodiagnosis of invasive amebiasis using a recombinant Entamoeba histolytica antigen-based ELISA. Arch Med Res 1992;23(2):285–8.
28. Lotter H, Mannweiler E, Schreiber M, et al. Sensitive and specific serodiagnosis of invasive amebiasis by using a recombinant surface protein of pathogenic Entamoeba histolytica. J Clin Microbiol 1992;30(12):3163–7.
29. Jackson T, Reddy S, Fincham J, et al. A comparison of cross-sectional and longitudinal seroepidemiological assessments of entamoeba-infected populations in South Africa. Arch Med Res 2000;31(4 Suppl):S36–7.
30. Abd-Alla MD, Wahib AA, Ravdin JI. Comparison of antigen-capture ELISA to stool-culture methods for the detection of asymptomatic Entamoeba species infection in Kafer Daoud, Egypt. Am J Trop Med Hyg 2000;62(5):579–82.
31. Haque R, Mondal D, Duggal P, et al. Entamoeba histolytica infection in children and protection from subsequent amebiasis. Infect Immun 2006;74(2):904–9.
32. Blessmann J, Van Linh P, Nu PA, et al. Epidemiology of amebiasis in a region of high incidence of amebic liver abscess in central Vietnam. Am J Trop Med Hyg 2002;66(5):578–83.
33. Acuna-Soto R, Maguire JH, Wirth DF. Gender distribution in asymptomatic and invasive amebiasis. Am J Gastroenterol 2000;95(5):1277–83.

34. Haque R, Huston CD, Hughes M, et al. Amebiasis. N Engl J Med 2003;348(16): 1565–73.
35. Gatti S, Swierczynski G, Robinson F, et al. Amebic infections due to the Entamoeba histolytica-Entamoeba dispar complex: a study of the incidence in a remote rural area of Ecuador. Am J Trop Med Hyg 2002;67(1):123–7.
36. Caballero-Salcedo A, Viveros-Rogel M, Salvatierra B, et al. Seroepidemiology of amebiasis in Mexico. Am J Trop Med Hyg 1994;50(4):412–9.
37. Haque R, Ali IM, Petri WA. Prevalence and immune response to Entamoeba histolytica infection in preschool children in Bangladesh. Am J Trop Med Hyg 1999; 60(6):1031–4.
38. Chen LH, Wilson ME, Davis X, et al. Illness in long-term travelers visiting GeoSentinel clinics. Emerg Infect Dis 2009;15(11):1773–82.
39. Lowther SA, Dworkin MS, Hanson DL. Entamoeba histolytica/Entamoeba dispar infections in human immunodeficiency virus-infected patients in the United States. Clin Infect Dis 2000;30(6):955–9.
40. Sexton DJ, Krogstad DJ, Spencer HC, et al. Amebiasis in a mental institution: serologic and epidemiologic studies. Am J Epidemiol 1974;100(5):414–23.
41. William DC, Shookhoff HB, Felman YM, et al. High rates of enteric protozoal infections in selected homosexual men attending a venereal disease clinic. Sex Transm Dis 1978;5(4):155–7.
42. Kean BH, William DC, Luminais SK. Epidemic of amoebiasis and giardiasis in a biased population. Br J Vener Dis 1979;55(5):375–8.
43. Escolà-Vergé L, Arando M, Vall M, et al. Outbreak of intestinal amoebiasis among men who have sex with men, Barcelona (Spain), October 2016 and January 2017. Euro Surveill 2017;22(30):30581.
44. Huang SH, Tsai MS, Lee CY, et al. Ongoing transmission of Entamoeba histolytica among newly diagnosed people living with HIV in Taiwan, 2009-2018. Plos Negl Trop Dis 2020;14(6):e0008400.
45. Zhou F, Li M, Li X, et al. Seroprevalence of Entamoeba histolytica infection among Chinese men who have sex with men. Plos Negl Trop Dis 2013;7(5): e2232.
46. Vreden SG, Visser LG, Verweij JJ, et al. Outbreak of amebiasis in a family in The Netherlands. Clin Infect Dis 2000;31(4):1101–4.
47. Spencer HC, Hermos JA, Healy GR, et al. Endemic amebiasis in an Arkansas community. Am J Epidemiol 1976;104(1):93–9.
48. Salit IE, Khairnar K, Gough K, et al. A possible cluster of sexually transmitted Entamoeba histolytica: genetic analysis of a highly virulent strain. Clin Infect Dis 2009;49(3):346–53.
49. Mahmoud AA, Warren KS. Algorithms in the diagnosis and management of exotic diseases. XVII. Amebiasis. J Infect Dis 1976;134(6):639–43.
50. Blessmann J, Ali IK, Nu PA, et al. Longitudinal study of intestinal Entamoeba histolytica infections in asymptomatic adult carriers. J Clin Microbiol 2003;41(10): 4745–50.
51. Braga LL, Gomes ML, Da Silva MW, et al. Household epidemiology of Entamoeba histolytica infection in an urban community in northeastern Brazil. Am J Trop Med Hyg 2001;65(4):268–71.
52. Gathiram V, Jackson TF. A longitudinal study of asymptomatic carriers of pathogenic zymodemes of Entamoeba histolytica. S Afr Med J 1987;72(10):669–72.
53. Haque R, Ali IM, Sack RB, et al. Amebiasis and mucosal IgA antibody against the Entamoeba histolytica adherence lectin in Bangladeshi children. J Infect Dis 2001;183(12):1787–93.

54. Espinosa-Cantellano M, Martínez-Palomo A. Pathogenesis of intestinal amebiasis: from molecules to disease. Clin Microbiol Rev 2000;13(2):318–31.
55. Adams EB, MacLeod IN. Invasive amebiasis. I. Amebic dysentery and its complications. Medicine (Baltimore) 1977;56(4):315–23.
56. Ravel A, Nesbitt A, Pintar K, et al. Epidemiological and clinical description of the top three reportable parasitic diseases in a Canadian community. Epidemiol Infect 2013;141(2):431–42.
57. Haque R, Mondal D, Karim A, et al. Prospective case-control study of the association between common enteric protozoal parasites and diarrhea in Bangladesh. Clin Infect Dis 2009;48(9):1191–7.
58. Jammal MA, Cox K, Ruebner B. Amebiasis presenting as rectal bleeding without diarrhea in childhood. J Pediatr Gastroenterol Nutr 1985;4(2):294–6.
59. Madden GR, Shirley DA, Townsend G, et al. Case Report: lower gastrointestinal bleeding due to entamoeba histolytica detected early by multiplex PCR: case report and review of the laboratory diagnosis of amebiasis. Am J Trop Med Hyg 2019;101(6):1380–3.
60. Merritt RJ, Coughlin E, Thomas DW, et al. Spectrum of amebiasis in children. Am J Dis Child 1982;136(9):785–9.
61. Long SS, Prober CG, Fischer M. Principles and practice of pediatric infectious diseases. Fifth edition. Elsevier; 2018. p. 1313.
62. Van Den Broucke S, Verschueren J, Van Esbroeck M, et al. Clinical and microscopic predictors of Entamoeba histolytica intestinal infection in travelers and migrants diagnosed with Entamoeba histolytica/dispar infection. PLoS Negl Trop Dis 2018;12(10):e0006892.
63. Anand AC, Reddy PS, Saiprasad GS, et al. Does non-dysenteric intestinal amoebiasis exist? Lancet 1997;349(9045):89–92.
64. Aristizábal H, Acevedo J, Botero M. Fulminant amebic colitis. World J Surg 1991;15(2):216–21.
65. Takahashi T, Gamboa-Dominguez A, Gomez-Mendez TJ, et al. Fulminant amebic colitis: analysis of 55 cases. Dis Colon Rectum 1997;40(11):1362–7.
66. Ortiz-Castillo F, Salinas-Aragón LE, Sánchez-Aguilar M, et al. Amoebic toxic colitis: analysis of factors related to mortality. Pathog Glob Health 2012;106(4):245–8.
67. Ravdin JI. Amebiasis: human infection by Entamoeba histolytica. New York: John Wiley & Sons; 1988. p. 650–719.
68. Shirley DA, Moonah S. Fulminant amebic colitis after corticosteroid therapy: a systematic review. PLoS Negl Trop Dis 2016;10(7):e0004879.
69. Cardoso JM, Kimura K, Stoopen M, et al. Radiology of invasive amebiasis of the colon. AJR Am J Roentgenol 1977;128(6):935–41.
70. Otan E, Akbulut S, Kayaalp C. Amebic acute appendicitis: systematic review of 174 cases. World J Surg 2013;37(9):2061–73.
71. Adams EB, MacLeod IN. Invasive amebiasis. II. Amebic liver abscess and its complications. Medicine (Baltimore) 1977;56(4):325–34.
72. Katzenstein D, Rickerson V, Braude A. New concepts of amebic liver abscess derived from hepatic imaging, serodiagnosis, and hepatic enzymes in 67 consecutive cases in San Diego. Medicine (Baltimore) 1982;61(4):237–46.
73. Knobloch J, Mannweiler E. Development and persistence of antibodies to Entamoeba histolytica in patients with amebic liver abscess. Analysis of 216 cases. Am J Trop Med Hyg 1983;32(4):727–32.
74. Lachish T, Wieder-Finesod A, Schwartz E. Amebic liver abscess in israeli travelers: a retrospective study. Am J Trop Med Hyg 2016;94(5):1015–9.

75. Haffar A, Boland FJ, Edwards MS. Amebic liver abscess in children. Pediatr Infect Dis 1982;1(5):322–7.
76. Nazir Z, Moazam F. Amebic liver abscess in children. Pediatr Infect Dis J 1993; 12(11):929–32.
77. Khotaii G, Hadipoor Z, Hadipoor F. Amebic liver abscess in Iranian children. Acta Med Iranica 2003;41(1):33–6.
78. Nazir Z, Qazi SH. Amebic liver abscesses among neonates can mimic bacterial sepsis. Pediatr Infect Dis J 2005;24(5):464–6.
79. Johnson JL, Baird JS, Hulbert TV, et al. Amebic liver abscess in infancy: case report and review. Clin Infect Dis 1994;19(4):765–7.
80. Shamsuzzaman SM, Hashiguchi Y. Thoracic amebiasis. Clin Chest Med 2002; 23(2):479–92.
81. Ibarra-Pérez C. Thoracic complications of amebic abscess of the liver: report of 501 cases. Chest 1981;79(6):672–7.
82. Lombardo L, Alonso P, Saenzarroyo L, et al. CEREBRAL AMEBIASIS: REPORT OF 17 CASES. J Neurosurg 1964;21:704–9.
83. Orbison JA, Reeves N, Leedham CL, et al. Amebic brain abscess; review of the literature and report of five additional cases. Medicine (Baltimore) 1951;30(3): 247–82.
84. Maldonado-Barrera CA, Campos-Esparza Mdel R, Muñoz-Fernández L, et al. Clinical case of cerebral amebiasis caused by E. Histolytica. Parasitol Res 2012;110(3):1291–6.
85. Petri WA, Haque R. Entamoeba histolytica brain abscess. Handb Clin Neurol 2013;114:147–52.
86. Rao S, Solaymani-Mohammadi S, Petri WA Jr, et al. Hepatic amebiasis: a reminder of the complications. Curr Opin Pediatr 2009;21(1):145–9.
87. Saidin S, Othman N, Noordin R. Update on laboratory diagnosis of amoebiasis. Eur J Clin Microbiol Infect Dis 2019;38(1):15–38.
88. González-Ruiz A, Haque R, Aguirre A, et al. Value of microscopy in the diagnosis of dysentery associated with invasive Entamoeba histolytica. J Clin Pathol 1994;47(3):236–9.
89. Fotedar R, Stark D, Beebe N, et al. Laboratory diagnostic techniques for Entamoeba species. Clin Microbiol Rev 2007;20(3):511–32, table of contents.
90. Leo M, Haque R, Kabir M, et al. Evaluation of Entamoeba histolytica antigen and antibody point-of-care tests for the rapid diagnosis of amebiasis. J Clin Microbiol 2006;44(12):4569–71.
91. Goñi P, Martín B, Villacampa M, et al. Evaluation of an immunochromatographic dip strip test for simultaneous detection of Cryptosporidium spp, Giardia duodenalis, and Entamoeba histolytica antigens in human faecal samples. Eur J Clin Microbiol Infect Dis 2012;31(8):2077–82.
92. Garcia LS, Shimizu RY, Bernard CN. Detection of Giardia lamblia, Entamoeba histolytica/Entamoeba dispar, and Cryptosporidium parvum antigens in human fecal specimens using the triage parasite panel enzyme immunoassay. J Clin Microbiol 2000;38(9):3337–40.
93. Ryan U, Paparini A, Oskam C. New Technologies for Detection of Enteric Parasites. Trends Parasitol 2017;33(7):532–46.
94. Ravdin JI, Jackson TF, Petri WA, et al. Association of serum antibodies to adherence lectin with invasive amebiasis and asymptomatic infection with pathogenic Entamoeba histolytica. J Infect Dis 1990;162(3):768–72.

95. Haque R, Mollah NU, Ali IK, et al. Diagnosis of amebic liver abscess and intestinal infection with the TechLab Entamoeba histolytica II antigen detection and antibody tests. J Clin Microbiol 2000;38(9):3235–9.
96. Paromomycin. Lexi-Drugs. Lexicomp. Available at: http://online.lexi.com. Accessed June 10, 2021.
97. Shirley DT, Farr L, Watanabe K, et al. A Review of the Global Burden, New Diagnostics, and Current Therapeutics for Amebiasis. Open Forum Infect Dis 2018;5(7):ofy161.
98. Metronidazole. Lexi-Drugs. Lexicomp. Available at: http://online.lexi.com. Accessed June 10, 2021.
99. Tinidazole. Lexi-Drugs. Lexicomp. Available at: http://online.lexi.com. Accessed June 10, 2021.
100. Gonzales MLM, Dans LF, Sio-Aguilar J. Antiamoebic drugs for treating amoebic colitis. Cochrane Database Syst Rev 2019;1:CD006085.
101. AAP. Amebiasis. Red book: *report of the committee on infectious diseases*. Elk Grove Village, IL: American Academy of Pediatrics; 2021.
102. Siegel JD, Rhinehart E, Jackson M, et al. Health Care Infection Control Practices Advisory Committee. 2007 Guideline for Isolation Precautions: Preventing Transmission of Infectious Agents in Health Care Settings. Am J Infect Control. 2007;35(10 Suppl 2):S65–164.
103. Quach J, St-Pierre J, Chadee K. The future for vaccine development against Entamoeba histolytica. Hum Vaccin Immunother 2014;10(6):1514–21.

Evaluation and Management of Traveler's Diarrhea in Children

Frank Zhu, MD

KEYWORDS

• Traveler's diarrhea • Children • Travel • Endemic infections

KEY POINTS

- Pretravel clinical consultation is essential to prevention of pediatric traveler's diarrhea.
- Most of pediatric traveler's diarrhea is self-limited.
- Oral rehydration is the mainstay of therapy for pediatric traveler's diarrhea.
- Antimicrobial therapy may be indicated in cases of moderate to severe disease.

INTRODUCTION

First described in 1958 by Kean,[1] traveler's diarrhea (TD) is defined as the passage of ≥3 unformed stools over 24 hours with or without additional symptoms (ie, abdominal cramps, tenesmus, nausea, vomiting, fever, or fecal urgency), which develops within 14 days of returning from travel to a typically resource-limited destination.[2,3] It accounts for nearly 335 out of every 1000 medical visits by returned travelers[4] and is the most common travel-related disease in both children and adults.[3] As children are less likely to have received pretravel health advice and are more likely to require hospitalization following return,[5] timely and accurate management of TD in children is essential in prevention of travel-related morbidity.

DEFINITION

The definition of TD in adults (≥3 unformed stools over 24 hours with or without additional symptoms within 14 days of travel) should be adapted to account for variable stooling patterns in the pediatric population. Indeed, multiple loose, unformed stools per day may be normal for a young, breast-fed infant. A commonly used pediatric definition is a change in normal stool pattern (typically increase in frequency to at least 3 stools over 24 hours) and a decrease in consistency to an unformed state.[6]

Department of Pediatrics, Division of Pediatric Infectious Diseases, Medical College of Wisconsin Suite 450C, 999 North 92nd Street, Wauwatosa, WI 53226, USA
E-mail address: frzhu@mcw.edu

Pediatr Clin N Am 69 (2022) 99–113
https://doi.org/10.1016/j.pcl.2021.08.004
pediatric.theclinics.com

DISCUSSION

Epidemiology

The reported rate of pediatric TD has varied considerably among publications (13.5%–39%), but a summary of 8 publications resulted in a rate of 28.6%.[7] Higher rates of TD were found in children who travel to visit friends or relatives compared with children who traveled for tourism.[8–10] In a prospective study of 606 pediatric travelers from Spain, 21.6% children who traveled to visit friends/family had developed TD compared with a rate of 5.6% of tourist children.[11]

In addition, travel to Africa, South Asia, and Latin America has been associated with the highest rates of TD.[12,13] Greenwood and colleagues[14] performed a multicenter, retrospective analysis of 6086 returning travelers who sought care at a GeoSentinal clinic. Country-specific reporting rate ratios (RRR) for gastrointestinal illnesses using western and northern Europe as a baseline destination region showed the highest RRR in South Asia (890), Sub-Saharan Africa (282), and South America (203). Moderate RRR were reported for Southeast Asia (104), Caribbean (94), Central America (87), North Africa (76), Middle East (60), and Oceania (41). The lowest RRR were Australasia (17), northeast Asia (10), southern Europe (7), central/east Europe (4), North America (2), and western and northern Europe (1).

However, the ultimate determination of risk is likely related to local hygiene conditions. Improved hygiene has reduced the risk of TD from 20% to 8-20% in some regions.[15] Indeed, income level of a country has been found to be inversely proportional to RRR of TD,[14] and ultimately, higher rates of TD in children who visit friends/relatives compared with tourism may be related to the increased hygiene present at many tourist destinations.

Clinical Manifestations

Of TD, 90% manifest within the first 2 weeks of travel, with an average onset of 8 days in children.[7] Diarrhea is usually watery, but dysentery (defined as the presence of blood or mucus in stool) with high fever may be present depending on the etiologic pathogen. Compared with adults, dysentery is seen more commonly in pediatric TD.[3,16] Most children present with 3 to 5 unformed stools daily (45.1%), followed by 1 to 2 unformed stools (31%), with a minority of children presenting with 6 to 9 (13.4%) or greater than 10 (4.9%) unformed stools. Additional symptoms accompany approximately two-thirds of pediatric patients. The most common symptoms are abdominal cramps (43%), vomiting (18.3%), and fever (14.1%).[16]

Most TD presents as a self-limited acute syndrome, but persistent (>2 weeks) or chronic (>4 weeks) may develop in some patients.[13,15–17] The reported incidence of persistent diarrhea in pediatric TD ranges from 14%[13] to 20%,[5] whereas the incidence of chronic diarrhea is significantly lower (5%).[18] However, younger children may be at significantly higher risk for the development of chronic diarrhea, with 1 prospective study reporting 11/12 of younger children developing TD lasting greater than 3 weeks. Indeed, the same study showed an average duration of diarrhea of 29.5 days in children less than 2 years of age, 8.4 days in children 3 to 6 years old, and 5.3 days in children 15 to 20 years old.[16] This is consistent with the more severe presentation of TD that is reported in infants and young children.[5,7,15]

The complications of TD in children closely mirror complications of acute gastroenteritis. The most common complication is dehydration, accounting for 40% of TD-related emergency department visits in children.[7] Dehydration manifests as decreased urine output, dry mucous membranes, reduced skin turgor, weight loss (in infants), reduced tearing, sunken eyes, weakness, tachycardia, orthostatic hypotension, and electrolyte imbalance.[19,20] Uncommon complications may also present based on etiologic pathogen (that is, hemolytic-uremic syndrome with Shiga toxin-producing *Escherichia coli* [STEC]).

Cause

The cause of TD is similar to other causes of infectious gastroenteritis present at the location and season of travel.[21] There are limited data on the cause of pediatric TD, and data are generally extrapolated from adult studies.[7] However, community-based studies of childhood diarrhea indicate that its cause is similar to that of diarrhea in adult travelers.[22]

Historically, the cause of TD was not detected in a significant proportion (28%–50%) of cases. However, use of stool culture and antigen detection may have resulted in a significantly lower sensitivity because of delays in stool sampling and transport to central laboratories.[7] The development and widespread implementation of multiplex polymerase chain reaction (PCR) have enhanced the detection of bacteria, parasites, and viruses in stool samples[23] and resulted in an increase in identification of etiologic agents. Indeed, use of these molecular methods has decreased the percentage of unexplained TD cases to 4% to 24%.[21] However, multiplex PCR has also detected high rates of coinfection (34% bacteria and viruses, 16% bacteria and parasites, 10% bacteria and viruses and parasites).[24] The detection of multiple agents may confound the true etiologic pathogen, as the high sensitivity of multiplex PCR may incidentally detect nonpathological organisms.

Bacterial endemic at the travel destination continues to be the predominant pathogen in TD.[19] First identified in the 1970s in returning travelers from Mexico,[25] enterotoxigenic *Escherichia coli* (ETEC) has been historically reported to be the predominant bacterial pathogen in most regions with the exception of southeast Asia.[15,21,26] However, Laaveri and colleagues[21] analyzed the stool samples of 459 prospectively recruited travelers via multiplex PCR and found enteropathogenic (EPEC) and enteroaggregative (EAEC) *Escherichia coli* to be the most frequent bacterial pathogen of TD, followed by ETEC and *Campylobacter* spp.

The predominant bacterial pathogen found varies significantly by travel destination. ETEC was seen at the highest rate in East Africa (38%), followed by South Asia (27%), West Africa (23%), and Latin America (13%). EPEC was seen at highest prevalence in South Asia (56%) followed by East Africa (58%), West Africa (40%), and Latin America (30%). EAEC was seen most frequently in South Asia (60%), followed by Latin America (54%), West Africa (47%), and East Africa (44%). *Campylobacter* spp remains a significant concern in South Asia, found in up to 20% of stool samples, but was seen extremely infrequently in other regions (2% West Africa, 7% East Africa, not detected in Latin America).[21] Less common bacterial causes of TD include STEC (includes enterohemorrhagic *E coli*, enteroinvasive *E coli*, *Salmonella* spp, *Shigella* spp [classically associated with travel to Africa and Latin America], *Aeromonas* spp, *Plesiomonas shigelloides*, and *Vibrio* spp).[5,7,15]

Viral causes of TD account for approximately 10% of TD and include norovirus, rotavirus, enteric adenovirus, and astrovirus.[27] Rotavirus remains the leading cause of severe, dehydrating diarrhea in hospitalized children under the age of 5 worldwide,[22] and the seasonality of rotavirus in the Americas (peaks in winter) is not reflected in other parts of the world. Indeed, there is often no seasonality in the tropics (within 10° of latitude of the equator), and peaks during other seasons (autumn, spring) are present in other parts of the world.[28] Therefore, a high index of suspicion should be maintained for rotavirus in pediatric TD regardless of season in pediatric patients who have not received the rotavirus vaccine.

Parasitic causes account for 12%[13] to 28%[5] of pediatric TD. However, lower rates of parasitic pathogens (0.7%) were found in a prospective study of 146 Finnish travelers and may indicate that higher rates of parasitic pathogens are historically reported by patients seeking medical care for prolonged or severe TD when compared with prospective studies.[29] The typical parasitic pathogens are protozoa: *Giardia lamblia*, *Entamoeba histolytica*, and less commonly, *Cryptosporidium parvum*.[5,13,24] The onset is typically more gradual, often resulting in prolonged or chronic TD.

Evaluation

A thorough history should be obtained during initial evaluation, including medical history of patient, duration and frequency of diarrhea, additional symptoms, medication, and travel history (including food history, location of travel, animal exposure).

Acute TD in adults is classified into mild, moderate, and severe, which is subsequently used for treatment guidelines.[30] Mild TD is classified as diarrhea that is tolerable, is not distressing, and does not interfere with planned activities. Moderate TD is classified as diarrhea that is distressing or interferes with planned activities. Severe TD is classified as diarrhea that is incapacitating or completely prevents planned activities. All dysentery is considered severe. As pediatric TD data are limited, a similar classification is used in pediatric TD, although treatment may differ significantly based on the patient's age. However, it should be noted this classification may be difficult to apply to young children/infants.

Careful attention should be given to signs and symptoms of dehydration in children (decreased urine output, decreased skin turgor, sunken anterior fontanelle, absent tears, dry mucous membranes, weight loss, tachycardia, orthostatic hypotension). Young infants are typically more susceptible to dehydration because of increased insensible fluid losses, higher severity/duration of diarrhea, increased rates of emesis, and infant dependence on milk (higher osmotic load). Risk factors for dehydration include age (<12 months), greater than 8 stools per day, greater than 2 emesis per day, undernutrition, discontinuation of breastfeeding during illness, and failure to give oral rehydration solution (ORS).[7,31]

Management

Rehydration through fluid administration is the mainstay of management for diarrhea, including pediatric TD.[20] ORS is preferred over intravenous (IV) rehydration. Breastfeeding should be continued during TD, as it has been shown to reduce the number and volume of diarrheal stools as well as reduce the duration of rotavirus gastroenteritis.[32] Hospitalization should be reserved for children that require hospital procedures, such as IV rehydration. Enteral rehydration is associated with significantly fewer major adverse events, including death and seizures, and shorter hospital stay.[33] When enteral rehydration is not feasible, use of oral rehydration therapy through a nasogastric tube is as effective and preferred over IV rehydration.[20]

Reduced osmolarity solution (sodium 75 mmol/L, glucose 75 mmol/L, potassium 20 mEq/L, chloride 65 mEq/L, citrate 10 mmol/L, and osmolarity 245 mOsmol/L) is recommended by the World Health Organization for noncholera diarrhea. However, limited data also suggest that reduced osmolarity ORS also appears safe for children with cholera. Rice/cereal-based ORS can be used as an alternative therapy for cholera diarrhea, as it may reduce diarrhea by adding more substrate to the gut lumen but should not be used for noncholera diarrhea given the lack of additional benefit.[20] Frequent administration of small-volume ORS is often necessary in an ill child with the goal of administering 50 mL/kg over 2 to 4 hours for mild dehydration or 100 mL/kg over 2 to 4 hours for moderate dehydration.[7]

Table 1
Pediatric dehydration assessment

	Mild Dehydration	Moderate Dehydration	Severe Dehydration
Weight loss (infants)	4%–5%	6%–9%	≥10% weight loss
Anterior fontanelle (infants)	Normal	Mildly sunken	Very sunken
Mental status	Normal	Irritable	Lethargic/somnolent
Tears	Normal	Decreased	Absent
Mucous membranes	Mildly dry	Dry	Very dry
Urine output	Normal or mildly decreased	Reduced/concentrated	Anuria >8 h
Respirations	Normal	Mildly rapid	Deep and rapid
Blood pressure	Normal	Normal to mild orthostatic hypotension (>10 mm Hg change)	Hypotension
Pulse	Normal	Rapid	Weak and rapid
Skin turgor	Normal	Decreased	Severely decreased/ tenting present
Capillary refill	Normal (<2 s)	Slowed (2–4 s)	Marked delayed (>4 s)

Although the use of pharmacologic agents has been recommended in treatment guidelines for adult TD,[30] these agents are typically not indicated for use in children. Bismuth subsalicylate prophylaxis/treatment is generally not recommended in children because of risk of Reye syndrome.[7] However, the American Academy of Pediatrics Red Book does state that it can be used in mild cases of TD in children 12 years and older.[34] Antimotility agents, such as loperamide, are contraindicated in children less than 3 years of age given concerns for central nervous system depression, ileus, and toxic megacolon. The Infectious Disease Society of America does not recommend use of loperamide in children less than 18 years of age for acute diarrhea.[35] Zinc supplementation is not recommended in children given lack of evidence for its efficacy.[7,19,20]

Antimicrobial therapy is not routinely recommended for treatment of TD. Antimicrobial use has been demonstrated to increase risk of colonization by extended-spectrum beta-lactamase-producing *Enterobacteriaceae*.[36,37] Intestinal colonization has been associated with subsequent onset of infection by gram-negative pathogens, raising the risk of development of multidrug-resistant organisms in these patients.[38,39] Azithromycin could be the empiric drug of choice for pediatric TD because of its coverage of most pathogens.[7] However, specific antimicrobial therapy should ultimately be tailored based on etiologic agent suspected/diagnosed and its associated complications, underlying medical condition of the patient, and severity of TD in the child (refer to Clinics Care Points for specific pathogens).

SUMMARY

TD is the most common travel-related disease in both children and adults. However, significant gaps persist regarding randomized controlled studies in the evaluation and management of pediatric TD,[7] which has resulted in significant variation in clinical practice in both pretravel health advice in children and management of pediatric

TD. There are often pitfalls when adapting adult guidelines for TD to pediatric TD.[40] Therefore, it is essential for clinicians to account for the differences in pediatric pathophysiology, clinical presentations, and treatment recommendations during the management of pediatric TD.

CLINICS CARE POINTS

- Pretravel clinic consultation
  - Prevent travel-related hazards, behavior, personal hygiene rules, administer appropriate travel vaccines and prophylactic medications.
  - Counsel caregivers to recognize acute signs and symptoms of dehydration in a child with diarrhea.
    - Counsel appropriate usage of oral rehydration solution and feeding.
    - Packets of oral rehydration salts can be obtained before travel in most pharmacies.
    - Seek medical attention for traveler's diarrhea with any signs of moderate or severe dehydration (see later discussion; assess hydration status).
  - Families may want to carry an antimicrobial agent (eg, 3-day course of azithromycin or fluoroquinolone) to provide self-treatment should TD develop.[41]
    - Counsel caregivers to reserve treatment for moderate to severe cases of traveler's diarrhea.
    - Counsel caregivers that use of antibiotic therapy may increase the risk of acquisition of multidrug-resistant bacteria.
    - Children typically prescribed azithromycin 10 mg/kg/d (maximum 500 mg) for 3 days.
    - Fluroquinolone should be limited in children less than 18 years of age unless no alternatives exist (no Food and Drug Administration approval for <18 years of age for a concern for cartilage toxicity).[42]
  - Hygiene recommendations with emphasis to avoid contaminated food and water[7]:
    - Counsel parents and children that most cases of traveler's diarrhea are caused by ingestion of contaminated food and water.
    - Avoid contaminated water.
      - Avoid tap water: Use only bottled or boiled water for drinking, tooth brushing.
      - Prepare all beverages and ice cubes with bottled or boiled water.
      - Avoid bathing in swimming pools or lakes of unknown microbiological quality because of risk of ingesting contaminated water.
    - Avoid contaminated food.
      - Consume only pasteurized or irradiated milk and dairy products.
      - Wash hands with soap or alcohol-based detergents before eating or preparing foods.
      - Eat only well-cooked food served hot.
      - Consume only peeled vegetables or fruits and cooked vegetables.
      - Avoid raw seafood or shellfish.
      - Avoid food from street vendors.
        - May carry readily available snacks to avoid buying street vendor food for children.
    - Continue breastfeeding throughout travel in breast-fed infants.
  - Pharmacologic prophylaxis is typically not recommended.
    - Bismuth subsalicylate (BSS) is generally not recommended in children because of risk of Reye syndrome (salicylate component).
      - May be considered in adults (2.1 g/d or 4.2 g/d in 4 divided doses) given strong evidence for protective effect (>60%).[43,44]
      - Approved for use in children older than 12 years of age.
      - May cause blackening of tongue and stool.
      - Caution should be taken in administering to children with viral infections (influenza, varicella) given concern for Reye syndrome.
      - Rare side effects: Nausea, constipation, tinnitus.
    - Antimicrobial prophylaxis.
      - Not routinely recommended in children or adults.
      - Prophylaxis with rifaximin is recommended for adults who are at high risk of health-related complications of traveler's diarrhea.[30]

- Rifaximin (200 mg 1–3 times per day)
  - Nonabsorbable antibiotic with favorable safety profile
  - Unknown impact on multidrug-resistant organism acquisition
  - No coverage of invasive enteropathogens, including the following:
    - *Campylobacter* spp are resistant, resulting in only moderate effectiveness in South and Southeast Asia
    - *Shigella* spp
    - *Salmonella* spp
  - Approved for use in children ≥12 years of age
- Fluoroquinolones no longer recommended
  - Rising rates of resistance from enteric pathogens (70% *Campylobacter* spp from Nepal/Thailand, 65% enterotoxigenic *Escherichia coli* and enteroaggregative *Escherichia coli* from India)

- Probiotics: Insufficient data for safety and efficacy for use in children or adults.
  - Significant variation in probiotic dosages/formulations, causes of diarrhea, setting, timing and administration, concurrent treatment with antimicrobials in studies of probiotic efficacy at preventing traveler's diarrhea.
  - Two meta-analyses have suggested marginal benefit but state there is insufficient evidence for extrapolation to global recommendations for use.[45,46]
- Pretravel vaccination
  - Routine vaccination schedule should be followed in all children with particular attention given to hepatitis A and rotavirus vaccines.
    - Rotavirus is a rare cause of TD, but vaccination is desirable given the potentially severe gastroenteritis in young infants.
  - Oral cholera vaccine is available for children ≥2 years of age.
    - World Health Organization states vaccine is generally not recommended for long-term or short-term travelers to cholera-affected countries.[47]
    - Can be considered in at-risk populations (pregnant/lactating women, HIV-infected individuals) or high-risk travelers likely to be directly exposed to contaminated food or water (eg, emergency/relief workers).
  - Typhoid fever vaccination is recommended for travelers to areas with increased risk of exposure to *Salmonella typhi* (East and Southeast Asia, Africa, Caribbean, Central and Southern America).[35]
    - Two formulations available:
      - Ty21a (live, attenuated, oral vaccine) for children ≥6 years of age.
      - Vi capsular polysaccharide vaccine (inactivated, intramuscular) for children ≥2 years of age.

- Evaluation
  - Careful history essential to determine most likely causative organism.
    - Medical history of patient (eg, immunocompromised status), duration and frequency of diarrhea, additional symptoms, medication history, and travel history (including food history, location of travel, animal exposure).
  - Time to onset of symptoms can be a valuable clue if specific exposure is identified (ie, street vendor food, water exposure).
    - Short duration (<48 hours): Norovirus, rotavirus, *Vibrio* spp, enterotoxigenic *Escherichia coli* (can be longer, incubation period 12 hours to 3 days), *Salmonella* spp.
    - Moderate duration (<1 week): Enterotoxigenic *Escherichia coli*, *Shigella* spp, *Campylobacter* spp, *Yersinia enterocolitica*, enterohemorrhagic *Escherichia coli*, protozoa is typically immunocompromised host (*Cryptosporidium* spp, *Cyclospora* spp).
    - Long duration (>12 days): Typically protozoa (*Giardia duodenalis*, *Entamoeba histolytica*).[48]
  - Exposures
    - Contaminated water is the most common exposure associated with traveler's diarrhea.
    - Contact with brackish rivers and coastal waters, ingestion of raw or undercooked shellfish: *Vibrio cholerae, Vibrio parahaemolyticus.*
    - Contact with fresh water or brackish water: *Plesiomonas shigelloides*, *Aeromonas* spp.
    - Birds, mammals, reptiles, amphibians: Nontyphoidal *Salmonella.*

- Raw leafy vegetables, undercooked ground beef, unpasteurized milk/juice: Shiga toxin-producing *Escherichia coli*.
- Contact with raw pork intestines (chitterlings): Often reported in caregivers of infants, ingestion of raw or incompletely cooked pork products, *Yersinia enterocolitica.*
- History of antibiotic usage: *Clostridium difficile.*

- Clinical presentation[48]
  - Few large-volume stools (small bowel origin).
    - *Vibrio cholerae, parahaemolyticus*: Stools tend to be watery and severe.
    - Enterotoxigenic *Escherichia coli*
    - *Shigella* spp (early)
    - *Giardia duodenalis*: Greasy/fatty with foul smell
  - Many small-volume stools (large bowel origin)
    - *Shigella* spp
    - *Salmonella* spp
    - *Campylobacter* spp
    - *Escherichia coli*
    - *Yersinia enterocolitica*, *Entamoeba histolytica*
  - Tenesmus, fecal urgency, dysentery (colitis)
    - *Shigella* spp
    - *Salmonella* spp
    - *Campylobacter* spp
    - Invasive *Escherichia coli* (enteroinvasive *Escherichia coli*, enterohemorrhagic *Escherichia coli*)
    - *Entamoeba histolytica*
    - *Vibrio parahaemolyticus* (rare)
  - Predominance of vomiting (early gastroenteritis)
    - Viral (rotavirus, norovirus) or food poisoning
  - Predominance of fever (mucosal invasion)
    - *Shigella* spp
    - *Campylobacter* spp
    - *Salmonella* spp
      - Enteric (typhoid) fever should be suspected in older children with gradual onset of fever, which typically plateaus at 39°C to 40°C at end of week, particularly if patients develop dactylitis or rose spots.
      - Constipation/diarrhea (pea soup) may be present early.
      - Nonspecific systemic features (headache, malaise, anorexia, lethargy, abdominal pain) may be present.
      - Younger children may present with fever alone.
    - Enteroinvasive *Escherichia coli*
  - Prolonged diarrhea (>2 weeks), protozoa
    - *Giardia duodenalis*
    - *Entamoeba histolytica*
    - *Cryptosporidium* spp
- Assess hydration status of child[7]
  - **Table 1** provides a pediatric dehydration assessment.
  - Signs of moderate or severe dehydration may require hospitalization

- Management
  - Adult guidelines on therapy based on classification are not applicable in most children.
    - Can be considered for older children/adolescents.
    - Adult therapy recommendations.[30]
      - Mild traveler's diarrhea (diarrhea that is tolerable, not distressing, and does not interfere with planned activities).
        - Antibiotic therapy not recommended.
        - Loperamide (patients >18 years) or bismuth subsalicylate may be considered.
      - Moderate traveler's diarrhea (diarrhea is distressing or interferes with planned activities).
        - Antibiotics may be used (weak recommendation).

- Loperamide (patients >18 years), may be used as monotherapy or adjunctive therapy.
- Severe traveler's diarrhea (diarrhea that is incapacitating or completely prevents planned activities, includes all dysentery).
  - Antibiotics should be used to treat severe traveler's diarrhea.

- Pharmacologic agents suggested in adult guidelines have limited use and increased risk in children.
  - Bismuth subsalicylate: Generally not recommended in children because of risk of Reye syndrome (salicylate component).
    - Approved for use in children older than 12 years of age.
      - Some clinicians use bismuth subsalicylate off label in younger children.
        - Should not be used in children less than 3 years of age.
    - Studies have not established safety of bismuth subsalicylate for use longer than 3 weeks.
    - May cause blackening of tongue and stool.
    - Caution should be taken in administering to children with viral infections (influenza, varicella) given concern for Reye syndrome.
    - Rare side effects: Nausea, constipation, tinnitus.
  - Loperamide: Locally acting opioid receptor agonist that decreases muscular tone and motility of intestinal wall.
    - Significant potential side effects in children (particularly young children/infants).
      - Toxic megacolon: Avoid use in children with bloody/mucous diarrhea.
      - Central nervous system depression: Has been associated with fatal overdoses, coma, respiratory depression.
    - Infectious Diseases Society of America does not recommend use in children with acute diarrhea less than 18 years of age.[35]
- Rehydration remains the mainstay of therapy[7]
  - Oral rehydration solution preferred over intravenous rehydration.
    - Intravenous rehydration may be necessary in persistent emesis/inability to tolerate oral intake.
  - Reduced osmolarity solution is recommended by World Health Organization for noncholera diarrhea.
    - Also appears safe for children with cholera diarrhea.
  - Rice-based oral rehydration solution can be used in cholera diarrhea to reduce diarrhea through addition of more substrates in gut lumen.
  - Frequent administration of small-volume oral rehydration solution is often necessary.
    - Goal of administering 50 mL/kg over 2 to 4 hours for mild dehydration or 100 mL/kg over 2 to 4 hours for moderate dehydration.
- Antimicrobial therapy
  - Antimicrobial therapy is not routinely recommended in pediatric traveler's diarrhea.
    - Antimicrobial therapy is typically considered when invasive enteropathogens are suspected.
      - Moderate to severe diarrhea ± blood or mucus.
      - Prolonged duration (protozoa infection).
    - Severely ill-appearing child
  - Azithromycin (10 mg/kg daily × 3 days) typically recommended as the empiric drug of choice for TD owing to broad coverage of most pathogens.
    - Rifaximin can be used in children greater than 12 years if a noninvasive enteropathogen is suspected (ie, nonbloody diarrhea).
  - Antimicrobial management should be guided by etiologic pathogens.
    - Etiologic diagnosis typically not available during acute infection via conventional culture methods.
    - Use of stool multiplex polymerase chain reaction may provide etiologic diagnosis in a timely manner (hours).
  - Organism-specific considerations
    - *Campylobacter* spp[49]
      - Antibiotic treatment reduces duration of intestinal symptoms by 1.3 days.

- More pronounced effect in children and when initiated within 3 days of illness onset.
- Increased resistance to macrolides is reported in Southeast Asia (12.5% Thailand, 21.8% China, 22.2% India).[50]
- Recommended regimen
  - Azithromycin (10 mg/kg/d) × 3 days
  - Alternative: Erythromycin 40 mg/kg/d divided in 4 doses × 5 days
  - Known susceptibility: Ciprofloxacin (20–30 mg/kg/d) × 3 days

- *Escherichia coli*[34]
  - Antimicrobial therapy not recommended in most cases of *Escherichia coli*
    - Consider in patients with moderate or severe illness with greater than 14 days of diarrhea attributable to diarrheagenic *Escherichia coli*
  - Recommend antibiotics
    - Azithromycin 10 mg/kg/d × 3 days
    - Alternative:
      - Ciprofloxacin in susceptible strains (20–30 mg/kg/d) × 3 days.
      - Rifaximin in children greater than 12 years (200 mg/dose 3 times a day × 3 days).
  - Antibiotic therapy not recommended in traveler's diarrhea due to Shiga toxin-producing *Escherichia coli*.
    - Increased risk of developing hemolytic uremic syndrome.
- *Salmonella* spp (nontyphoid)[51]
  - Treatment does not significantly affect duration of fever or diarrhea in healthy children.
  - Treatment recommended in all children at risk for invasive disease (<3 months of age, chronic gastrointestinal disease, malignant neoplasms, hemoglobinopathies, HIV infection, other immunosuppressive illnesses, or therapies).
  - All ill-appearing children should have blood and stool cultures obtained before antibiotics and started on IV ceftriaxone.
  - Well-appearing children can be discharged on oral azithromycin.
  - Disseminated disease (meningitis, osteoarticular infection, endocarditis) should be excluded in all bacteremic patients.
- *Salmonella* spp (typhoid)[51]
  - Travel history and regional antibiotic resistance patterns should be carefully considered.
    - Pakistan
      - Since 2016, extensively drug-resistant *Salmonella typhi* (resistant to ceftriaxone, ampicillin, ciprofloxacin, and trimethoprim-sulfamethoxazole) reported.
      - Isolates are sensitive to carbapenems and azithromycin.
  - Empiric therapy with parenteral third-generation cephalosporin or azithromycin recommended.
  - Corticosteroids may be beneficial in children with severe enteric fever (delirium, obtundation, stupor, coma, or shock).
    - Initial dose: 3 mg/kg followed by 1 mg/kg every 6 hours for a total of 48 hours.
  - Relapse occurs in up to 17% of patients within 4 weeks.
    - Rates appear lower in those treated with azithromycin.
  - Chronic carrier state (typically within gall bladder) may develop.
    - Requires prolonged antimicrobial therapy.
      - 4 weeks of oral ciprofloxacin or norfloxacin.
    - Parenteral ampicillin can be used as an alternative if train is susceptible.
    - Cholecystectomy may be indicated if antimicrobial therapy fails.
  - Stool culture should be performed on all people who travel with index cases, and treatment should be initiated in positive travelers.
    - Asymptomatic people with contact with index case should be evaluated on a case-by-case basis to determine necessity for stool culture.
- *Shigella* spp[52]

- Antibiotic therapy significantly shortens duration of fever, diarrhea, fecal excretion.
- Rising rates of antimicrobial resistance among travelers, particularly to tetracycline, cotrimoxazole, ampicillin.[53]
- Antimicrobial therapy recommended in severe disease or children with underlying immunosuppressive conditions.
- Recommended antibiotic
  - Azithromycin (10 mg/kg/d) × 3 days
  - Parental ceftriaxone (50 mg/kg/d) × 2 to 5 days
  - Known susceptibility
    - Ciprofloxacin (20–30 mg/kg/d) × 3 days
    - Oral ampicillin or trimethoprim-sulfamethoxazole × 5 days in susceptible strains

- *Vibrio cholera*[54]
  - Appropriate antibiotic treatment reduces duration of diarrhea by 50% and fecal shedding by 1 day.
  - Antimicrobial therapy considered in moderately to severely ill children.
  - Recommended antibiotic
    - Azithromycin 20 mg/kg, single dose
    - Doxycycline 4.4 mg/kg, single dose (>8 years of age)
- Prolonged diarrhea owing to protozoa
  - *Giardia duodenalis*[55]
    - Treatment warranted in prolonged diarrhea course (>1–2 weeks).
    - Symptoms may reoccur following treatment with variety of causes.
      - Reinfection/recurrence
      - Post-*Giardia* irritable bowel
      - Residual lactose intolerance
    - Immunocompromised children are at particular risk (hypogammaglobulinemia, lymphoproliferative disease, HIV).
      - May require prolonged courses for refractory disease.
    - Treatment of asymptomatic carriers is controversial but recommended in the United States and other areas of low prevalence.
    - Recommend antimicrobial
      - Metronidazole 5 mg/kg/dose 3 times a day × 5 to 7 days orally
      - Nitazoxanide (children >1 years)
        - 1 to 3 years: 100 mg twice a day × 3 days orally
        - 4 to 11 years: 200 mg twice a day × 3 days orally
        - ≥12 years: 500 mg twice a day × 3 days orally
      - Tinidazole (≥3 years): 50 mg/kg (maximum: 2 g) orally × 1 dose
  - *Entamoeba histolytica*[56]
    - Progressive involvement can result in toxic megacolon, fulminant colitis, ulceration of colon, and rarely, perforation.
    - Extraintestinal disease may occur (liver abscess, central nervous system, lungs, pericardium).
    - Treatment should be prioritized for all patients given propensity to spread to other contacts and cause invasive infection.
      - Liver abscesses may require aspiration and take months to resolve on therapy.
      - Colectomy may be necessary in toxic megacolon.
    - Recommended antimicrobial
      - Initial regimen (metronidazole or tinidazole)
        - Metronidazole 30 to 50 mg/kg/d divided 3 times per day × 7 to 10 days
        - Tinidazole (≥3 years of age): 50 mg/kg (maximum, 2 g) daily × 3 days
        - Followed by iodoquinol or paromomycin
      - Iodoquinol 30 to 40 mg/kg/d (maximum, 650 mg per dose) divided 3 times per day × 20 days
      - Paromomycin 25 to 35 mg/kg/d divided 3 times per day × 7 days
    - Asymptomatic intestinal colonization treatment (choose 1 option)

- Iodoquinol 30 to 40 mg/kg/d (maximum, 650 mg per dose) divided 3 times per day × 20 days (not available in United States).
- Paromomycin 25 to 35 mg/kg/d divided 3 times per day × 7 days.
- Diloxanide furoate 20 mg/kg/d (maximum, 500 mg per dose) divided 3 times a day × 10 days (not available in United States)

DISCLOSURE

The author has nothing to disclose.

REFERENCES

1. Kean BH. The Diarrhea of Travelers to Mexico. Summary of Five-Year Study. Ann Intern Med 1963;59:605–14.
2. Hill DR, Beeching NJ. Travelers' diarrhea. Curr Opin Infect Dis 2010;23(5):481–7.
3. Fox TG, Manaloor JJ, Christenson JC. Travel-related infections in children. Pediatr Clin North Am 2013;60(2):507–27.
4. Harvey K, Esposito DH, Han P, et al. Surveillance for travel-related disease–GeoSentinel Surveillance System, United States, 1997-2011. MMWR Surveill Summ 2013;62:1–23.
5. Hagmann S, Neugebauer R, Schwartz E, et al. Illness in children after international travel: analysis from the GeoSentinel Surveillance Network. Pediatrics 2010;125(5):e1072–80.
6. Alam NH, Ashraf H. Treatment of infectious diarrhea in children. Paediatr Drugs 2003;5(3):151–65.
7. Ashkenazi S, Schwartz E. Traveler's diarrhea in children: New insights and existing gaps. Travel Med Infect Dis 2020;34:101503.
8. Hagmann S, LaRocque RC, Rao SR, et al. Pre-Travel Health Preparation of Pediatric International Travelers: Analysis From the Global TravEpiNet Consortium. J Pediatr Infect Dis Soc 2013;2(4):327–34.
9. Hagmann S, Benavides V, Neugebauer R, et al. Travel health care for immigrant children visiting friends and relatives abroad: retrospective analysis of a hospital-based travel health service in a US urban underserved area. J Travel Med 2009; 16(6):407–12.
10. Leder K, Tong S, Weld L, et al. Illness in travelers visiting friends and relatives: a review of the GeoSentinel Surveillance Network. Clin Infect Dis 2006;43(9): 1185–93.
11. Soriano-Arandes A, Garcia-Carrasco E, Serre-Delcor N, et al. Travelers' Diarrhea in Children at Risk: An Observational Study From a Spanish Database. Pediatr Infect Dis J 2016;35(4):392–5.
12. Hill DR. Occurrence and self-treatment of diarrhea in a large cohort of Americans traveling to developing countries. Am J Trop Med Hyg 2000;62(5):585–9.
13. Herbinger KH, Drerup L, Alberer M, et al. Spectrum of imported infectious diseases among children and adolescents returning from the tropics and subtropics. J Travel Med 2012;19(3):150–7.
14. Greenwood Z, Black J, Weld L, et al. Gastrointestinal infection among international travelers globally. J Travel Med 2008;15(4):221–8.
15. Steffen R, Hill DR, DuPont HL. Traveler's diarrhea: a clinical review. JAMA 2015; 313(1):71–80.
16. Pitzinger B, Steffen R, Tschopp A. Incidence and clinical features of traveler's diarrhea in infants and children. Pediatr Infect Dis J 1991;10(10):719–23.

17. Duplessis CA, Gutierrez RL, Porter CK. Review: chronic and persistent diarrhea with a focus in the returning traveler. Trop Dis Travel Med Vaccin 2017;3:9.
18. Chong CH, McCaskill ME, Britton PN. Pediatric travelers presenting to an Australian emergency department (2014-2015): A retrospective, cross-sectional analysis. Travel Med Infect Dis 2019;31:101345.
19. Ashkenazi S, Schwartz E, O'Ryan M. Travelers' Diarrhea in Children: What Have We Learnt? Pediatr Infect Dis J 2016;35(6):698–700.
20. Guarino A. Foreword: ESPGHAN/ESPID evidence-based guidelines for the management of acute gastroenteritis in children in Europe. J Pediatr Gastroenterol Nutr 2008;46(Suppl 2):vii–viii.
21. Laaveri T, Vilkman K, Pakkanen SH, et al. A prospective study of travellers' diarrhoea: analysis of pathogen findings by destination in various (sub)tropical regions. Clin Microbiol Infect 2018;24(8):908.e9-16.
22. Mackell S. Traveler's diarrhea in the pediatric population: etiology and impact. Clin Infect Dis 2005;41(Suppl 8):S547–52.
23. McAuliffe GN, Anderson TP, Stevens M, et al. Systematic application of multiplex PCR enhances the detection of bacteria, parasites, and viruses in stool samples. J Infect 2013;67(2):122–9.
24. Pouletty M, De Pontual L, Lopez M, et al. Multiplex PCR reveals a high prevalence of multiple pathogens in traveller's diarrhoea in children. Arch Dis Child 2019; 104(2):141–6.
25. Gorbach SL, Kean BH, Evans DG, et al. Travelers' diarrhea and toxigenic Escherichia coli. N Engl J Med 1975;292(18):933–6.
26. Shah N, DuPont HL, Ramsey DJ. Global etiology of travelers' diarrhea: systematic review from 1973 to the present. Am J Trop Med Hyg 2009;80(4):609–14.
27. Leung AKC, Leung AAM, Wong AHC, et al. Travelers' diarrhea: a clinical review. Recent Pat Inflamm Allergy Drug Discov 2019;13(1):38–48.
28. Cook SM, Glass RI, LeBaron CW, et al. Global seasonality of rotavirus infections. Bull World Health Organ 1990;68(2):171–7.
29. Laaveri T, Antikainen J, Mero S, et al. Bacterial, viral and parasitic pathogens analysed by qPCR: Findings from a prospective study of travellers' diarrhoea. Travel Med Infect Dis 2021;40:101957.
30. Riddle MS, Connor BA, Beeching NJ, et al. Guidelines for the prevention and treatment of travelers' diarrhea: a graded expert panel report. J Travel Med 2017;24(suppl_1):S57–74.
31. Murphy MS. Guidelines for managing acute gastroenteritis based on a systematic review of published research. Arch Dis Child 1998;79(3):279–84.
32. Khin MU, Nyunt Nyunt W, Myo K, et al. Effect on clinical outcome of breast feeding during acute diarrhoea. Br Med J (Clin Res Ed) 1985;290(6468):587–9.
33. Fonseca BK, Holdgate A, Craig JC. Enteral vs intravenous rehydration therapy for children with gastroenteritis: a meta-analysis of randomized controlled trials. Arch Pediatr Adolesc Med 2004;158(5):483–90.
34. American Academy of Pediatrics. Escherichia coli Diarrhea (Including Hemolytic-Uremic Syndrome). In: Red book: 2021–2024 report of the committee on infectious diseases. American Academy of Pediatrics; 2021. p. 322–8.
35. Shane AL, Mody RK, Crump JA, et al. 2017 Infectious Diseases Society of America clinical practice guidelines for the diagnosis and management of infectious diarrhea. Clin Infect Dis 2017;65(12):e45–80.
36. Kantele A, Laaveri T, Mero S, et al. Antimicrobials increase travelers' risk of colonization by extended-spectrum betalactamase-producing Enterobacteriaceae. Clin Infect Dis 2015;60(6):837–46.

37. Kantele A, Mero S, Kirveskari J, et al. Increased Risk for ESBL-Producing Bacteria from Co-administration of Loperamide and Antimicrobial Drugs for Travelers' Diarrhea. Emerg Infect Dis 2016;22(1):117–20.
38. Zhu FH, Rodado MP, Asmar BI, et al. Risk factors for community acquired urinary tract infections caused by extended spectrum beta-lactamase (ESBL) producing Escherichia coli in children: a case control study. Infect Dis (Lond) 2019; 51(11–12):802–9.
39. Donskey CJ. Antibiotic regimens and intestinal colonization with antibiotic-resistant gram-negative bacilli. Clin Infect Dis 2006;43(Suppl 2):S62–9.
40. Hagmann SHF, Christenson JC, Fischer PR, et al. Travelers' diarrhea in children: a blind spot in the expert panel guidelines on prevention and treatment. J Travel Med 2018;25(1).
41. American Academy of Pediatrics. International Travel. In: Red book: 2021–2024 report of the committee on infectious diseases. American Academy of Pediatrics; 2021. p. 99–105.
42. Patel K, Goldman JL. Safety Concerns Surrounding Quinolone Use in Children. J Clin Pharmacol 2016;56(9):1060–75.
43. DuPont HL, Sullivan P, Evans DG, et al. Prevention of traveler's diarrhea (emporiatric enteritis). Prophylactic administration of subsalicylate bismuth). JAMA 1980; 243(3):237–41.
44. Steffen R, DuPont HL, Heusser R, et al. Prevention of traveler's diarrhea by the tablet form of bismuth subsalicylate. Antimicrob Agents Chemother 1986;29(4): 625–7.
45. McFarland LV. Meta-analysis of probiotics for the prevention of traveler's diarrhea. Travel Med Infect Dis 2007;5(2):97–105.
46. Sazawal S, Hiremath G, Dhingra U, et al. Efficacy of probiotics in prevention of acute diarrhoea: a meta-analysis of masked, randomised, placebo-controlled trials. Lancet Infect Dis 2006;6(6):374–82.
47. Cholera vaccines: WHO position paper - August 2017. Wkly Epidemiol Rec 2017; 92(34):477–98.
48. Goldsmid JM, Leggat PA. The returned traveller with diarrhoea. Aust Fam Physician 2007;36(5):322–7.
49. American Academy of Pediatrics. Campylobacter Infections. In: Red book: 2021–2024 report of the committee on infectious diseases. American Academy of Pediatrics; 2021. p. 243–6.
50. Schiaffino F, Colston JM, Paredes-Olortegui M, et al. Antibiotic resistance of campylobacter species in a pediatric cohort study. Antimicrob Agents Chemother 2019;63(2).
51. American Academy of Pediatrics. Salmonella Infections. In: Red book: 2021–2024 report of the committee on infectious diseases. American Academy of Pediatrics; 2021. p. 655–63.
52. American Academy of Pediatrics. Shigella Infections. In: Red book: 2021–2024 report of the committee on infectious diseases. American Academy of Pediatrics; 2021. p. 668–72.
53. Pons MJ, Gomes C, Martinez-Puchol S, et al. Antimicrobial resistance in Shigella spp. causing traveller's diarrhoea (1995-2010): a retrospective analysis. Travel Med Infect Dis 2013;11(5):315–9.
54. American Academy of Pediatrics. Cholera (Vibrio cholerae). In: Red book: 2021–2024 report of the committee on infectious diseases. American Academy of Pediatrics; 2021. p. 843–7.

55. American Academy of Pediatrics. Giardia duodenalis (formerly Giardia lamblia and Giardia intestinalis) Infections (Giardiasis). In: Red book: 2021–2024 report of the committee on infectious diseases. American Academy of Pediatrics; 2021. p. 335–8.
56. American Academy of Pediatrics. Amebiasis. In: Red book: 2021–2024 report of the committee on infectious diseases. American Academy of Pediatrics; 2021. p. 190–3.

Neurocysticercosis in Children

Montida Veeravigrom, MD[a,*], Lunliya Thampratankul, MD[b]

KEYWORDS

• Neurocysticercosis • Pediatric • Seizure • Critical care

KEY POINTS

- Neurocysticercosis is one of the most common acquired causes of new-onset focal seizure in children, especially in endemic areas and among immigrant populations.
- Neurocysticercosis has multiple clinical manifestations depending on the size, number, and location of cysts.
- The initial management should pay attention to managing critical neurologic symptoms including the use of antiepileptic drugs and neurocritical care strategy.

INTRODUCTION

Neurocysticercosis (NCC) is the central nervous system (CNS) infestation caused by the encysted larval stage of *Taenia solium* (pork tapeworm) called cysticercus. NCC is the most common parasitic infection in the CNS worldwide, especially in Southeast Asian, the Indian subcontinent, Latin America, and sub-Saharan Africa.[1] Pediatricians in nonendemic countries including the United States should be aware of this disease in high-risk immigrant children or travelers.[1,2] Recently, NCC has become more common in other countries because of ease of international travel and high migration rate of people from endemic countries.[3] NCC sometimes has a long incubation period of several years and may not be detected at initial screening. NCC in children has a wide spectrum of clinical manifestation from asymptomatic infestation to severe disease. The clinical manifestation depends on the number, size, location, viability of cysts, and host response.[4]

Statement of financial support: This work was not supported by any grants and funding sources.

[a] Section of Child Neurology, Department of Pediatrics, The University of Chicago Biological Sciences, 5841 South Maryland Avenue, Room C-526, MC 3055, Chicago, IL 60637, USA; [b] Department of Pediatrics, Faculty of Medicine Ramathibodi Hospital, Mahidol University, 270 Rama VI Road, Ratchathewi, Bangkok 10400, Thailand
* Corresponding author.
E-mail address: mveeravigrom@uchicago.edu

Pediatr Clin N Am 69 (2022) 115–127
https://doi.org/10.1016/j.pcl.2021.09.005
0031-3955/22/

There are case reports of NCC in infants and toddlers. In these cases, the search for *T solium* carriers in family members and domestic employees is important and mandatory.[5]

LIFE CYCLE OF THE PARASITE

To summarize the *T solium* life cycle, there are three phases including egg, larva, and adult. Humans are the definitive hosts for the adult tapeworm. When humans eat uncooked or undercooked larva-infested pork, this allows the adult tapeworm to form in the intestinal tract, the eggs are then produced and shed in stool, allowing the cycle to complete. The human intestinal infection by adult form is called taeniasis.[4,6] Moreover, pigs and humans are the intermediate host for the larval form (cysticercosis). Eating the eggs leads to development of the larva in the soft tissue of the intermediate host. Ingestion by fecal-oral contamination is the main mechanism through which humans acquire NCC. When *T solium* eggs are ingested, the embryos are released from the eggs in the intestines and actively cross the intestinal mucosa to the bloodstream and lodge as the larva form (cysticerci) in human tissues, predominantly muscle, soft tissues, and the CNS. Most cysts are destroyed by the host's immune response and die within weeks or months. When cysticerci are implanted in the brain or its coverings, this is called NCC.[4,6]

EPIDEMIOLOGY

NCC is the well-recognized parasitic infection in the CNS in children worldwide especially in Southeast Asian, the Indian subcontinent, Latin America, and sub-Saharan Africa.[1] This is particularly true in rural communities where raising pigs is a common practice. In a study in rural northern India, 54.4% of children with first-onset seizure were diagnosed with NCC based on MRI findings.[7] Humans develop NCC after ingestion of *T solium* eggs, which mostly occurs via the fecal-oral route from close contact with a tapeworm carriage.

The dramatic increase in incidence of NCC in nonendemic countries, especially in the United States and European countries, has been caused by travel or immigration and widespread access to neuroimaging.[8] NCC has become an emerging health problem in developed countries and affects poor hygienic communities. The parasite can subsequently transmit from human to human through eggs even with absence of travel to endemic areas.[9]

PATHOGENESIS AND CLASSIFICATION

The cysticerci evolve through four important stages. The first stage is a live or active cyst (vesicular stage) where parasite resides in a clear fluid and can initiate inflammatory response with edema once degenerating. A thin-walled cyst contains the fluid and live larva with a tapeworm head (protoscolex) inside. The parasite escapes the host immune surveillance by secreting a serine proteinase inhibitor, called taenia statin, which inhibits the complement activation, lymphocytic migration, and cytokine formation. The second stage is when the cyst undergoes degenerative changes with wall thickening and transformation of clear fluid to whitish gel (colloidal stage). In the third stage, an inflammatory reaction surrounds and damages the cyst, filling with the caseous material while the larva degenerates and dies (granular stage). Finally, in the fourth stage the degenerated cyst is replaced by fibrotic tissue and becomes calcified (calcified nodular stage). The patient may be asymptomatic for years and the clinical symptoms usually occur during the third stage when the cysticerci degenerate and the inflammatory reaction occurs (**Table 1**).[4,6]

The clinical type described next is established by the location of the parasite in the CNS, which determines its effect toward clinical manifestations. Some patients may have mixed forms of NCC.

1. *Parenchymal NCC:* Parenchymal NCC is the most common type in children. As cysticerci reaches the brain via hematogenous spread, most of them are at gray-white junctions. Initially viable cysts were in brain parenchyma with a clear liquid content. Cysts may survive for many years until the hosts immune response detects the parasite. The cellular immune response disrupts the cysts membrane and its homeostasis leading to increasing density of cyst contents with local inflammation. Then the cyst degenerates into a granulomatous lesion that is later completely clear or replaced by a calcified lesion. Seizures are the most common presenting features. The other manifestations are headache, altered mental status, and focal neurologic deficits.[10]
2. *Intraventricular NCC:* About 20% of NCC in children fall into this category and it is frequently found in conjunction with subarachnoid NCC. Ventricular cysts frequently cause cerebrospinal fluid (CSF) obstruction, hydrocephalus, and increased intracranial pressure. Some of the cysts, those attached to a ventricular wall and not blocking CSF flow, follow evolutive course as parenchymal cysts.[11] Migrating intraventricular NCC is a unique clinical entity and presents with the fluctuation of clinical symptoms caused by mobility of intraventricular cyst and position changes of cyst within the ventricular system. The migrating factors include gravity and CSF pressure.[12]
3. *Subarachnoid NCC (cysticercosis arachnoiditis):* This type is rare in children. However, it is progressive and associated with significant morbidity and mortality.[13,14] Cysts in subarachnoid space tend to grow and expand their membranes forming vesicular clusters like a bunch of grapes (racemus). This type of lesion is known as racemose NCC, which may grow as large cystic masses and involve the neighboring space. The cysts may locate within the basal cisterns, sylvian fissures, and cortical and spinal subarachnoid spaces. The basal cistern NCC is associated with extensive parasitic infestation and marked inflammation. Patients usually present with the symptoms and signs of meningitis and increased intracranial pressure.[15] Headaches, papilledema, optic atrophy, vomiting, coma, and cranial nerve deficits may occur. Basal subarachnoid NCC is associated with spinal involvement in about 60% of the cases.[16]

Table 1
The stages of cysticerci[46]

Stage	Description
1. Vesicular (metacestode)	Viable cyst with clear liquid content, thin semitransparent wall, and an eccentric protoscolex seen as a 4- to 5-mm nodule adjacent to the wall
2. Colloidal	Increased density of cyst content from hyaline degeneration of the larva
3. Granular nodular	The cyst being degenerated into granulomatous lesion
4. Nodular calcified	The degenerated granular tissue being replaced by calcification

4. *Spinal NCC:* Spinal cysticercosis is subdivided into leptomeningeal (subarachnoid) and intramedullary (parenchymal) forms. Leptomeningeal spinal cysts are the most prevalent type of spinal parasitic infestation. Cysticerci reach spinal cord parenchyma or CSF space by hematogenous, ventriculoependymal route, or subarachnoid space, followed by migration into the spinal cord. This is rare and it may cause spinal compression, nerve root pain, or cauda equina syndrome.[17]
5. *Ocular cysticercosis:* The most common location is the subretina, with the clinical presentation of visual disturbance. Other involvements are subconjunctival space, anterior chamber, vitreous, retina, and extraocular muscle.[18,19]

CLINICAL MANIFESTATION

Clinical manifestations can vary from asymptomatic infection to severe diseases, depending on the characteristics of the infection (number, size, location, and stage of cyst lesions) and intensity of host immune response. Seizure is the most common clinical presentation of parenchymal NCC. NCC is a common cause of focal seizure in endemic areas and among immigrants and travelers. Moreover, the symptoms are associated with local mass effects or secondary to inflammatory change in the brain parenchyma and/or subarachnoid space.[21]

Seizure and Epilepsy

Seizure is the most common presentation of intraparenchymal cyst. It often presents as focal seizure but sometimes progresses to generalized tonic-clonic seizure. The semiology of seizure correlates with the anatomic location of the parasite. Children with NCC may present as a single seizure episode or recurrent epilepsy.

Headache and Intracranial Hypertension

Headache is usually secondary to increase in intracranial pressure from extraparenchymal NCC. However, headache may also occur as a postictal manifestation. Increased intracranial pressure develops by diverse mechanisms, such as CSF pathway obstruction (intraventricular cysts), mass effects (large cysts in sylvian fissure or interhemispheric fissure), or arachnoiditis in chronic cases.[11,12]

Meningitis or Encephalitis

This is a rare presentation that occurs more frequently in adolescent female patients and termed "cysticercotic encephalitis."[20] The patient presents with headache and alteration of consciousness, and it may be life-threatening. The symptoms are caused by diffuse immune response to massive cyst infections. Cysticercotic encephalitis should be considered in the differential diagnosis of acute encephalitis especially in endemic areas or with a history of intake of raw pork. Infrequently, fever with nuchal rigidity is the first presentation as acute cysticercal meningitis. CSF eosinophilia assists in differentiation from acute bacterial meningitis.[22,23]

Transverse Myelitis

Cysticercus lesions in the spinal cord can mimic acquired demyelinating syndrome.[24] NCC should be considered in the differential diagnosis of myelopathy in endemic or tropical areas.

Radiculopathy

Cysts in intradural extramedullary space cause the symptoms of radiculitis or radiculopathy, such as numbness, tingling, pain, or weakness in the distribution area of affected nerve.[25]

Mass Effect and Focal Neurologic Deficit

Racemose cysticercosis or large cysts in subarachnoid space can cause mass effect and focal neurologic deficit mimics brain or spinal cord tumor. Symptoms depend on the size and the location of the lesions.

Decrease Visual Acuity, Ptosis, Eye Pain

Ocular cysticercosis is one of the preventable causes of blindness. Clinical presentations were varied depend on the site of involvement, the number and size of cysts, and host immune response. It must be differentiated with other causes of ocular mass.[18]

DIAGNOSIS

The diagnosis of NCC needs a high index of suspicion because the disease has a variety of clinical manifestations (**Box 1**) and can mimic other diseases (**Box 2**).

Diagnosis is a challenge because of nonspecific clinical and neuroimaging findings and suboptimal predictive values in immunodiagnostic tests, particularly in endemic settings. The first diagnostic criteria for NCC were developed in 1996 using objective evaluation of clinical, radiologic, immunologic, and epidemiologic data. An updated version using the same category structure (absolute, major, minor, and epidemiologic) was proposed in 2001. Recent revised diagnostic criteria that are simpler with operational definition and integrate the advancement of diagnosis was published in 2017 (**Box 3**).[26,27]

Neuroimaging

MRI is the most useful neuroimaging of brain and/or spinal cord. MRI provides information regarding the characteristics of the cysts, location, and degree of edema or inflammation. A protoscolex, characterized by a 4- to 5-mm nodule within the cyst, is pathognomonic sign of NCC (**Fig. 1**). MRI is also sensitive for detection of basal arachnoiditis, posterior fossa lesions, and extraparenchymal NCC. The MRI finding of cysticercotic encephalitis called "starry-sky" appearance shows multiple parenchymal cysts with white matter edema.

Box 1
Clinical manifestation of NCC[20]

Seizure and epilepsy

Headache and intracranial hypertension

Encephalitis

Transverse myelitis

Radiculopathy

Mass effect and focal neurologic deficits

Abnormal vision and eye pain

Box 2
Differential diagnosis of NCC

Brain abscess

Brain granulomas (tuberculomas, fungal infections, Langerhans histiocytosis, toxoplasmosis)

Brain tumor (low-grade astrocytoma)

Arachnoid/colloid cysts

Acute bacterial meningitis

Each sequence of MRI is useful for different cysticercus stages. Calcified lesions are better seen in susceptibility-weighted images.[28] Fluid-attenuated inversion recovery and diffusion-weighted image is for visualization of scolex as an internal asymmetric nodule in the cysts ("hole with dot" appearance). Proton magnetic resonance spectroscopy is used for differentiation from tuberculoma. There is the presence of lactate, alanine, lipids, and acetate in cysticercal cyst. Pyruvate is a noninvasive marker of parasitic infection in subarachnoid cyst (racemose cyst). Three-dimensional constructive interference in steady state is helpful for differentiating a cyst lesion from CSF.[29] Subarachnoid cysticercosis is frequently associated with hydrocephalus, widespread arachnoiditis, or mass effects. Racemose form of the NCC is a large, multilobe appearance in the basal CSF cisterns. Intraventricular and cisternal cysts are better visualized on MRI with fluid-attenuated inversion recovery sequences, fast imaging using steady state acquisition sequence, constructive interference in steady state, or balanced fast filled echo protocols.[30–32]

Computed tomography (CT) scan is the imaging of choice in resource-limited countries, because of the availability, less imaging duration, and cost. CT is helpful in detecting intracranial calcification in the nodular calcified stage (**Fig. 2**).[33] Cyst is solitary or multiple and are usually 5 to 20 mm in diameter. It might have a punctate high density within the ring scolex. Intraventricular and cisternal cysts are infrequently visualized on CT because they are isodense with CSF. CT can detect the edema around the cyst, which indicates the inflammatory response to the organism death.[20]

Cerebrospinal Fluid Analysis

CSF shows mild pleocytosis (often lymphocytic, but occasionally eosinophilic profile), decreased glucose, increased protein, and elevated opening pressure. In addition, CSF analysis can help exclude other infectious or malignant diagnoses.[21,22] CSF examination with Wright-Giemsa staining to avoid misdiagnosis of eosinophilia in CSF is needed.[11]

Immunodiagnostic Test

Enzyme-linked immunoelectrotransfer blot assay

Enzyme-linked immunoelectrotransfer blot assay is currently the best documented serologic test to detect antibodies to *T solium*. The sensitivity of antibody detection in the serum is around 98% for patients with two or more live parasites in the nervous system and the sensitivity of antibody detection in the CSF was slightly lower.[34,35] However, the sensitivity is lower (50%–70%) in patients with solitary lesions and with calcified NCC. It should be noted that a positive enzyme-linked immunoelectrotransfer blot assay test indicates exposure to the *T solium* larval antigen and does not necessarily indicate an active disease. Positive antibodies to *T solium* are frequently

Box 3
Revised diagnostic criteria and degrees of diagnostic certainty for neurocysticercosis[26]

Diagnostic Criteria

Absolute criteria

- Histologic demonstration of the parasite from biopsy of a brain or spinal cord lesion.
- Visualization of subretinal cysticercus.
- Conclusive demonstration of a scolex within a cystic lesion on neuroimaging studies.

Neuroimaging criteria

Major neuroimaging criteria

- Cystic lesions without a discernible scolex.
- Enhancing lesions.[a]
- Multilobulated cystic lesions in the subarachnoid space.
- Typical parenchymal brain calcifications.[a]

Confirmative neuroimaging criteria

- Resolution of cystic lesions after cysticidal drug therapy.
- Spontaneous resolution of single small enhancing lesions.[b]
- Migration of ventricular cysts documented on sequential neuroimaging studies.[a]

Minor neuroimaging criteria

- Obstructive hydrocephalus (symmetric or asymmetric) or abnormal enhancement of basal leptomeninges.

Clinical/exposure criteria

Major clinical/exposure

- Detection of specific anticysticercal antibodies or cysticercal antigens by well-standardized immunodiagnostic tests.[a]
- Cysticercosis outside the central nervous system.[a]
- Evidence of a household contact with *T solium* infection.

Minor clinical/exposure

- Clinical manifestations suggestive of neurocysticercosis.[a]
- Individuals coming from or living in an area where cysticercosis is endemic.[a]

Degrees of Diagnostic Certainty

Definitive diagnosis

- One absolute criterion.
- Two major neuroimaging criteria plus any clinical/exposure criteria.
- One major and one confirmative neuroimaging criteria plus any clinical/exposure criteria.
- One major neuroimaging criteria plus two clinical/exposure criteria (including at least one major clinical/exposure criterion), together with the exclusion of other pathologies producing similar neuroimaging findings.

Probable diagnosis

- One major neuroimaging criteria plus any two clinical/exposure criteria.
- One minor neuroimaging criteria plus at least one major clinical/exposure criteria.

[a]Operational definitions. Cystic lesions: rounded, well-defined lesions with liquid contents of signal similar to that of CSF on computed tomography (CT) or MRI. Enhancing lesions: single or multiple, ring- or nodular-enhancing lesions of 10 to 20 mm in diameter, with or without surrounding edema, but not displacing midline structures. Typical parenchymal brain calcifications: single or multiple, solid, and most usually less than 10 mm in diameter. Migration of ventricular cyst: demonstration of a different location of ventricular cystic lesions on sequential CT or MRI. Well-standardized immunodiagnostic tests: so far, antibody detection by enzyme-linked immunoelectrotransfer blot assay using lentil lectin-purified *T solium* antigens, and detection of cysticercal antigens by monoclonal antibody-based enzyme-linked immunosorbent assay. Cysticercosis outside the CNS: demonstration of cysticerci from biopsy of subcutaneous nodules, radiographs, or CT showing cigar-shape calcifications in soft tissues, or visualization of the parasite in the anterior chamber of the eye. Suggestive clinical manifestations: mainly seizures (often starting in individuals aged 20–49 years; the diagnosis of seizures in this context is not excluded if patients are outside of the typical age range), but other manifestations include chronic headaches, focal neurologic deficits, intracranial hypertension, and cognitive decline. Cysticercosis-endemic area: a place where active transmission is documented.

[b]The use of corticosteroids makes this criterion invalid.

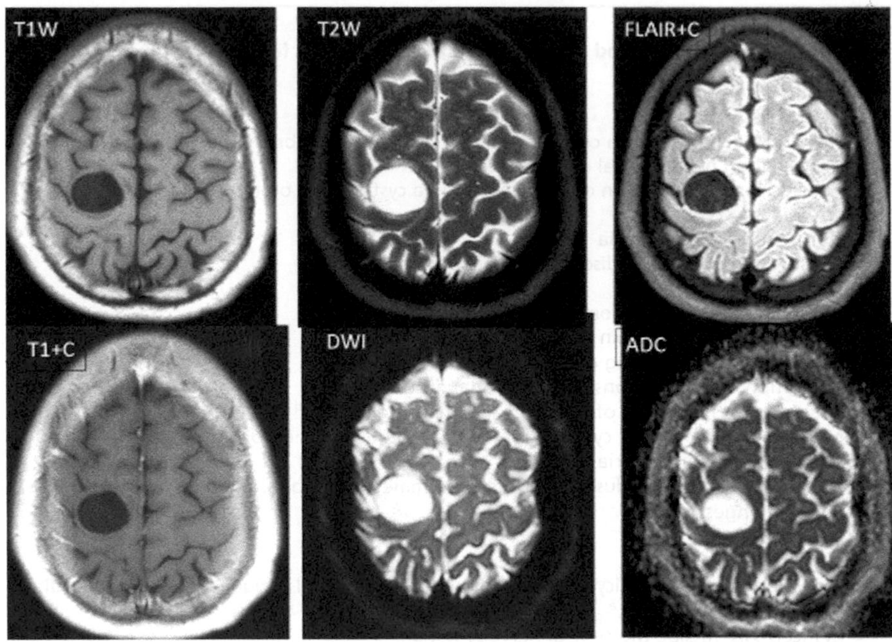

Fig. 1. Axial MRI shows well-defined round lesion with CSF-intensity intraparenchymal lesion at right parietal area with eccentric scolex. No enhancement on postcontrast sequence. DWI, diffusion-weighted imaging; FLAIR, fluid-attenuated inversion recovery; T1W, T1-weighted; T2W, T2-weighted. (Figure courtesy of Professor Anannit Visudtibhan.)

reported in asymptomatic general populations in endemic regions; this might represent asymptomatic, current, or past infection.

Enzyme-linked immunosorbent assay

Detection of antibodies in the CSF by enzyme-linked immunosorbent assay (ELISA) is 89% sensitive and 93% specific in patients with viable NCC infection.[36] ELISA is more reliable in CSF than in serum. ELISA is frequently negative in patients with a few parenchymal cysts and in those with only calcified disease. There might be cross reactivity in serum in patients with other helminthic infections.[37]

In addition, detection of parasitic antigens in serum by ELISA with monoclonal antibodies has been used. The sensitivity of this test in serum for parenchymal NCC is poor and is commonly negative in patients with one or few live cysts. Circulating antigens are almost always present in patients with basal subarachnoid NCC and in most patients with racemose involvement of the subarachnoid spaces. Circulating antigens are present in the serum of patients with viable parasitic tissue, and serum concentrations rapidly decrease after successful antiparasitic treatment. Quantitative serial serum ELISA assays are helpful to determine a response to treatment in subarachnoid NCC.[38,39]

Others

Peripheral eosinophilia may be noted. In addition, concurrent intestinal taeniasis was reported in less than 5%. The greater the infestation of the brain, the greater the chance that the patient also has taeniasis through self-infection, which is detected by a stool examination.

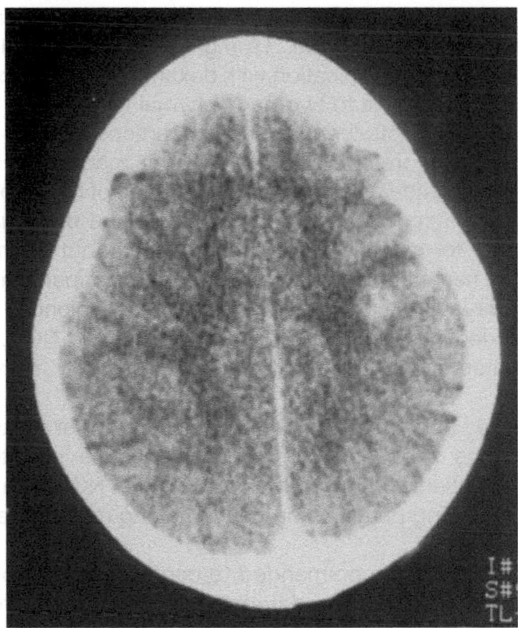

Fig. 2. Contrast-enhanced computed tomography scan shows a single small enhancing lesion with ring enhancement at grey-white junction of left parietal area with perilesional edema. (Figure courtesy of Professor Anannit Visudtibhan.)

MANAGEMENT

Antiparasitic medication for cysticerci has been available since 1978. In the past, there were conflicting results and hypotheses regarding using antiparasitic medication.[40] A well-designed double-blind, placebo-controlled trial in 2004 demonstrated strong evidence supporting antiparasitic treatment to reduce the rate of seizure in cerebral cysticercosis.[41] However, antiparasitic medication is not the key part of the initial management. The initial approach to a patient with NCC should be critical symptom management with antiepileptic drugs and neuroprotective strategy. Steroids might be used in combination with an antiparasitic drug to minimize the inflammatory reaction, vasculitis, or cerebral edema. Other treatments, including acetazolamide or hypertonic solution, should be considered for treatment of intracranial hypertension as appropriate. Surgical removal of large lesions with mass effects and intraventricular cysts causing hydrocephalus might be considered and ventriculoperitoneal shunt insertion is needed for obstructive or severe hydrocephalus. An ophthalmic examination should always precede treatment to exclude intraocular cysts because the inflammatory response after treatment can cause ocular damage and result in blindness. Intraocular cyst is usually treated with surgical treatment.[1]

ANTIPARASITIC TREATMENT

Cyst death after antiparasitic treatment is a result of the medication and the host immune system in response to the release of antigen associated with cell damage after treatment.[41] Albendazole has been shown to be beneficial in a double-blinded, placebo-controlled trial in 2004.[42] Mechanism of action of albendazole is selective binding of the nematode β-tubulin, which prevents the formation of microtubules, which stops cell division. Albendazole, 15 mg/kg/d, in two divided doses per day for 10 to 14 days with food in combination with dexamethasone or prednisolone is recommended for patients with one to two parenchymal NCC cases.[42] A meta-analysis showed that dual treatment of albendazole and corticosteroid is the most effective regimen.[43] Albendazole is preferred as the first-line medication because it is less expensive, with fewer side effects and better penetration of blood-brain barrier.[6] There is recent evidence that a combination of albendazole and praziquantel (50 mg/kg/d) increases the efficacy for multiple cysticercal cysts without an increase in side effects.[44] Worsening of neurologic status may occur after antiparasitic therapy because of host inflammatory response against dying parasites. Prolonged course of antiparasitic therapy is needed in patients with basal subarachnoid NCC. Antiparasitic therapy is contraindicated in ophthalmic lesion and severely increased intracranial pressure.[4]

Some cysts resolve spontaneously with time. Treatment of an asymptomatic case with incidental findings has been controversial because post-treatment seizures have been reported. Patients with inactive parenchymal NCC with evidence of calcified lesions or degenerating parasites on neuroimaging may not require antiparasitic treatment.

Antiepileptic medication is recommended to continue until resolution of the acute lesion. CT or MRI is the useful tool to determine the duration of an antiepileptic drug until its resolution. Around 40% of newly diagnosed NCC patients have seizure recurrence after first seizure. Antiparasitic medication did not influence the recurrence of seizure. The persistence of abnormalities with unchanged number of cyst or persistent cyst with calcification in the follow-up CT scan predicts high risk of recurrence. Long-term antiepileptic drug use is needed in patients who have seizures after the resolution of the cysts or brain edema or calcification of the cyst. The seizure in this category is considered as unprovoked seizure or truly epilepsy.[45]

PROGNOSIS

Epilepsy related to NCC responds well to antiepileptic treatment. The resolution of the lesions is associated with improvement in seizure. Extraparenchymal NCC is associated with higher mortality, mainly because of intracranial hypertension, whereas mortality in parenchymal NCC is associated with epilepsy-related deaths or high burden of the cysts.[4,6]

PREVENTION

NCC is a preventable and eradicative disease. Preventive measures included improvement in sanitation; elimination of intestinal tapeworms; improvement in sewage disposal system; and consumption of properly cooked, clean, vegetables and pork. Taeniasis should be assessed in patients and household members.[6] Health education is certainly critical to increase awareness about burden and impact of the disease among community stakeholders to provide strategies on cross-sectoral collaboration to control and eradicate the disease.[46]

SUMMARY

NCC is a common helminthic CNS infection. The common manifestations are seizures, headache, and focal neurologic deficit. Recent advances in neuroimaging and serology facilitate the accurate diagnosis. Treatment should be individualized based on the location, number of cysticerci, and host response. Antiparasitic treatment is safely used for treatment in combination with other symptomatic management.

DISCLOSURE

There is no potential conflict of interest related to this work.

REFERENCES

1. White AC Jr, Fischer PR. Cysticercosis. In: Kliegman R, Geme JS, editors. Nelson textbook of pediatrics. 21st Edition. Philadelphia: Elsevier; 2019. p. 7539–45.
2. Del Brutto OH, García HH. Neurocysticercosis in nonendemic countries: time for a reappraisal. Neuroepidemiology 2012;39(2):145–6.
3. Garcia HH, Gonzalez AE, Evans CA, et al. Cysticercosis Working Group in Peru. *Taenia solium* cysticercosis. Lancet 2003;362:547–56.
4. de Oliveira RS, Viana DC, Colli BO, et al. Pediatric neurocysticercosis. Childs Nerv Syst 2018;34(10):1957–65.
5. Del Brutto OH. Neurocysticercosis in infants and toddlers: report of seven cases and review of published patients. Pediatr Neurol 2013;48(6):432–5.
6. Singhi P, Saini AG. Pediatric neurocysticercosis. Indian J Pediatr 2019;86(1): 76–82.
7. Mital AK, Choudhary P, Jain RB. Prevalence and risk factors for neurocysticercosis in children with a first-onset seizure in rural North India. Paediatr Int Child Health 2020;40(3):158–65.
8. Serpa JA, White AC Jr. Neurocysticercosis in the United States. Pathog Glob Health 2012;106(5):256–60.
9. Fabiani S, Bruschi F. Neurocysticercosis in Europe: still a public health concern not only for imported cases. Acta Trop 2013;128(1):18–26.
10. Wallin MT, Kurtzke JF. Neurocysticercosis in the United States. Review of an important emerging infection. Neurology 2004;63:1559–64.
11. Kalra V, Mishra D, Suri A, et al. Intraventricular neurocysticercosis. Indian J Pediatr 2009;76(4):420–3.
12. Baro V, Anglani M, Martinolli F, et al. The rolling cyst: migrating intraventricular neurocysticercosis. A case-based update. Childs Nerv Syst 2020;36(4):669–77.
13. DeGiorgio CM, Houston I, Oviedo S, et al. Deaths associated with cysticercosis. Report of three cases and review of the literature. Neurosurg Focus 2002;12:e2.
14. Fleury A, Carrillo-Mezo R, Flisser A, et al. Subarachnoid basal neurocysticercosis: a focus on the most severe form of the disease. Expert Rev Anti Infect Ther 2011; 9:123–33.
15. Lobato RD, Lamas E, Portillo JM, et al. Hydrocephalus in cerebral cysticercosis. Pathogenic and therapeutic considerations. J Neurosurg 1981;55:786–93.
16. Callacondo D, Garcia HH, Gonzales I, et al. High frequency of spinal involvement in patients with basal subarachnoid neurocysticercosis. Neurol 2012;78: 1394–400.
17. Colli BO, Valença MM, Carlotti CG Jr, et al. Spinal cord cysticercosis: neurosurgical aspects. Neurosurg Focus 2002;12(6):e9.
18. Dhiman R, Devi S, Duraipandi K, et al. Cysticercosis of the eye. Int J Ophthalmol 2017;10:1319–24.
19. Kumar V, Surve A, Kumar P, et al. Submacular cysticercosis. Eur J Ophthalmol 2020;30(5):NP58–61.
20. Garcia HH, Nash TE, Del Brutto OH. Clinical symptoms, diagnosis, and treatment of neurocysticercosis. Lancet Neurol 2014;13(12):1202–15.

21. Rangel R, Torres B, Del Bruto O, et al. Cysticercotic encephalitis: a severe form in young females. Am J Trop Med Hyg 1987;36(2):387–92.
22. Mishra D, Sharma S, Gupta S, et al. Acute cysticercal meningitis: missed diagnosis. Indian J Pediatr 2006;73(9):835–7.
23. Visudhiphan P, Chiemchanya S. Acute cysticercal meningitis in children: response to praziquantel. Ann Trop Paediatr 1997;17(1):9–13.
24. O'Mahony J, Shroff M, Banwell B. Mimics and rare presentations of pediatric demyelination. Neuroimaging Clin N Am 2013;23(2):321–36.
25. Pérez-Jacoiste Asín MA, Calleja-Castaño P, Hilario A. Lumbosacral radiculopathy as the clinical presentation of neurocysticercosis. Am J Trop Med Hyg 2020; 102(6):1166–7.
26. Del Brutto OH, Nash TE, White AC Jr, et al. Revised diagnostic criteria for neurocysticercosis. J Neurol Sci 2017;372:202–10.
27. Del Brutto OH. Diagnostic criteria for neurocysticercosis, revisited. Pathog Glob Health 2012;106(5):299–304.
28. Lerner A, Shiroishi MS, Zee CS, et al. Imaging of neurocysticercosis. Neuroimag Clin N Am 2012;22:659–76.
29. do Amaral LL, Ferreira RM, da Rocha AJ, et al. Neurocysticercosis: evaluation with advanced magnetic resonance techniques and atypical forms. Top Magn Reson Imaging 2005;16(2):127–44.
30. Govindappa SS, Narayanan JP, Krishnamoorthy VM, et al. Improved detection of intraventricular cysticercal cysts with the use of three-dimensional constructive interference in steady state MR sequences. AJNR Am J Neuroradiol 2000;21: 679–84.
31. Mont'Alverne Filho FE, Machado Ldos R, Lucato LT, et al. The role of 3D volumetric MR sequences in diagnosing intraventricular neurocysticercosis: preliminary results. Arq Neuropsiquiatr 2011;69:74–8.
32. Neyaz Z, Patwari SS, Paliwal VK. Role of FIESTA and SWAN sequences in diagnosis of intraventricular neurocysticercosis. Neurol India 2012;60:646–7.
33. Nash TE, Del Brutto OH, Butman JA, et al. Calcified neurocysticercosis and epileptogenesis. Neurology 2004;62(11):1934–8.
34. Tsang VC, Brand JA, Boyer AE. An enzyme-linked immunoelectrotransfer blot assay and glycoprotein antigens for diagnosing human cysticercosis (*Taenia solium*). J Infect Dis 1989;159:50–9.
35. Rodriguez S, Dorny P, Tsang VC, et al. Detection of *Taenia solium* antigens and anti-*T. solium* antibodies in paired serum and cerebrospinal fluid samples from patients with intraparenchymal or extraparenchymal neurocysticercosis. J Infect Dis 2009;199:1345–52.
36. Odashima NS, Takayanagui OM, Figueiredo JF. Enzyme linked immunosorbent assay (ELISA) for the detection of IgG, IgM, IgE and IgA against cysticercus cellulosae in cerebrospinal fluid of patients with neurocysticercosis. Arq Neuropsiquiatr 2002;60:400–5.
37. Rodriguez S, Wilkins P, Dorny P. Immunological and molecular diagnosis of cysticercosis. Pathog Glob Health 2012;106:286–98.
38. Zamora H, Castillo Y, Garcia HH, et al. Drop in antigen levels following successful treatment of subarachnoid neurocysticercosis. Am J Trop Med Hyg 2005;73:s41.
39. Fleury A, Garcia E, Hernandez M, et al. Neurocysticercosis: HP10 antigen detection is useful for the follow-up of the severe patients. Plos Negl Trop Dis 2013;7: e2096.
40. Maguire JH. Tapeworms and seizures: treatment and prevention. N Engl J Med 2004;350(3):215–7.

41. Garcia HH, Pretell EJ, Gilman RH, et al. Cysticercosis Working Group in Peru. A trial of antiparasitic treatment to reduce the rate of seizures due to cerebral cysticercosis. N Engl J Med 2004;350(3):249–58.
42. White AC Jr, Coyle CM, Rajshekhar V, et al. Diagnosis and treatment of neurocysticercosis: 2017 Clinical Practice Guidelines by the Infectious Diseases Society of America (IDSA) and the American Society of Tropical Medicine and Hygiene (ASTMH). Clin Infect Dis 2018;66(8):e49–75.
43. Zhao B-C, Jiang H-Y, Ma W-Y, et al. Albendazole and corticosteroids for the treatment of solitary cysticercus granuloma: a network meta-analysis. Plos Negl Trop Dis 2016;10(2):e0004418.
44. Garcia HH, Gonzales I, Lescano AG, et al. Cysticercosis Working Group in Peru. Efficacy of combined antiparasitic therapy with praziquantel and albendazole for neurocysticercosis: a double-blind, randomised controlled trial. Lancet Infect Dis 2014;14(8):687–95.
45. Carpio A, Hauser WA. Prognosis for seizure recurrence in patients with newly diagnosed neurocysticercosis. Neurology 2002;59(11):1730–4.
46. Ngowi HA, Winkler AS, Braae UC, et al. *Taenia solium* taeniosis and cysticercosis literature in Tanzania provides research evidence justification for control: a systematic scoping review. PLoS One 2019;14(6):e0217420.

Important Nematodes in Children

Angela F. Veesenmeyer, MD, MPH

KEYWORDS

• Soil-transmitted helminths • Ascariasis • Trichuriasis • Hookworm

KEY POINTS

- Soil-transmitted helminth infections affect the world's poorest populations.
- Helminth infections disproportionately negatively impact the development and potential of children.
- Progress in the prevention of helminth infections has been stagnant, and the effectiveness of public health measures is controversial.

INTRODUCTION

Intestinal nematode infections caused by soil-transmitted helminths (STH), such as the roundworm *Ascaris lumbricoides*, the whipworm *Trichuris trichiura*, and the hookworms *Ancylostoma duodenale* and *Necator americanus*, infect more than 1 billion people throughout the world. It is estimated that between 4.5 and 39 million disability-adjusted life-years are attributable to STH infections.[1] These infections are considered "neglected tropical diseases" and "neglected infections of poverty," a group of diseases that disproportionately impact those in poverty but are also poverty-promoting chronic and disabling infections. Helminth infections are among the most common diseases of children, particularly those living in extreme poverty in the developing countries of Asia, Africa, and Latin America, although many children in the United States and Europe are also infected (**Table 1**).[2,3] Helminths are not a source of mortality in children but are a major contributor to morbidity. School-aged children tend to harbor the greatest numbers of intestinal worms, and as a result, experience more adverse health consequences.[4] They cause chronic disability that often lasts throughout childhood into adolescence and adulthood. For example, worms can stunt growth, cause intellectual and cognitive deficits, and produce damage to major organs, such as the heart, liver, and brain. These in turn impair childhood educational performance and reduce school attendance, thereby negatively impacting future wage-earning capacity.[4] The Global Burden of Diseases, Injuries, and

Department of Child Health, University of Arizona College of Medicine-Phoenix, Pediatric Infectious Disease, Valleywise Health Medical Center, 2601 East Roosevelt Street, Phoenix, AZ 85008, USA

E-mail address: Angela_veesenmeyer@dmgaz.org

Pediatr Clin N Am 69 (2022) 129–139
https://doi.org/10.1016/j.pcl.2021.08.005

Table 1
Soil-transmitted helminth infections in children

Intestinal Helminth Infections	Species	Estimated Number of Cases, Global	Leading Geographic Area
Ascariasis	*Ascaris lumbricoides*	800 million	South Asia, East Asia
Trichuriasis	*Trichuris trichiura*	450 million	Southeast Asia South Asia
Hookworm	*Necator americanus* *Ancylostoma duodenale*	450 million	South Asia, Southeast Asia

Risk Factors Study 2016 estimates that around 800 million people have ascariasis, whereas approximately 450 million people each have trichuriasis or hookworm infection.[5] It is common for children especially, to have simultaneous infections with 2 or even all 3 of these helminth infections.[6]

Worm intensity, which refers to the average number of worms per individual, seems to be greatest in children and adolescents for reasons that are not well understood. Ascariasis and trichuriasis reach maximum intensities among school-aged children, and hookworm intensity is maximal among older adolescents and those in early adulthood.[7] Because of the increased worm intensity in adolescents and young adults and the propensity of hookworm to cause anemia, women of childbearing age and pregnant women are especially vulnerable to this health threat. In Africa, almost 40 million women of childbearing age are infected with hookworms, thus putting them at risk for severe anemia and their infants at risk for reduced birth weight and higher mortality.[8]

EPIDEMIOLOGY

The human roundworm *A lumbricoides* is one of the most common parasites in the world, with an estimated 800 million, and possibly up to 1.2 billion, people worldwide infected.[2,9] Infections are most commonly documented in sub-Saharan Africa, the Americas, China, and southeast Asia.[9] Studies in host populations find that a range of socioeconomic factors, such as housing, environmental conditions, and cultural practices, such as unhygienic sanitation, influence infection intensity with *Ascaris*.[10] Adults are known to harbor *A lumbricoides* at a lower intensity than children. This may suggest that there is a gradual development of specific immunity over time. However, it is known that hosts with prior infection can also become reinfected.[11]

Hosts contract *Ascaris* infection via the fecal-oral route. Following the ingestion of infective ova, larvae hatch in the small intestine and migrate to the colon. From there, they penetrate the mucosa and migrate to the portal blood to reach the liver and lungs. This hepatotracheal migration takes place over a 10- to 14-day period after the ingestion of eggs.[12] Male and female adult worms measure 15 to 35 cm. Female *Ascaris* daily egg production is around 200,000 eggs, but this decreases with increased worm burden.[12] Eggs can remain viable in soil for years.

T trichiura, the human whipworm, infects an estimated 477 million individuals worldwide, with the highest infection prevalence and intensity in children.[5] Like *Ascaris*, *T trichiura* is transmitted through the fecal-oral route with embryonated eggs ingested via food or hands, which then hatch into larvae in the small intestine. Unlike *Ascaris*, *Trichuris* does not migrate through the lungs. The larvae attach to the intestinal villi and develop into adult worms, which remain in the colon. Female worms lay thousands of eggs daily for several years. The eggs pass in the stool and embryonate in warm, moist soil, where they can survive for months.[7]

The hookworms *A duodenale* and *N americanus* infect an estimated 472 million people globally.[7] In contrast to ascariasis and trichuriasis, hookworm prevalence and infection intensity are highest in adults, although children are commonly infected.[7] *N americanus* is the most widespread hookworm, found across sub-Saharan Africa, the Americas, and Asia. Both species of hookworm can coexist in the same area and within the same individual. Hookworm morbidity is mostly due to anemia. Given the extensive disease burden, morbidity, predilection for young adults, and the economic cost, hookworm is regarded as the most important of all human parasitic infections.[13] Humans acquire hookworm infection when larvae living in the soil or on blades of grass burrow into exposed skin. *A duodenale* larvae can also be transmitted via the oral routes. Upon entering a human host, the larvae travel through the bloodstream to the lungs, burrow into the alveolar spaces, and are coughed up and swallowed by the host. They eventually mature into adults in the host small intestine. Most adult hookworms are eliminated from the host in 1 to 2 years, but *A duodenale* can live in the intestine for up to 7 years, whereas *N americanus* can persist for 4 to 20 years. Hookworms use a cutting apparatus to disrupt capillaries in the intestine and secrete an anticoagulant substance to sustain blood flow, contributing to chronic anemia of infection. Male and female worms mate in the intestines, after which the female worms will produce up to 20,000 eggs per day, which are passed into the host feces. The eggs will hatch in suitable conditions after 24 to 48 hours and continue to develop into mature larvae ready to infect a new human host.[14]

CLINICAL PRESENTATION

Adult *Ascaris* infections can present as acute abdomen, upper gastrointestinal (GI) bleeding, small bowel obstruction, volvulus, and intussusception when worm burdens are severe. Intestinal obstruction most often occurs in the ileum, especially in younger children. They can also enter the common bile duct and cause a blockage leading to cholangitis and pancreatitis, although this is more common in adults.[15] Clinicians should maintain a high degree of suspicion in endemic areas when patients present with surgical abdomens, particularly children. More indolent symptoms include asthenia, lack of appetite, abdominal discomfort, diarrhea, and weight loss.[16]

A lumbricoides, as with all STH, can alter nutrition and intestinal microbiota.[17] Helminth-induced chronic malnutrition may result in growth stunting and decreased physical fitness that may resolve after effective treatment, although some deficits may be permanent.[15] *A lumbricoides* can cause a type 1 hypersensitivity reaction to the larval stages that occurs about 10 to 14 days after infection. This condition, called Loeffler syndrome, is a self-limited disease with transient respiratory symptoms occurring in sensitized hosts during larval migration through the lungs. This follows a mostly benign course and resolves within a period of 2 to 3 weeks. Peripheral eosinophilia may be present during this stage as well. In most worm infections, the host immune system elicits a Th2 response with increased production of cytokines. The increased cytokine release triggers an immune response comprising eosinophils and mast cells in tissue and serum and immunoglobulin E (IgE) antibodies in the serum.[18,19] When the patient is symptomatic with Loeffler syndrome (eosinophilic pneumonia), they may have urticaria, cough, dyspnea, and hemoptysis. In rare instances, a pleural effusion may develop.[20]

T trichiura has a slender anterior allowing it to burrow into the intestinal mucosa, causing petechial lesions, mucosal hemorrhage, and oozing. It can also cause colonic mucosal inflammation seen on endoscopy.[21] Anemia can be severe because of the chronic oozing but not as pronounced as with hookworm. Eosinophilia stimulated by cytokine responses are also typical of trichuriasis.[22] *T trichiura* embeds into the colonic mucosa and causes local inflammation at the point of attachment. This causes colitis, abdominal pain, diarrhea, and decreased nutrient intake. This can become chronic, leading to impaired growth and anemia of chronic disease.[15] Trichuris colitis can lead to a chronic dysentery syndrome that presents as bloody diarrhea, abdominal pain, tenesmus, severe anemia, protein-calorie malnutrition, and cachexia, mimicking inflammatory bowel disease. A heavy worm burden is also associated with rectal prolapse, likely related to straining with defecation and increased peristalsis associated with irritation of colonic nerve endings.[23]

A duodenale and *N americanus* infections are commonly asymptomatic but may cause a type 1 hypersensitivity reaction during pulmonary migration (Loeffler syndrome). As with other helminths, hookworm infection is associated with a Th2 cell-mediated response. Elevated IgE and eosinophilia are common but, unlike other helminth infections, repeated exposure does not seem to stimulate immunity to reinfection.[24,25] Once in the small intestine, adult worms burrow their teeth into the mucosa, causing blood loss, leading to anemia. In fact, hookworm infection is a major cause of anemia globally, particularly for children and pregnant women.[8,26] Following penetration by a hookworm, a local pruritic, papular rash called "ground itch" may develop. Ground itch appears most frequently on the hands and feet, although the entire body surface is susceptible. Within 10 days of penetration of the skin, larvae migrate to the lungs, causing cough, sore throat, and in some cases pneumonitis. The larvae leave the lungs and enter the GI tract. Infection with *A duodenale* can rarely occur by the oral route and cause a syndrome known as Wakana disease, characterized by nausea, vomiting, pharyngeal irritation, cough, dyspnea, and hoarseness.[27] The most devastating effect of hookworm infection is intestinal blood loss and anemia. The term "hookworm disease" refers primarily to the iron-deficiency anemia that results from moderate to heavy worm burden. The worms not only puncture the mucosa using their cutting apparatus but also secrete hydrolytic enzymes and anticlotting agents to ensure continuous blood flow.[26] Iron-deficiency anemia and hypoalbuminemia develop when blood loss exceeds the intake and reserves of host iron and protein. *A duodenale* causes greater blood loss than does infection with *N americanus*.[28] Most of the physical signs of chronic hookworm infection reflect the presence of anemia. Other than anemia, the most common laboratory finding is eosinophilia. A moderate or heavy hookworm burden results in recurrent epigastric pain, nausea, exertional dyspnea, pain in the lower extremities, palpitations, joint and sternal pain, headache, and fatigue. In children, the presence of chronic anemia and hypoproteinemia leads to slowing of physical growth, becoming most apparent at puberty.[26] Evidence suggests that hookworm infection has adverse impacts on memory, reasoning ability, and reading comprehension in childhood.[29]

DIAGNOSIS

Diagnosis of the STH requires a basic knowledge of the parasites' geographic distributions and an understanding of the various clinical presentations of disease. Most visitors who return from endemic areas typically present with low worm burden infections. Individuals living in endemic areas, and those who emigrate from those areas, are more likely to present with high worm burdens because of repeated exposure and chronic infections. The most widely used and gold-standard diagnostic method for *A lumbricoides*, hookworm, and *T trichiura* is microscopy for direct egg detection in the stool. The Kato-Katz technique, whereby a thick smear of a defined volume of stool (41.7 mg) is stained and cleared with a malachite green or methylene blue and glycerol-soaked cellophane coverslip, is the most widely used technique. The eggs are enumerated under a microscope by a laboratory technician. This method is particularly useful in resource-limited settings for the quantitative diagnosis of worms when intensity of infection measurement is desired.[1,15,30,31] The flotation translation and centrifugation (FLOTAC) technique is a newer microscopic detection technique of helminth eggs in host samples. The FLOTAC technique uses the ability of the parasitic elements, such as eggs, to gather in the apical portion of a flotation column and can then be cut to view under a microscope. This allows parasitic elements to be separated from fecal debris and eggs to be enumerated more readily. A single FLOTAC examination is usually able to analyze 1 g of stool, a 24-fold higher amount of stool than the Kato-Katz technique, making FLOTAC more sensitive for diagnosis of an STH infection.[30] Unfortunately, FLOTAC requires more expensive laboratory equipment, including a centrifuge and specific flotation solutions to facilitate separation of parasitic elements.

Because of limitations of sensitivity of microscopy, polymerase chain reaction (PCR) -based assays for STH infections are becoming widely available.[31,32] PCR has been shown to be more sensitive than microscopy for detection of *A lumbricoides, T trichiura*, and *A duodenale*.[33] PCR-based techniques require high costs for equipment, reagents, and training. However, the advantages, other than increased sensitivity, include the ability to detect multiple coexisting pathogens, distinguishing among multiple STH species, and allowing for the detection of mutation in genes that has been implicated in helminth resistance to available therapies.[34,35]

Diagnosis of *A lumbricoides* requires the identification of parasite eggs, larvae, or adult worms. In Loeffler syndrome, examination of sputum, bronchoalveolar lavage, or gastric aspirate might reveal filariform larvae. Eosinophilia and increased IgE are associated with acute larval infections but are nonspecific.[36] Although *A lumbricoides* eggs can be detected under light microscopy of stool samples, egg enumeration techniques are limited by variability and uneven distribution of eggs in stool, which might provide false negative results, especially in low-intensity infections and infections in nonendemic regions. In visitors returning from endemic areas, eggs may not appear in appreciable quantities in the stool for several months.[37,38] In patients with an acute abdomen, although plain films might identify *Ascaris* or signs of obstruction (air-fluid levels, dilated loops of bowel), ultrasound remains the diagnostic tool of choice for hepatobiliary and pancreatic ascariasis. Upper endoscopy might identify duodenal *Ascaris*, and endoscopic retrograde cholangiopancreatography (ERCP) can be used to remove worms from ducts and duodenum.[16] Stool microscopy using the above techniques is sufficient for detecting *T trichiura.* Patients may also have accompanying iron-deficiency anemia.[38] Stool microscopy is also the mainstay of diagnosis for *A duodenale* and *N americanus* with similar sensitivity as for *A lumbricoides*. As with any hookworm infection, it is important to determine the severity of anemia, particularly in children and women of child-bearing age.

THERAPEUTIC OPTIONS

In nonendemic countries, such as the United States and Europe, children with helminth infections are generally treated after establishing a specific diagnosis based on symptoms and diagnostic testing (**Table 2**). For *A lumbricoides*, albendazole 400 mg or mebendazole 500 mg in a single oral dose, mebendazole 100 mg twice daily for 3 days, or ivermectin 200 μg/kg orally once is recommended for patients older than

Table 2
Medications recommended for treatment of soil-transmitted helminth infection in children

Disease	First-Line Medications
Ascariasis	Albendazole 400 mg po once OR Mebendazole 100 mg po bid × 3 d OR Mebendazole 500 mg po once
Trichuriasis	Albendazole 400 mg po × 3–7 d OR Mebendazole 100 mg po × 3–7 d
Hookworm	Albendazole 400 mg po once OR Mebendazole 100 mg po × 3 d

12 months of age with uncomplicated infections.[39] Alternatively, pyrantel pamoate or nitazoxanide can be used. Albendazole may be slightly more efficacious than mebendazole, but both show a fecal egg count reduction rate of greater than 95% after a single dose.[40,41] In addition, albendazole is metabolized after absorption and can distribute widely in human tissues, making it a drug of choice for the larval helminth infections (toxocariasis, cysticercosis) as well as for the intestinal helminth infections if more than 1 infection is suspected.[3] Both albendazole and mebendazole can cause transient abdominal pain, nausea, or diarrhea in children who are infected with large numbers of worms.[3] Patients with intestinal obstruction can be managed with conservative measures, such as nasogastric suction and intravenous fluids, in addition to antihelminthics once bowel motility is restored. In uncomplicated small bowel obstruction owing to heavy worm burden, orally administered contrast or mineral oil can be used to relax a bolus of worms and may expel worms more rapidly than does conservative management alone.[39] In extreme cases, laparotomy may be necessary to surgically remove worms and accompanying gangrenous tissue. ERCP has also been used to remove worms from the biliary tree. The effectiveness of treatment should be evaluated in cases requiring surgery or with high worm burden with up to 3 stool samples examined 2 weeks after treatment. Relevant imaging, such as ultrasonography, should also be considered during follow-up when appropriate.

In contrast to ascariasis, both benzimidazoles (albendazole, mebendazole) show low efficacy against *T trichiura*. Current recommended therapies are albendazole 400 mg orally for 3 days, mebendazole 100 mg orally twice daily for 3 days, or ivermectin 200 μg/kg/d orally for 3 days. Single albendazole and mebendazole treatments have limited efficacy, especially with high worm burdens, with cure rates of 28% and 36%, respectively.[42] A recent meta-analysis found pooled cure rates for albendazole and mebendazole of 30% and 42%, respectively.[41] The rate of egg reduction was significantly higher for mebendazole (66%) than albendazole (49%).[41] More worrisome, over a 20-year period from 1995 to 2015, there was a significant decrease in cure rates for albendazole from 38.6% to 16.4% and in egg reduction rates for albendazole from 72.6% to 43.4% and mebendazole from 91.4% to 54.7%.[41] These findings illustrate the urgent need for new drugs with higher efficacy against *T trichiura*, especially for preventive chemotherapy programs. A randomized controlled trial investigated various combination therapies for trichuriasis in children and found the highest efficacy for albendazole and oxantel pamoate (68.5%). Most common side effects were abdominal cramps in 18% of patients and headaches reported by 10% of patients.[43] A current phase 3 trial is investigating the efficacy and safety of coadministered albendazole and ivermectin in children and adults with infected with *T trichiura*.[44] Because of the incomplete effectiveness of drugs for *T trichiura*, treatment outcome should be monitored at suggested intervals of 3 weeks, 3 months, and 12 months after therapy is completed.[44,45] In addition to supportive therapy for patients with dysentery, iron supplementation should be considered in patients with severe or symptomatic anemia.

For the hookworms, *A duodenale* and *N americanus*, treatment with albendazole 400 mg orally once or mebendazole 100 mg orally twice daily for 3 days or 500 mg orally once is recommended. Pyrantel pamoate 11 mg/kg (up to a maximum of 1 g) orally once daily for 3 days can also be effective.[39] These are generally safe in children younger than 2 years, but the World Health Organization (WHO) recommends a half dose of albendazole for this age group.[46] Efficacy of albendazole single dose is significantly more efficacious against hookworm when compared with mebendazole single dose (96% vs 79%).[40] This finding is consistent with the findings of a meta-analysis comparing albendazole and mebendazole.[41] However, a 3-dose regimen of mebendazole (100 mg once daily for 3 days) is superior to a single dose (500 mg once).[47] Although the multiple-dose regimen is more complex, when feasible, it is preferable to use the 3-dose regimen when in hookworm endemic areas. Tribendimidine, a broad-spectrum antihelminthic developed in China and approved for use in children, has a different mechanism of action than the benzimidazole drugs, albendazole and mebendazole.[45] Tribendimidine has shown an egg reduction rate of around 90% at a dose of 400 mg and is well tolerated.[47] Tribendimidine is not currently approved for use in the United States by the Food and Drug Administration.

In endemic countries, one of the mainstays of STH control is organized programs of mass drug administration. Mass drug administration with a single annual dose of either albendazole or mebendazole, together with praziquantel, has become standard practice over the past 20 years. The WHO recommends annual or biannual preventive chemotherapy (deworming) for all children 1 to 12 years of age living in areas where the baseline prevalence of any STH infection is 20% or more among children. Biannual administration is encouraged in areas where the baseline prevalence is more than 50%.[46] Preventive chemotherapy bypasses the need to have trained microscopists for diagnosis or medical personnel for administration of the medicines. Because the antihelminthics have an excellent safety profile, they can be administered by schoolteachers or community health workers.[7] Both mebendazole and albendazole are currently donated free of charge for mass drug administration of at-risk school-aged children. Drugs are often coadministered with vitamin A during child health drug distribution days.[48] Periodic mass drug administration with single doses reduces infection intensity and prevalence. However, as discussed previously, single doses of albendazole and mebendazole are often inadequate for those with heavy worm burdens of *T trichiura* or hookworms. A recent Cochrane review found that in studies published over the last 20 years, there was little impact of regular deworming programs on the height, weight, cognitive performance, hemoglobin, and mortality of children, whether they were given a single dose or multiple doses of antihelminthics.[49,50]

Because of the past success of mass deworming efforts and the known health benefits of treating STH infections, mass drug administration for children is still recommended by most experts.

PREVENTION

Prevention efforts have focused on increased access to improved water, sanitation, and hygiene (WASH) infrastructure and services. However, many people lack access to these basic WASH services with many lacking adequate sanitation services, lacking clean water, and practicing open defecation. The success of WASH efforts varies with the level of the intervention, the prevalent species of worm, and the underlying intensity of helminth infection.[51]

Hookworm infection also can be prevented by reducing skin contact with infected soil by wearing closed shoes or gloves.

Effective vaccines against the STH are unlikely to be available for large-scale use soon, although there are vaccines in development for hookworm and a pan-helminthic (targeting *Ascaris*, *Trichuris*, and hookworms) vaccine.[4,5]

SUMMARY

Infections with the STH *A lumbricoides*, *A duodenale*, *N americanus*, and *T trichiura* impact populations whereby access to WASH is poor. Children are disproportionately impacted because of the negative effect of long-term infection on future development and productivity. Clinicians should be aware of the presentation of helminthiasis in children from endemic areas and should have a general idea of diagnostic and treatment strategies. Eradication of STH as a public health problem requires a global effort to provide all individuals access to improved WASH facilities.

CLINICS CARE POINTS

- Soil-transmitted helminth infections are considered "neglected tropical diseases" or "neglected infections of poverty."
- The most common soil-transmitted helminth infections are ascariasis, trichuriasis, and hookworms.
- Children and adolescents are at high risk for acquiring large worm burdens (high-intensity infections).
- Helminth infections can cause stunted growth, anemia, and poor cognitive function in children.
- Preventive chemotherapy (mass deworming) is standard practice in many endemic areas, but recent studies have found questionable benefit of this practice.

DISCLOSURE

The author has nothing to disclose.

REFERENCES

1. Knopp S, Steinmann P, Keiser J, et al. Nematode infections. Soil-transmitted helminths and trichinella. Infect Dis Clin North Am 2012;26(2):341–58.
2. Pullan RL, Smith JL, Jasrasaria R, et al. Global numbers of infection and disease burden of soil transmitted helminth infections in 2010. Parasites and Vectors 2014;7(1). https://doi.org/10.1186/1756-3305-7-37.
3. Weatherhead JE, Hotez PJ. Worm infections in children. Pediatr Rev 2015;36(8): 341–54. Available at: http://pedsinreview.aappublications.org/.
4. Hotez PJ, Brindley PJ, Bethony JM, et al. Helminth infections: the great neglected tropical diseases. J Clin Invest 2008;118(4):1311–21.
5. Vos T, Abajobir AA, Abate KH, et al. Global, regional, and national incidence, prevalence, and years lived with disability for 328 diseases and injuries for 195

countries, 1990–2016: a systematic analysis for the Global Burden of Disease Study 2016. Lancet 2017;390(10100):1211–59.
6. McCarty TR, Turkeltaub JA, Hotez PJ. Global progress towards eliminating gastrointestinal helminth infections. Curr Opin Gastroenterol 2014;30(1):18–24.
7. Jourdan PM, Lamberton PHL, Fenwick A, et al. Soil-transmitted helminth infections. Lancet 2018;391(10117):252–65.
8. Brooker S, Hotez PJ, Bundy DAP. Hookworm-related anaemia among pregnant women: a systematic review. PLoS Negl Trop Dis 2008;2(9). https://doi.org/10.1371/journal.pntd.0000291.
9. Centers for Disease Control. 2021. Available at: cdc.gov/parasites/ascariasis. Accessed June 10, 2021.
10. Haswell-Elkins M, Elkins D, Anderson RM. The influence of individual, social group and household factors on the distribution of *Ascaris lumbricoides* within a community and implications for control strategies. Parasitology 1989;98(1). https://doi.org/10.1017/S003118200005976X.
11. Bundy D. Population ecology of intestinal helminth infections in human communities. Philos Trans R Soc Lond B Biol Sci 1988;321(1207). https://doi.org/10.1098/rstb.1988.0100.
12. Dold C, Holland C v. Ascaris and ascariasis. Microbes Infect 2011;13(7):632–7.
13. Hotez P. Forgotten people, forgotten diseases. 2nd edition. Washington, DC: ASM Press; 2013.
14. Haldeman MS, Nolan MS, Ng'habi KRN. Human hookworm infection: is effective control possible? A review of hookworm control efforts and future directions. Acta Tropica 2020;201. https://doi.org/10.1016/j.actatropica.2019.105214.
15. Bethony J, Brooker S, Albonico M, et al. Soil-transmitted helminth infections: ascariasis, trichuriasis, and hookworm. Lancet 2006;367(9521). https://doi.org/10.1016/S0140-6736(06)68653-4.
16. Khuroo MS. Ascariasis. Gastroenterol Clin North Am 1996;25(3). https://doi.org/10.1016/S0889-8553(05)70263-6.
17. Strunz EC, Suchdev PS, Addiss DG. Soil-transmitted helminthiasis and vitamin A deficiency: two problems, one policy. Trends Parasitol 2016;32(1). https://doi.org/10.1016/j.pt.2015.11.007.
18. MacDonald AS, Araujo MI, Pearce EJ. Immunology of parasitic helminth infections. Infect Immun 2002;70(2). https://doi.org/10.1128/IAI.70.2.427-433.2002.
19. Klion AD, Nutman TB. The role of eosinophils in host defense against helminth parasites. J Allergy Clin Immunol 2004;113(1). https://doi.org/10.1016/j.jaci.2003.10.050.
20. Lal C, Huggins JT, Sahn SA. Parasitic diseases of the pleura. Am J Med Sci 2013;345(5). https://doi.org/10.1097/MAJ.0b013e318266e984.
21. Khuroo MS, Khuroo MS, Khuroo NS. Trichuris dysentery syndrome: a common cause of chronic iron deficiency anemia in adults in an endemic area (with videos). Gastrointest Endosc 2010;71(1). https://doi.org/10.1016/j.gie.2009.08.002.
22. Wright VJ, Ame SM, Haji HS, et al. Early exposure of infants to GI nematodes induces Th2 dominant immune responses which are unaffected by periodic anthelminthic treatment. PLoS Negl Trop Dis 2009;3(5). https://doi.org/10.1371/journal.pntd.0000433.
23. Stephenson LS, Holland CV, Cooper ES. The public health significance of *Trichuris trichiura*. Parasitology 2000;121(S1). https://doi.org/10.1017/S0031182000006867.

24. Loukas A, Constant SL, Bethony JM. Immunobiology of hookworm infection. FEMS Immunol Med Microbiol 2005;43(2). https://doi.org/10.1016/j.femsim.2004.11.006.
25. Geiger SM, Caldas IR, McGlone BE, et al. Stage-specific immune responses in human Necator americanus infection. Parasite Immunol 2007;29(7). https://doi.org/10.1111/j.1365-3024.2007.00950.x.
26. Hotez PJ, Brooker S, Bethony JM, et al. Hookworm infection. N Engl J Med 2004; 351(8). https://doi.org/10.1056/NEJMra032492.
27. Schad GA, Nutman TB, Poindexter RW, et al. The clinical and immunologic responses of normal human volunteers to low dose hookworm (Necator americanus) infection. Am J Trop Med Hyg 1987;37(1). https://doi.org/10.4269/ajtmh.1987.37.126.
28. Albonico M. Epidemiological evidence for a differential effect of hookworm species, Ancylostoma duodenale or Necator americanus, on iron status of children. Int J Epidemiol 1998;27(3). https://doi.org/10.1093/ije/27.3.530.
29. Sakti H, Nokes C, Hertanto W, et al. Evidence for an association between hookworm infection and cognitive function in Indonesian school children. Trop Med Int Health 1999;4(5). https://doi.org/10.1046/j.1365-3156.1999.00410.x.
30. Glinz D, Silué KD, Knopp S, et al. Comparing diagnostic accuracy of Kato-Katz, Koga Agar plate, ether-concentration, and FLOTAC for Schistosoma mansoni and soil-transmitted helminths. PLoS Negl Trop Dis 2010;4(7). https://doi.org/10.1371/journal.pntd.0000754.
31. Knopp S, Salim N, Schindler T, et al. Diagnostic accuracy of Kato-Katz, FLOTAC, Baermann, and PCR methods for the detection of light-intensity hookworm and Strongyloides stercoralis infections in Tanzania. Am J Trop Med Hyg 2014; 90(3). https://doi.org/10.4269/ajtmh.13-0268.
32. Mejia R, Vicuña Y, Vaca M, et al. A novel, multi-parallel, real-time polymerase chain reaction approach for eight gastrointestinal parasites provides improved diagnostic capabilities to resource-limited at-risk populations. Am J Trop Med Hyg 2013;88(6). https://doi.org/10.4269/ajtmh.12-0726.
33. Cools P, Vlaminck J, Albonico M, et al. Diagnostic performance of a single and duplicate Kato-Katz, Mini-FLOTAC, FECPAKG2 and qPCR for the detection and quantification of soil-transmitted helminths in three endemic countries. PLoS Negl Trop Dis 2019;13(8). https://doi.org/10.1371/journal.pntd.0007446.
34. Diawara A, Drake LJ, Suswillo RR, et al. Assays to detect β-tubulin codon 200 polymorphism in Trichuris trichiura and Ascaris lumbricoides. PLoS Negl Trop Dis 2009;3(3). https://doi.org/10.1371/journal.pntd.0000397.
35. Diawara A, Halpenny CM, Churcher TS, et al. Association between response to albendazole treatment and β-tubulin genotype frequencies in soil-transmitted helminths. PLoS Negl Trop Dis 2013;7(5). https://doi.org/10.1371/journal.pntd.0002247.
36. Akuthota P, Weller PF. Eosinophilic pneumonias. Clin Microbiol Rev 2012;25(4). https://doi.org/10.1128/CMR.00025-12.
37. Nikolay B, Brooker SJ, Pullan RL. Sensitivity of diagnostic tests for human soil-transmitted helminth infections: a meta-analysis in the absence of a true gold standard. Int J Parasitol 2014;44(11). https://doi.org/10.1016/j.ijpara.2014.05.009.
38. Speich B, Ali SM, Ame SM, et al. Quality control in the diagnosis of Trichuris trichiura and Ascaris lumbricoides using the Kato-Katz technique: experience from three randomised controlled trials. Parasites Vectors 2015;8(1). https://doi.org/10.1186/s13071-015-0702-z.

39. Committee on Infectious Diseases AA of P. RedBook. 31st ed. (Kimberlin D, ed.).; Itasca, IL: American Academy of Pediatrics; 2018.
40. Levecke B, Montresor A, Albonico M, et al. Assessment of anthelmintic efficacy of mebendazole in school children in six countries where soil-transmitted helminths are endemic. PLoS Negl Trop Dis 2014;8(10). https://doi.org/10.1371/journal.pntd.0003204.
41. Moser W, Schindler C, Keiser J. Efficacy of recommended drugs against soil transmitted helminths: systematic review and network meta-analysis. BMJ (Online) 2017;358. https://doi.org/10.1136/bmj.j4307.
42. Keiser J, Utzinger J. Efficacy of current drugs against soil-transmitted helminth infections. JAMA 2008;299(16). https://doi.org/10.1001/jama.299.16.1937.
43. Speich B, Ali SM, Ame SM, et al. Efficacy and safety of albendazole plus ivermectin, albendazole plus mebendazole, albendazole plus oxantel pamoate, and mebendazole alone against Trichuris trichiura and concomitant soil-transmitted helminth infections: a four-arm, randomised controlled trial. Lancet Infect Dis 2015;15(3):277–84.
44. Patel C, Hürlimann E, Keller L, et al. Efficacy and safety of ivermectin and albendazole co-administration in school-aged children and adults infected with Trichuris trichiura: study protocol for a multi-country randomized controlled double-blind trial. BMC Infect Dis 2019;19(1). https://doi.org/10.1186/s12879-019-3882-x.
45. Coulibaly JT, Hiroshige N, N'gbesso YK, et al. Efficacy and safety of ascending dosages of tribendimidine against hookworm infections in children: a randomized controlled trial. Clin Infect Dis 2019;69(5):845–52.
46. WHO. Preventive chemotherapy to control soil-transmitted helminth infections in at-risk population groups. Geneva (Switzerland): World Health Organization; 2017. Available at: http://www.who.int/nutrition/publications/guidelines/deworming/en/.
47. Eshetu T, Aemero M, Zeleke AJ. Efficacy of a single dose versus a multiple dose regimen of mebendazole against hookworm infections among school children: a randomized open-label trial. BMC Infect Dis 2020;20(1). https://doi.org/10.1186/s12879-020-05097-1.
48. Kumapley RS, Kupka R, Dalmiya N. The role of child health days in the attainment of global deworming coverage targets among preschool-age children. PLoS Negl Trop Dis 2015;9(11). https://doi.org/10.1371/journal.pntd.0004206.
49. Taylor-Robinson DC, Maayan N, Donegan S, et al. Public health deworming programmes for soil-transmitted helminths in children living in endemic areas. Cochrane Database Syst Rev 2019. https://doi.org/10.1002/14651858.cd000371.pub7.
50. Taylor-Robinson DC, Maayan N, Soares-Weiser K, et al. Deworming drugs for soil-transmitted intestinal worms in children: effects on nutritional indicators, haemoglobin, and school performance. Cochrane Database Syst Rev 2015;2015(7). https://doi.org/10.1002/14651858.CD000371.pub6.
51. Vaz Nery S, Pickering AJ, Abate E, et al. The role of water, sanitation and hygiene interventions in reducing soil-transmitted helminths: interpreting the evidence and identifying next steps. Parasites and Vectors 2019;12(1). https://doi.org/10.1186/s13071-019-3532-6.

Multidrug-Resistant Infections in the Developing World

Prachi Singh, DO*, Jenna Holmen, MD, MPH

KEYWORDS

• LMIC • Multidrug resistant • Antimicrobial resistance • AMR
• Global antimicrobial use

KEY POINTS

- There is an emerging concern for increase in antimicrobial resistance globally, with a greater burden in low- and middle-income countries.
- Emergence of antimicrobial resistance is associated with antimicrobial overuse and lack of effective surveillance.
- Antimicrobial stewardship interventions such as close monitoring and surveillance of antimicrobial use at local and national levels can combat antimicrobial resistance.

INTRODUCTION

Antimicrobials are important tools in reducing morbidity and mortality globally. Severe bacterial infections such as pneumonia, meningitis, and sepsis continue to burden South Asia, sub-Saharan Africa, and Latin America.[1,2] Within these regions, 7.6 million deaths were reported in children younger than 5 years in 2010, 64% of which were attributable to infectious diseases.[2] Access to antimicrobials is critical in helping reduce the burden of mortality from infectious diseases. Improved access to penicillin alone reduced mortality from pneumococcal bacteremia from 50% to 80% to 18% to 20%.[3,4] Unfortunately, antimicrobial resistance (AMR) is increasing globally. Resource distribution and wealth per capita are important factors contributing to this increase in AMR.

Low- and middle-income countries (LMICs) as defined by the World Bank (**Table 1**) have a significantly higher burden of infectious disease.[5,6] According to the World Health Organization (WHO)-led Global Antimicrobial Resistance and Use Surveillance System (GLASS), a surveillance system for AMR since 2015, there is a confirmed increase of AMR, especially in LMICs.[7]

Department of Pediatrics, Division of Pediatric Infectious Diseases and Global Health, UCSF Benioff Children's Hospital, Oakland, 747 52nd Street, Oakland, CA 94609, USA
* Corresponding author.
E-mail address: Prachi.singh@ucsf.edu

Pediatr Clin N Am 69 (2022) 141–152
https://doi.org/10.1016/j.pcl.2021.09.003

Table 1
World Bank definitions of countries by resource distribution

GNI per Capita 2020 US Dollar	World Bank Classification
Low-middle income	$1046–$4095
Upper-middle income	$4096–$12,695
High-income	≥$12,696

Abbreviation: GNI, gross national income.
From Worldbank.org, Last accessed August 23, 2021.

DRIVERS FOR ANTIMICROBIAL RESISTANCE

Antimicrobial Consumption

Overuse of antimicrobials is a major factor of AMR; this is a rising challenge in both high-income countries (HICs) and LMICs. Global antibiotic consumption increased by 65% between 2005 and 2015.[5,8] Efforts to mitigate AMR antibiotic consumption in HICs has been effective in slowing antimicrobial consumption in these regions.[9]

In 2019, the WHO developed a framework to categorize antibiotics called AWaRE (Access, Watch, and Reserve).[10] Antibiotics classified in the Access group are considered first- or second-choice antibiotics that maximize therapeutic value and minimize the risk potential for development of resistance. Antibiotics classified in the Watch group are first- or second-choice antibiotics for specific, limited infections that are also more prone to the development of resistance. Antibiotics classified in the Reserve group are those that are considered last resort and are to be reserved for highly specific patient scenarios and warrant close monitoring of their use. Between 2000 and 2015 Watch antibiotics consumption increased by 90%; in contrast, Access antibiotic use increased by 26.2% globally, with a greater increase noted in LMICs.[11]

Evaluation of global antibiotic use by class of antibiotics has noted a sharp increase in the use of broad-spectrum antimicrobials.[12] Carbapenem use increased by 45%, glycopeptide (vancomycin) use increased by 232%, and broad-spectrum penicillin antibiotic use increased by 94% between 2000 and 2010.[9] The increase in broad-spectrum antimicrobial use has been particularly pronounced in LMICs (**Fig. 1**).

Antimicrobial Access

Access to appropriate antimicrobials is critical, especially in LMICs where there is a higher burden of infectious diseases. Many people in LMICs do not have access to essential antimicrobials that can be lifesaving. In addition, in many parts of Africa and Asia antimicrobials are available without prescription or oversight from trained clinicians, thereby encouraging inappropriate use. Pharmacies are often a family-run operation without appropriately trained pharmacists who can guide patients regarding the appropriate use of antimicrobials. The scale of nonprescription-based use of antimicrobials has not been well evaluated in LMICs. Reports suggest that more than 50% of antibiotics used in these countries is secondary to self-prescription.[13] One study evaluated 73 pharmacies across Zambia and noted that 97% of requests for antimicrobials were nonprescribed.[14] A review of 22 studies across the Middle East found the prevalence of self-prescribed antibiotics to be 19% to 82% of total antibiotic consumption there. [15] Another study showed that 55.2% and 45.7% of antibiotics used in Vietnam and Bangladesh, respectively, were self-prescribed.[16]

Lack of Effective Surveillance

One of the greatest challenges in understanding and addressing AMR in LMICs is effective surveillance of resistance and antibiotic consumption. WHO's GLASS was

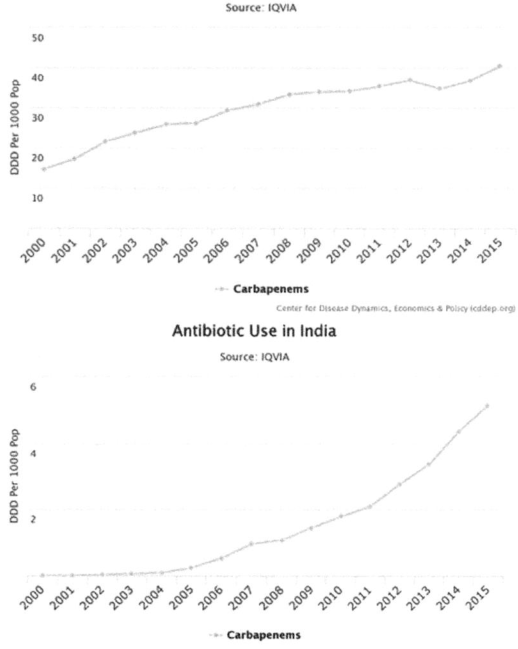

Fig. 1. Antibiotic use trend across high-income country (United States) and LMIC (India) for carbapenems from 2000 to 2015. DDD, daily defined doses. (*From* Center for Disease Dynamic Economics and Policy. Resistance Map. Available at: https:/resistancemap.cddep.org/. Accessed June 18, 2021.)

established in 2015 to address this. As of April 30, 2021, 109 countries are enrolled in GLASS.[7] GLASS provides a standardized method of data collection, analysis, and interpretation; however, intercountry comparisons are not always possible due to inconsistent data from source countries. Diagnostic laboratories in LMICs often lack infrastructure and quality assurance to provide reliable information about the antimicrobial susceptibility of pathogens.[17,18] Environmental factors such as heat and humidity play a significant role maintaining sustainability of laboratory equipment.[17] Other sources of data including pharmacies and academic networks have limited use because of lack of sustainability.[17]

Lack of National Surveillance Programs

Programs such as GLASS have helped establish surveillance programs for LMICs; however, there continues to be a lack of support at government levels. Lack of government oversight allows for many unchecked regulations, including self-prescription of antimicrobials, substandard quality assurance in laboratories analyzing susceptibility data, and suboptimal training of microbiologists as well as health care professionals.[17] In recent years, several countries have made progress through the development of a national action plan for surveillance of AMR. India, for example, developed a national policy for containment of AMR as well as various programs to promote awareness about the appropriate use of antimicrobials.[12,19]

Antibiotic Use in Agriculture and Aquaculture

AMR extends beyond human overuse and consumption. The Centers for Disease Control and Prevention (CDC) and WHO established the One Health initiative to address the linkage between human and animal health. Antibiotics are commonly used in livestock to promote growth, and this overuse drives the selection of antimicrobial-resistant organisms, which can then spread to humans.[20] There is minimal oversight of the use of antimicrobials in animals and agriculture in LMICs. By 2030, the greatest increase in veterinary antibiotic use is predicted to be in 5 LMIC countries: Myanmar, Indonesia, Nigeria, Peru, and Vietnam.[21] A Point prevalence survey collected from LMICs reporting AMR in animals noted a greater than 50% increase in AMR patterns in chickens and pigs from 2000 to 2018.[22] Seafood is also a problem because fish do not effectively metabolize antibiotics and large portion of the antimicrobials are excreted in the environment.[23] There has additionally been an increase in global consumption of seafood.[24] Antimicrobial consumption in aquaculture is driven by the Asia-Pacific region, with China contributing to 57.9% of global aquaculture antimicrobial consumption in 2017.[24] Antimicrobials are used in 70% of aquaculture in Vietnam and Thailand.[25] Approximately 27% of fish and shrimp samples from local markets in Vietnam contained antimicrobial residuals.[23] Resistance to antimicrobials will spread as long as the widespread use of antimicrobials continues in humans and animals. Therefore, reducing antimicrobial use in both animals and humans is critical to reduce the spread of AMR.

MECHANISMS OF ANTIMICROBIAL RESISTANCE

Bacterial pathogens develop resistance to antimicrobials by selective pressure. This process is accelerated by the overuse and misuse of antibiotics. Antibiotics work by several different mechanisms, which include inhibition of cell wall synthesis, cell membrane depolarization, inhibition of protein synthesis, inhibition of nucleic acid synthesis, and inhibition of metabolic pathways.[26] Bacteria can develop resistance to antibiotics either through intrinsic mechanisms or through acquired processes. Intrinsic resistance occurs within bacterial species, and examples include reduced permeability of the outer membrane as well as the production of efflux pumps. Acquired resistance is conferred by transference of genetic material, which can occur either through plasmid transfer from one bacterium to another or through bacteriophage transmission.

There are 6 primary different mechanisms by which bacteria can develop resistance to antibiotics, and these can occur concurrently. These mechanisms include (1) enzymatic inactivation, (2) alteration of antimicrobial binding sites, (3) active efflux, (4) alterations in membrane permeability to prevent antimicrobial entry, (5) alterations in enzymatic pathways, and (6) overproduction of antimicrobial targets.[27]

Multidrug-resistant (MDR) bacteria express more than one mechanism of antibiotic resistance, and one of the most concerning resistance patterns has been the emergence of coproduction of β-lactamases and carbapenemases. β-Lactamases are enzymes produced by bacteria that inactivate β-lactam drugs through hydrolysis of the β-lactam peptide bond; this is the most common mechanism of resistance against penicillins and cephalosporins. Carbapenemases are specialized β-lactamases produced by bacteria that are able to hydrolyze several different β-lactam antibiotics, including carbapenems, through various different mechanisms.

There are several mechanisms of resistance of high concern globally. The ceftriaxone (CTX) family of enzymes is responsible for the worldwide dissemination of extended spectrum beta lactamase (ESBL) organisms.[28] There also has been an alarming spread of *Klebsiella pneumoniae* carbapenemases (KPCs). KPCs are concerning because they can hydrolyze all β-lactams and have been found in multiple gram-negative species, including *Eschersichia coli, Citrobacter, Enterobacter,*

Salmonella, Serratia, and Pseudomonas aeruginosa.[29,30] The New Delhi metallo-β-lactamases-1 (NMD-1), which were first described in a *K pneumoniae* isolate from India in 2008, are also of concern.[31,32] Metallo-β-lactamases use a Zn^{2+} cation for the hydrolysis of the β-lactam ring, making them resistant to clavulanic acid, tazobactam, and sulbactam.[30] NMDs are present mainly in Enterobacteriaceae, and also in nonfermenters and Vibrionaceae.[32]

Bacterial pathogens contain a complex aggregation of genetic material, allowing for the development of resistance to antibiotics. New mechanisms of resistance will evolve with the use of newer antimicrobial agents through selective pressure. The only way to preserve antibiotic efficacy toward bacterial pathogens is to use them judiciously.

BLOODSTREAM INFECTIONS

Bloodstream infections (BSI) carry significant morbidity and mortality in pediatrics and adults.[33,34] WHO's GLASS collects information on key pathogens causing BSI, including *Acinetobacter spp, E coli, K pneumoniae, Salmonella spp, Staphylococcus aureus,* and *Streptococcus pneumoniae*. GLASS has noted a significant difference in resistance patterns across LMICs and HICs.[7] Gram-negative organisms, *E coli* in particular, are the predominant BSI in children.[33] There is a concerning trend toward community-acquired MDR organisms as a cause of BSI.[35] In one prospective cohort study of children in Tanzania, only 20% of community-acquired isolates of Enterobacteriaceae were susceptible to ampicillin, and just two-thirds of isolates were susceptible to gentamicin.[36] A review of blood culture data over a period of 20 years from a large referral center in Malawi noted an overall decrease in the incidence of BSI in children; however, there was an increase in resistance to all first-line empirical antibiotics from 7% to 68% for gram-negative infections in young infants.[37] In Asia, the organisms associated with and resistance patterns of BSI in children vary by region. In a retrospective surveillance study from 2015 through 2018 that included 8365 children in China, gram-positive bacteria accounted for most BSI (70.6%).[38] There was no significant change over time in resistance patterns for gram-positive bacteria; however, for gram-negative infections there was a concerning increase in resistance in *K pneumoniae* with up to 43% of isolates demonstrating resistance to fourth-generation cephalosporins.[38] In a surveillance study across pediatric intensive care units in India, *Salmonella typhi* and non-typhi were the leading causes of BSI. About 90% of *Salmonella* isolates in this study exhibited resistance to the first-line antibiotics ampicillin and cefotaxime.[39]

Acinetobacter spp have been a significant pathogen in health care-associated infections, and the increase of drug resistance in this pathogen has led to significantly limited therapeutic treatment options. Surveillance data on *Acinetobacter spp* in pediatric populations across Asia and Africa are largely missing or combined with adults. GLASS noted high resistance to carbapenems with a median of 64% of *Acinetobacter* isolates exhibiting resistance to meropenem.[7] Across Asia, *Acinetobacter spp* resistance to imipenem/meropenem ranged from 12% in Cambodia to 73% in India.[40]

There are limited data on *S aureus* BSI in pediatrics. One surveillance report from Thailand, including neonates (0–28 days), children (1 month–15 years), and adults, reported a stable incidence rate of methicillin-resistant *S aureus* (MRSA) bacteremia from 2006 through 2014.[41] In a cross-sectional study in Rwanda from 2014, which included children, 50% of blood cultures positive for *S aureus* isolates were methicillin resistant.[42] These reports are particularly concerning because there is evidence that MRSA BSI in HICs has been decreasing.[7]

S pneumoniae, an important pathogen as a cause of BSI and other invasive infections including meningitis, osteomyelitis, and pneumonia in children, has displayed a concerning trend of resistance profiles in children in Asia and Africa. A retrospective study in children across 10 hospitals in China reported that 46.1% of isolates from invasive *Streptococcus* infections to be multidrug resistant.[43] In India, surveillance of invasive pneumococcal disease found 59.7% of isolates to display penicillin resistance and 18% of isolates to display cefotaxime resistance in children younger than 5 years.[44] Finally, a cross-sectional study evaluating BSI in malnourished children in Tanzania found 60% of *S pneumoniae* isolates to be resistant to oxacillin.[45]

Gastrointestinal Infections

Salmonella infections are responsible for a large disease burden worldwide. Most infections secondary to both *S typhi* and non-typhi are reported out of the Indian subcontinent, whereas the disease burden from Africa is less well understood.[46] There is an emerging concern for an increase of MDR *Salmonella* infections globally, and this is of grave concern, because without treatment, mortality from typhoid fever can be as high as 26%.[47] A surveillance study from 2007 through 2009 in rural Ghana revealed 77% of non-typhi *Salmonella* and 65% of *S typhi* isolates to be multidrug resistant, defined as resistant to amoxicillin, cotrimoxazole, and chloramphenicol.[48] More recently, there have been reports of further development of diminished susceptibility to third-generation cephalosporins from Malawi and Kenya.[49–51] A recent systematic review of AMR across India revealed a decrease in overall multidrug-resistant *Salmonella* infections; however, it also found a significant increase in fluroquinolone resistance from 10% (2001–2005) to 66% (2011–2015).[52]

Genital Infections

Gonorrhea

Sexually transmitted diseases also carry a high global burden of disease. In 2016, there were 87 million new cases of gonorrhea worldwide.[53] *Neisseria gonorrhoeae* commonly causes urethritis in men and cervicitis in women and can result in severe sequalae such as infertility.[54] Emergence of AMR in gonorrhea is concerning because it would severely impact the ability to effectively treat this infection. Multiple mechanisms of resistance such as inactivation of drugs, efflux pumps, and reduction of drug influx have all been described in the development of resistance to antimicrobials in gonorrhea. Over the past 70 to 80 years, resistance has been reported to nearly all previously considered first-line antimicrobials including penicillin, first- and second-generation cephalosporins, and tetracyclines.[55] Recently, resistance to the third-generation cephalosporin ceftriaxone has also been reported. The burden of resistance has been reported to be the highest in LMICs.[53] In addition, the burden of disease is higher in sexually active young adults in LMICs when compared with HICs.[56] Treatment based on only clinical signs and symptoms in LMICs as opposed to confirmatory testing has led to widespread overuse of antimicrobials, contributing in part to the emergence of resistance.[57] Because there are challenges in culturing *N gonorrhoeae,* diagnosis is often made based on nucleic acid amplification testing, which does not allow for susceptibility testing, which can exacerbate the problem.

In recent years, however, there has been progress in combating resistance. WHO's Global Gonococcal Surveillance Program (GASP) was established initially in the 1990s and revitalized in 2009.[55,58] GASP strives to increase surveillance by supporting gonococcal cultures and early detection of resistance patterns. A surveillance study done in Côte d'Ivoire, Africa, from 2014 through 2017 revealed 84.9% of isolates to have resistance to tetracyclines, 68.9% resistance to penicillins, and 62.7% resistance to ciprofloxacin; no resistance was reported to ceftriaxone or cefixime.[59] A similar susceptibility pattern was demonstrated from South Africa in a cross-sectional study with high rates of resistance to tetracyclines (74%) and fluroquinolones (78%) and no resistance to ceftriaxone or cefixime.[60] Predominant reports of ceftriaxone-resistant gonorrhea have been from the Western Pacific and East Asian regions.[61] A surveillance study from the Asia Pacific region from 2011 to 2016 reported increasing minimum inhibitory concentrations to ceftriaxone, azithromycin, and ciprofloxacin.[62] Emerging resistance in gonococcal disease in LMICs needs to be closely monitored.

Coronavirus Disease 2019 Pandemic and Antimicrobial Resistance

The coronavirus disease 2019 (COVID-19) pandemic has placed an enormous stress on health care worldwide. Reports of widespread use of antimicrobials during COVID-19 pandemic has only exacerbated the threat of AMR. A meta-analysis of prevalence of bacterial coinfections in patients with COVID-19 reported up to 71.9% of severe acute respiratory syndrome coronavirus 2 (SARS-CoV-2)-infected patients received antibiotics, of whom only 6.9% had a documented bacterial co-infection.[63] The overwhelming burden and stress on the health care system due to the COVID-19 pandemic is thought to have attributed to an outbreak of MDR *K pneumoniae* at a Peruvian hospital.[64] The COVID-19 pandemic has also placed an additional strain on various resources including infection prevention measures, personal protective equipment supply, and divergence of diagnostic technologies from testing for antimicrobial susceptibility, thereby furthering the risk for development of AMR.[65]

WHO issued guidance for the treatment of COVID-19 that discouraged the routine use of antimicrobials.[66] Despite this, a rapid review of national treatment guidelines from 10 African countries revealed the recommended use of a wide range of antibiotics for patients with COVID-19, including recommendations to use azithromycin, vancomycin, and meropenem.[67(p19)] A time-interrupted series from India revealed increased sales in antibiotics during the pandemic, with 216.4 million excess doses.[68] There is also concern for overuse of biocidal agents that would be selective for MDR organisms.[69–71] Last, vaccines have been crucial in reducing the burden of infectious diseases, but the pandemic has caused disruptions in vaccine campaigns.[72]

In summary, the COVID-19 pandemic has led to widespread disruptions in efforts to curb AMR, and there remains a knowledge gap regarding the impact of the pandemic on AMR in LMICs.

Combating Antimicrobial Resistance with Antimicrobial Stewardship

Several studies have demonstrated that antimicrobial stewardship programs (ASPs) lead to a reduction in morbidity and mortality.[73] ASPs have demonstrated cost-effectiveness, which has been even more pronounced in LMICs when compared with HICs.[74] The most effective ASP interventions in LMICs are guideline development, prospective audit feedback, and provider education.[75] In Asia, ASP interventions have demonstrated a 10% reduction in carbapenem use and have led to decreases in overall antimicrobial consumption.[76]

ASPs will be more effective in LMICs at reducing AMR if there is also development of other infrastructure projects to include monitoring surveillance in agriculture and aquaculture, quality assurance of antimicrobials, and development of national plans and support health policies.[58]

DISCLOSURE

The authors have no financial disclosures.

REFERENCES

1. Seale AC, Blencowe H, Zaidi A, et al. Neonatal severe bacterial infection impairment estimates in South Asia, sub-Saharan Africa, and Latin America for 2010. Pediatr Res 2013;74(Suppl 1):73–85.
2. Liu L, Johnson HL, Cousens S, et al. Global, regional, and national causes of child mortality: an updated systematic analysis for 2010 with time trends since 2000. Lancet 2012;379(9832):2151–61.
3. Örtqvist Å, Hedlund J, Kalin M. Streptococcus pneumoniae: epidemiology, risk factors, and clinical features. Semin Respir Crit Care Med 2005;26(06):563–74.
4. Tomasz A. Antibiotic resistance in Streptococcus pneumoniae. Clin Infect Dis 1997;24(Suppl 1):S85–8.
5. Laxminarayan R, Duse A, Wattal C, et al. Antibiotic resistance-the need for global solutions. Lancet Infect Dis 2013;13(12):1057–98.
6. World Bank Country and Lending Groups – World Bank Data Help Desk. Available at: https://datahelpdesk.worldbank.org/knowledgebase/articles/906519-world-bank-country-and-lending-groups. Accessed August 23, 2021.
7. GLASS | Global antimicrobial resistance and use surveillance system (GLASS) report. WHO. Available at: http://www.who.int/glass/resources/publications/early-implementation-report-2020/en/. Accessed June 6, 2021.
8. Klein EY, Van Boeckel TP, Martinez EM, et al. Global increase and geographic convergence in antibiotic consumption between 2000 and 2015. Proc Natl Acad Sci U S A 2018;115(15):E3463–70.
9. The state of the World's antibiotics report in 2021. Center for Disease Dynamics, Economics & Policy (CDDEP); 2021. Available at: https://cddep.org/blog/posts/the-state-of-the-worlds-antibiotics-report-in-2021/. Accessed July 6, 2021.
10. Essential Medicines. Available at: https://essentialmeds.org/. Accessed June 21, 2021.
11. Klein EY, Milkowska-Shibata M, Tseng KK, et al. Assessment of WHO antibiotic consumption and access targets in 76 countries, 2000–15: an analysis of pharmaceutical sales data. Lancet Infect Dis 2021;21(1):107–15.
12. Antimicrobial Resistance (AMR) Containment: National Centre for Disease Control (NCDC). Available at: https://ncdc.gov.in/index1.php?lang=1&level=1&sublinkid=145&lid=74. Accessed June 21, 2021.
13. Ocan M, Obuku EA, Bwanga F, et al. Household antimicrobial self-medication: a systematic review and meta-analysis of the burden, risk factors and outcomes in developing countries. BMC Public Health 2015;15:742.
14. Kalungia AC, Burger J, Godman B, et al. Non-prescription sale and dispensing of antibiotics in community pharmacies in Zambia. Expert Rev Anti Infect Ther 2016;14(12):1215–23.
15. Alhomoud F, Aljamea Z, Almahasnah R, et al. Self-medication and self-prescription with antibiotics in the Middle East—do they really happen? A systematic review of the prevalence, possible reasons, and outcomes. Int J Infect Dis 2017;57:3–12.
16. Do NTT, Vu HTL, Nguyen CTK, et al. Community-based antibiotic access and use in six low-income and middle-income countries: a mixed-method approach. Lancet Glob Health 2021;9(5):e610–9.

17. Iskandar K, Molinier L, Hallit S, et al. Surveillance of antimicrobial resistance in low- and middle-income countries: a scattered picture. Antimicrob Resist Infect Control 2021;10(1):63.
18. Ombelet S, Ronat J-B, Walsh T, et al. Clinical bacteriology in low-resource settings: today's solutions. Lancet Infect Dis 2018;18(8):e248–58.
19. AMRSN Network. Available at: https://iamrsn.icmr.org.in/index.php/amrsn/amrsn-network. Accessed June 21, 2021.
20. Nadimpalli M, Delarocque-Astagneau E, Love DC, et al. Combating global antibiotic resistance: emerging one health concerns in lower- and middle-income countries. Clin Infect Dis 2018;66(6):963–9.
21. Van Boeckel TP, Brower C, Gilbert M, et al. Global trends in antimicrobial use in food animals. Proc Natl Acad Sci U S A 2015;112(18):5649–54.
22. Van Boeckel TP, Pires J, Silvester R, et al. Global trends in antimicrobial resistance in animals in low- and middle-income countries. Science 2019; 365(6459):eaaw1944.
23. Leano E, Weimin M, editors. Regional Consultative Workshop on antimicrobial resistance risk associated with aquaculture in the Asia-Pacific: Bangkok, Thailand, 4–6 September 2018. FAO; 2021. Available at: fao.org.
24. Schar D, Klein EY, Laxminarayan R, et al. Global trends in antimicrobial use in aquaculture. Sci Rep 2020;10:21878.
25. Pham DK, Chu J, Do NT, et al. Monitoring antibiotic use and residue in freshwater aquaculture for domestic use in vietnam. Ecohealth 2015;12(3):480–9.
26. Reygaert WC. An overview of the antimicrobial resistance mechanisms of bacteria. AIMS Microbiol 2018;4(3):482–501.
27. Tenover FC. Mechanisms of antimicrobial resistance in bacteria. Am J Infect Control 2006;34(5):S3–10.
28. Banerjee R, Johnson JR. A new clone sweeps clean: the enigmatic emergence of escherichia coli sequence type 131. Antimicrob Agents Chemother 2014;58(9): 4997–5004.
29. Landman D, Bratu S, Kochar S, et al. Evolution of antimicrobial resistance among Pseudomonas aeruginosa, Acinetobacter baumannii and Klebsiella pneumoniae in Brooklyn, NY. J Antimicrob Chemother 2007;60(1):78–82.
30. Cherry, J. Feigin and Cherry's textbook of pediatric infectious diseases. 8th edition. p. 234, 2320-2339.e10.
31. Yong D, Toleman MA, Giske CG, et al. Characterization of a new Metallo-β-Lactamase Gene, blaNDM-1, and a novel erythromycin esterase gene carried on a unique genetic structure in Klebsiella pneumoniae sequence type 14 from India. Antimicrob Agents Chemother 2009;53(12):5046–54.
32. Nordmann P, Poirel L, Walsh TR, et al. The emerging NDM carbapenemases. Trends Microbiol 2011;19(12):588–95.
33. Dramowski A, Cotton MF, Rabie H, et al. Trends in paediatric bloodstream infections at a South African referral hospital. BMC Pediatr 2015;15(1):33.
34. Obeng-Nkrumah N, Labi A-K, Addison NO, et al. Trends in paediatric and adult bloodstream infections at a Ghanaian referral hospital: a retrospective study. Ann Clin Microbiol Antimicrob 2016;15:49.
35. Musicha P, Cornick JE, Bar-Zeev N, et al. Trends in antimicrobial resistance in bloodstream infection isolates at a large urban hospital in Malawi (1998–2016): a surveillance study. Lancet Infect Dis 2017;17(10):1042–52.
36. Blomberg B, Manji KP, Urassa WK, et al. Antimicrobial resistance predicts death in Tanzanian children with bloodstream infections: a prospective cohort study. BMC Infect Dis 2007;7:43.

37. Iroh Tam P-Y, Musicha P, Kawaza K, et al. Emerging resistance to empiric antimicrobial regimens for pediatric bloodstream infections in Malawi (1998–2017). Clin Infect Dis 2019;69(1):61–8.
38. Wang C, Hao W, Yu R, et al. Analysis of pathogen distribution and its antimicrobial resistance in bloodstream infections in hospitalized children in East China, 2015–2018. J Trop Pediatr 2020;67(1):fmaa077.
39. Wattal C, Goel N. Pediatric blood cultures and antibiotic resistance: an overview. Indian J Pediatr 2020;87(2):125–31.
40. Gandra S, Alvarez-Uria G, Turner P, et al. Antimicrobial resistance surveillance in low- and middle-income countries: progress and challenges in eight South Asian and Southeast Asian Countries. Clin Microbiol Rev 2020;33(3):e00048.
41. Jaganath D, Jorakate P, Makprasert S, et al. Staphylococcus aureus bacteremia incidence and methicillin resistance in Rural Thailand, 2006–2014. Am J Trop Med Hyg 2018;99(1):155–63.
42. Masaisa F, Kayigi E, Seni J, et al. Antibiotic resistance patterns and molecular characterization of methicillin-resistant staphylococcus aureus in clinical settings in Rwanda. Am J Trop Med Hyg 2018;99(5):1239–45.
43. Wang C, Chen Y-H, Fang C, et al. Antibiotic resistance profiles and multidrug resistance patterns of Streptococcus pneumoniae in pediatrics. Medicine (Baltimore) 2019;98(24):e15942.
44. Verghese VP, Veeraraghavan B, Jayaraman R, et al. Increasing incidence of penicillin- and cefotaxime-resistant Streptococcus pneumoniae causing meningitis in India: time for revision of treatment guidelines? Indian J Med Microbiol 2017; 35(2):228–36.
45. Ahmed M, Mirambo MM, Mushi MF, et al. Bacteremia caused by multidrug-resistant bacteria among hospitalized malnourished children in Mwanza, Tanzania: a cross sectional study. BMC Res Notes 2017;10:62.
46. Wain J, Hendriksen RS, Mikoleit ML, et al. Typhoid fever. Lancet 2015;385(9973): 1136–45.
47. van den Bergh ET, Gasem MH, Keuter M, et al. Outcome in three groups of patients with typhoid fever in Indonesia between 1948 and 1990. Trop Med Int Health 1999;4(3):211–5.
48. Nielsen MV, Sarpong N, Krumkamp R, et al. Incidence and characteristics of bacteremia among children in Rural Ghana. PLoS One 2012;7(9):e44063.
49. Feasey NA, Cain AK, Msefula CL, et al. Drug resistance in Salmonella enterica ser. Typhimurium bloodstream infection, Malawi. Emerg Infect Dis 2014;20(11): 1957–9.
50. Oneko M, Kariuki S, Muturi-Kioi V, et al. Emergence of community-acquired, multidrug-resistant invasive nontyphoidal salmonella disease in Rural Western Kenya, 2009-2013. Clin Infect Dis 2015;61(Suppl 4):S310–6.
51. Sah R, Donovan S, Seth-Smith HMB, et al. A novel lineage of ceftriaxone-resistant Salmonella Typhi from India that is closely related to XDR S. Typhi Found in Pakistan. Clin Infect Dis 2020;71(5):1327–30.
52. Britto CD, John J, Verghese VP, et al. A systematic review of antimicrobial resistance of typhoidal Salmonella in India. Indian J Med Res 2019;149(2):151–63.
53. Rowley J, Vander Hoorn S, Korenromp E, et al. Chlamydia, gonorrhoea, trichomoniasis and syphilis: global prevalence and incidence estimates, 2016. Bull World Health Organ 2019;97(8):548–62.
54. Unemo M, Jensen JS. Antimicrobial-resistant sexually transmitted infections: gonorrhoea and Mycoplasma genitalium. Nat Rev Urol 2017;14(3):139–52.

55. Unemo M, Nicholas RA. Emergence of multidrug-resistant, extensively drug-resistant and untreatable gonorrhea. Future Microbiol 2012;7(12):1401–22.
56. Kirkcaldy RD, Weston E, Segurado AC, et al. Epidemiology of gonorrhea: a global perspective. Sex Health 2019;16(5):401–11.
57. Ferreyra C, Redard-Jacot M, Wi T, et al. Barriers to access to new gonorrhea point-of-care diagnostic tests in low- and middle-income countries and potential solutions: a qualitative interview-based study. Sex Transm Dis 2020;47(10):698–704.
58. Cox JA, Vlieghe E, Mendelson M, et al. Antibiotic stewardship in low- and middle-income countries: the same but different? Clin Microbiol Infect 2017;23(11):812–8.
59. Yéo A, Kouamé-Blavo B, Kouamé CE, et al. Establishment of a gonococcal antimicrobial surveillance programme, in accordance with World Health Organization Standards, in Côte d'Ivoire, Western Africa, 2014–2017. Sex Transm Dis 2019;46(3):179–84.
60. Maduna LD, Kock MM, van der Veer BMJW, et al. Antimicrobial resistance of neisseria gonorrhoeae isolates from high-risk men in Johannesburg, South Africa. Antimicrob Agents Chemother 2020;64(11):e00906–20.
61. Unemo M, Bradshaw CS, Hocking JS, et al. Sexually transmitted infections: challenges ahead. Lancet Infect Dis 2017;17(8):e235–79.
62. George CRR, Enriquez RP, Gatus BJ, et al. Systematic review and survey of Neisseria gonorrhoeae ceftriaxone and azithromycin susceptibility data in the Asia Pacific, 2011 to 2016. PLoS One 2019;14(4):e0213312.
63. Langford BJ, So M, Raybardhan S, et al. Bacterial co-infection and secondary infection in patients with COVID-19: a living rapid review and meta-analysis. Clin Microbiol Infect 2020. https://doi.org/10.1016/j.cmi.2020.07.016.
64. Arteaga-Livias K, Pinzas-Acosta K, Perez-Abad L, et al. A multidrug-resistant Klebsiella pneumoniae outbreak in a Peruvian hospital: another threat from the COVID-19 pandemic. Infect Control Hosp Epidemiol 2021;1–2. https://doi.org/10.1017/ice.2020.1401.
65. Subramanya SH, Czyż DM, Acharya KP, et al. The potential impact of the COVID-19 pandemic on antimicrobial resistance and antibiotic stewardship. Virusdisease 2021;1–8. https://doi.org/10.1007/s13337-021-00695-2.
66. COVID-19 Clinical management: living guidance. Available at: https://www.who.int/publications-detail-redirect/WHO-2019-nCoV-clinical-2021-1. Accessed July 6, 2021.
67. Adebisi YA, Jimoh ND, Ogunkola IO, et al. The use of antibiotics in COVID-19 management: a rapid review of national treatment guidelines in 10 African countries. Trop Med Health 2021;49(1):51.
68. Sulis G, Batomen B, Kotwani A, et al. Sales of antibiotics and hydroxychloroquine in India during the COVID-19 epidemic: an interrupted time series analysis. PLoS Med 2021;18(7):e1003682.
69. Ansari S, Hays JP, Kemp A, et al. The potential impact of the COVID-19 pandemic on global antimicrobial and biocide resistance: an AMR Insights global perspective. JAC Antimicrob Resist 2021;3(2):dlab038.
70. Buffet-Bataillon S, Tattevin P, Bonnaure-Mallet M, et al. Emergence of resistance to antibacterial agents: the role of quaternary ammonium compounds—a critical review. Int J Antimicrob Agents 2012;39(5):381–9.
71. Pal C, Bengtsson-Palme J, Kristiansson E, et al. Co-occurrence of resistance genes to antibiotics, biocides and metals reveals novel insights into their co-selection potential. BMC Genomics 2015;16:964.

72. Din M, Ali H, Khan M, et al. Impact of COVID-19 on polio vaccination in Pakistan: a concise overview. Rev Med Virol 2021;31(4):e2190.
73. Schuts EC, Hulscher MEJL, Mouton JW, et al. Current evidence on hospital antimicrobial stewardship objectives: a systematic review and meta-analysis. Lancet Infect Dis 2016;16(7):847–56.
74. Boyles TH, Naicker V, Rawoot N, et al. Sustained reduction in antibiotic consumption in a South African public sector hospital; four year outcomes from the Groote Schuur Hospital antibiotic stewardship program. S Afr Med J 2017;107(2):115–8.
75. Wilkinson A, Ebata A, MacGregor H. Interventions to reduce antibiotic prescribing in LMICs: a scoping review of evidence from human and animal health systems. Antibiotics 2018;8(1):2.
76. Honda H, Ohmagari N, Tokuda Y, et al. Antimicrobial Stewardship in inpatient settings in the asia pacific region: a systematic review and meta-analysis. Clin Infect Dis 2017;64(suppl_2):S119–26.

Pediatric Care for Immigrant, Refugee, and Internationally Adopted Children

Aimee Abu-Shamsieh, MD, MPH*, Soe Maw, MD, MPH

KEYWORDS

• Immigrant children • Refugee • Internationally adopted children
• Infectious diseases

KEY POINTS

- Immigrant children are a diverse group, coming from a variety of countries, and spanning a broad age range.
- Immigrant children include refugees, asylum seekers, unaccompanied minors, and internationally adopted children.
- Infectious risks are determined by a child's country of origin, respective journey, and various social determinants and behaviors; these should be elicited to guide any testing.
- Tuberculosis, hepatitis B, hepatitis C, HIV, and syphilis testing, and a screening complete blood count and stool examination for ova and parasites should be strongly considered for every immigrant child.
- In the presence of risk factors, unavailability of documentation, and/or when relevant history is unknown, testing is particularly important.

INTRODUCTION

An increasing number of people worldwide are leaving their country of birth in search of a new place to call home, with the hope of finding safe refuge, freedom from oppression, or economic opportunity. Among these people are children, some accompanied by their families and others making the journey alone. Political upheaval, war and conflict, social and economic inequities and instability, lack of opportunity, and natural disasters and climate change-related phenomena, with many of these factors exacerbated by the severe acute respiratory syndrome coronavirus 2 (SARS-CoV-2) pandemic, all serve as push factors in the increased movement of people across the globe.

The United States is home to more than 44 million immigrants, when counting all people residing in the country who were not citizens at birth, such as naturalized

Department of Pediatrics, University of California San Francisco (UCSF) Fresno Medical Education Program, 155 North Fresno Street, Suite 218, Fresno, CA, 93701, USA
* Corresponding author.
E-mail address: aimee.abu-shamsieh@ucsf.edu

Pediatr Clin N Am 69 (2022) 153–170
https://doi.org/10.1016/j.pcl.2021.09.006 pediatric.theclinics.com

citizens, lawful permanent residents, those on student or work visas, refugees and asylum seekers, and unauthorized immigrants.[1–3] Indeed, the United States remains a top destination for immigrants of all types. In 2019, approximately 1 million people became new legal permanent residents and more than 800,000 became naturalized citizens. Currently, 3% of children are born outside the United States, and 26% of children in the United States have at least 1 foreign-born parent.[1–3] The population of unauthorized immigrants in the United States is estimated to be almost 11 million, with nearly 1 in 5 of those being children or young adults.[1–3] Refugees and asylum seekers constitute only a small proportion of the immigrants relocating to the United States. In 2018, only 22,491 refugees were admitted to the United States, approximately one-tenth of the number admitted in 1980, the peak of refugee admissions into this country.[1–3] In 2020, this number had dropped even further, owing to the pandemic as well as trends in US immigration policy, to 11,814; falling short of the annual refugee ceiling set at 18,000.[1–3] In general, most refugees come from low- and middle-income countries and are most likely to flee to geographically nearby countries, which are likewise low to middle income; fewer find safe haven in higher income nations. Internationally adopted children make up another subgroup of children whose origins lie outside of the country in which they live. The US Department of State's 2019 Annual Report on Intercountry Adoptions lists the total number of international adoptions as 2971, significantly less than its peak of 22,986 in 2004.[4] The countries of origin of immigrant families in the United States are diverse and differ according to type of immigrant (**Table 1**).

Thus, pediatric providers in receiving countries need to be knowledgeable in the care of immigrant children from a variety of backgrounds. Providers will not only need to be aware of the country or region from which the child has come, but the details of their journey (where and how they traveled and with whom), as well as the various social determinants that impact their family of origin (such as socioeconomic status and education) and their current living conditions, including housing, poverty, and access to health care.

There is a relative lack of evidence-based guidelines supporting the provision of care to immigrant and refugee children, although research on this topic has been increasing in recent years, mostly from the receiving countries in Europe. A related issue is the lack of definitions used when describing immigrant populations. The most basic, and one of the most common, definitions of an *immigrant* is a person who is living in a country other than the country in which they were born. This term can apply to a person who leaves their respective homeland for any reason, by choice or otherwise. It can apply to a person of any age, gender, socioeconomic status or country of origin and, therefore, as a population, encompasses an extremely diverse

Table 1
Countries of origin of Immigrant families in the United States (2018–2020)

Legal Permanent Residents[6]	Refugees[7]	Unauthorized immigrants[8]	Internationally Adopted Children[4]
India	Democratic Republic of Congo	Mexico	China
Mexico	Burma	El Salvador	Ukraine
China	Ukraine	Guatemala	India
Dominican Republic	Afghanistan	India	Colombia
Philippines	Iraq	Honduras	South Korea
Brazil			Bulgaria

group. For the pediatric population, the term children in immigrant families refers to a child who has at least one parent born outside the country, regardless of the child's own nativity. The term migrant does not have a legal definition and at times is used interchangeably with immigrant; however, a more specific use refers to a person who is actively on the move, such as a migrant farmworker, who could thus be considered both an immigrant and a migrant. Unaccompanied immigrant minors are youth less than 18 years who are entering a country or seeking asylum, without a parent or guardian. The terms refugee and asylum seeker have specific legal definitions; both refer to a person outside of his country of origin who is unable to return to that country owing to a well-founded fear of persecution for their social identity or beliefs. Although a refugee would be screened for resettlement while outside the United States, an asylum seeker would be in the United States when submitting their application.[5] Undocumented immigrants, also called irregular migrants, fall into the category of unauthorized immigrants, which includes those who were in the country legally but whose paperwork subsequently lapsed. Refugees, asylum seekers, unaccompanied minors, and internationally adopted children could each be considered to fall under the umbrella of immigrant.

The focus of this article is on caring for immigrant children, particularly how to screen for and treat the myriad infectious diseases that these children may have encountered in the course of their respective journeys. We start by looking at some guidelines for their care, including reviewing the key components of history taking, the physical examination, and diagnostic testing or screening procedures. We then review the most clinically significant pathogens, their testing and treatment, before discussing immunization considerations and the impact of the coronavirus disease 2019 (COVID-19) pandemic on immigrant children and their families.

CLINICAL TOOLS, GUIDELINES, AND POLICIES

Several clinical tools are available to guide the pediatrician in the care of immigrant children. The three most widely used and readily accessible resources are the American Academy of Pediatrics (AAP) Immigrant Child Health Toolkit, which includes the latest AAP Policy Statement "Providing Care for Children in Immigrant Families,"[9] the AAP Red Book: 2021 Report of the Committee on Infectious Diseases,[10,11] and the Centers for Disease Control and Prevention (CDC) Immigrant and Refugee Health Guidelines.[5] In addition, the CDC Yellow Book 2020 is an authoritative resource on Health Information for International Travel and includes chapters on newly arrived immigrants and refugees as well as international adoption.[12] Compiled by the Canadian Pediatric Society, the website https://www.kidsnewtocanada.ca is a comprehensive guide for health professionals who care for immigrant and refugee children. These resources provide the pediatrician with guidelines for evaluation, screening and treatment of newly arrived immigrant children and include specific recommendations for recently arrived refugee or internationally adopted children. Recognizing the many vulnerabilities associated with being an immigrant, most of these sources address not only epidemiology (including regions affected and risk factors) and the screening and treatment of infectious diseases, but also lay out comprehensive care plans that address the child's physical, emotional, and social well-being.

PROVISION OF CARE TO IMMIGRANT CHILDREN

Medical care accessed by immigrant children before immigration is varied; many of these children may not have had access to regular health services, including screenings and preventive care, in their country of origin. Medical records, including immunization records, may not always be available. It should be noted that many immigrants, such as undocumented immigrants and asylum seekers, will not have had a predeparture medical screening or immunizations.

The Immigration and Naturalization Act requires all immigrants including refugees and internationally adopted children to undergo a medical screening examination before departing for the United States. Performed by a panel physician authorized by the US Embassy or Consulate, this examination is limited in scope with its sole purpose being the identification of inadmissible health conditions. The treatment of some communicable diseases may take place before immigration; it is mandated only for tuberculosis, syphilis, gonorrhea, and Hansen's disease (leprosy). Immunizations based on Advisory Committee on Immunization Practices (ACIP) recommendations are provided with some modifications for specific populations. Technical Instructions guiding these examinations are issued by the CDC Division of Global Migration and Quarantine and can be found at https://www.cdc.gov/immigrantrefugeehealth/panel-physicians.html.[5]

The CDC also provides guidelines for screening refugees upon arrival in the United States.[5,13,14] Although such an examination is not required, it was established under the Refugee Act of 1980 as a benefit for refugees provided by the Department of Health and Human Services' Office of Refugee Resettlement. This examination should take place within 90 days of arrival and includes screening for infectious diseases. In addition to these postarrival recommendations, many states have developed their own protocols for the initial evaluation of refugees. Others with humanitarian-based immigration status, such unaccompanied refugee minors and asylees, are eligible for this examination and other medical and social benefits as well. For immigrants pursuing adjustment of their status to become a permanent resident, a civil surgeon is authorized by the US Citizenship and Immigration Services to perform an official immigration medical examination.[12]

Internationally adopted children similarly have a limited screening examination by an authorized panel physician in their country of origin. Prospective parents can also have a preadoption medical review, which can be done by the family's own pediatrician, but may also be performed by a pediatrician with expertise in international adoption who is often part of a multispecialty team in a clinic specializing in the evaluation of international adoptees. Such practices often provide both preadoption and postadoption evaluations of the child, but subsequent care is assumed by the child's primary care provider. The assessment includes evaluations of photographs, videos, and medical records, and later the child in person, and focuses on assessing growth, development, infectious disease screening, immunizations, and prenatal exposures, especially fetal alcohol exposure. Such centers are often affiliated with academic centers and found in large urban areas and services are often paid for out of pocket. The CDC provides a resource for families at www.cdc.gov/immigrantrefugeehealth/adoption/, which includes a list of such practices. For international adoptees, an initial visit to a physician should take place within the first 2 weeks, sooner if the child exhibits signs of acute illness. Preadoption visits for prospective parents and other household members can take place at a travel medicine clinic to ensure immunizations are up to date for travel as well as to protect against exposure through direct contact with the child once the family is home.[15–17]

Because these initial examinations in the preimmigration and immediate postimmigration period may be limited, the results may not be available to subsequent providers, and they lack opportunity for the child and family to establish an ongoing therapeutic provider–patient relationship with the examiner, it becomes highly important for the immigrant or internationally adopted child to establish care in a medical home. The AAP describes the care provided in a medical home as accessible, continuous, comprehensive, family centered, coordinated, compassionate, and culturally effective[18]; it is also important that the medical home of the immigrant child emphasize collaboration with community partners, including schools, houses of worship, legal agencies, social services, and community-based organizations providing support to immigrant families.[11] The components of care in the medical home have been delineated and emphasize the importance of creating a culturally safe and effective space that includes access to interpreter services.[19] Explaining the role of the provider, the role of others on the health care team, clinic logistics, and an explanation of components of the evaluation including sensitive questions, a complete physical examination and any necessary laboratory work, will help to build trust.

After these issues are addressed, the comprehensive medical examination for a newly arrived immigrant starts with age-based well child care practices, such as those described in AAP Bright Futures including screening for nutrition, growth and development and a physical examination.[20] The components of this evaluation are summarized in **Table 2**. Any available medical records, immunization records or results available from the predeparture screening examination should be reviewed.

Because of the inconsistent use of the hepatitis B vaccine at birth; inconsistent perinatal screening for hepatitis B, syphilis, and HIV; and the high prevalence of certain intestinal parasites and tuberculosis, screening for these diseases should be considered for all immigrant children.[10] Hepatitis C screening should be done for those with risk factors or if their history is unknown. In addition, a complete blood count should be performed looking for eosinophilia, which can suggest parasitic disease; anemia, which can also be associated with parasitosis (as well as other conditions); and leukopenia, leukocytosis, or thrombocytopenia, which could be associated with viral and other infectious conditions. Details of testing are discussed elsewhere in this article. Additional infectious disease screening laboratory tests are guided by the identification of risk factors through history taking as well as information available in previous medical records.

PATHOGEN-SPECIFIC REVIEW ON PREVENTION, SCREENING, DIAGNOSIS, AND TREATMENT OF INFECTIOUS DISEASES IN IMMIGRANT CHILDREN

Tuberculosis

Testing and treating latent tuberculosis infection are crucial in this population. Children can manifest severe symptoms and are at high risk for reactivation in subsequent years. Predeparture screening algorithms differ based on low versus high tuberculosis burden countries. For immigrant children from countries with 20 or more cases per 100,000 population, screening requirements before departure set forth by the CDC include:

- Tuberculin skin test or interferon gamma release assay (IGRA) for children 2 to 14 years of age.[14,21]
- Chest radiographs for immigrants 15 years and older.[14,21]
- Sputum cultures and drug susceptibility testing.[14,21]
- Completion of directly observed treatment for tuberculosis before immigration for those with pulmonary involvement.[14,21]

Children less than 2 years of age are generally not tested unless they have known exposure to an active case, concomitant HIV infection, or symptoms of active tuberculosis. In the latter 2 instances, IGRA may be used if available; otherwise, a tuberculin skin test is the preferred test in this age group. For those 2 years of age and older, a tuberculin skin test or IGRA may be used, but the IGRA is the preferred method to avoid a false-positive result, especially if the BCG vaccine has been given previously. Upon arrival in the United States, children 2 years and older should undergo repeat testing if they do not have a negative test result within the previous 6 months. To avoid a false negative, which can occur with a recently acquired infection or anergy owing to malnutrition, some investigators recommend repeat testing 3 to 6 months after arrival. Because both malnutrition and HIV infection can give false-negative results owing to an anergic state, additional testing is warranted to rule out active tuberculosis in these cases.[14,15,17,21,22]

Hepatitis A, B, and C

The number of cases of hepatitis A virus has increased since 2016.[14,21] Immigrant children carrying hepatitis A may be asymptomatic. Hence, screening is important in high-

Table 2
Components of the initial evaluation of the pediatric patient in the medical home[10,11,19,20]

Domain	Guidelines and Tools	Comments
History History of immigration journey HEADSS[a] examination Review medical records, if available	–	May need a follow-up visit to complete history and physical once rapport is built and child more adjusted
Complete physical examination Check for dysmorphology Special attention to eye, skin, genitourinary examinations	–	Referral to dental home
Developmental and educational	Vision and hearing screen; ASQ[b] M-CHAT-R/F[c]	Refer for vision/audiology testing if indicated Culturally and linguistically appropriate assessment Link to school district or early childhood education services (eg, Head Start)
Mental and emotional health	PHQ-2/9[d]; ASQ-SE[b]; SWYC™ [e]; EPDS [f](for mothers); ACEs (adverse childhood experiences) screening (child or parent); Refugee Health Screener (RHS-15[g]); Pediatric Symptom Checklist[h]	–
Social determinants	SEEK,[i] food insecurity screen, assessment of need for legal assistance	Link to community-based organizations, community centers, houses of worship, local organizations serving immigrants/refugees. social services (WIC, Food Bank); language/literacy classes for parents; legal aid.

(continued on next page)

Table 2
(continued)

Domain	Guidelines and Tools	Comments
Laboratory testing Review results from predeparture screening if available	Complete blood count; lead level (≤6 y); Fasting lipid screen ± fasting glucose, liver function tests (if indicated by age or body mass index) Consider other laboratory tests for growth/nutrition concerns including: thyroid studies, vitamin D, metabolic panel, urinalysis. Infectious disease screening: tuberculosis screening (if no documentation) HIV (recommended for <13 y if perinatal exposure unknown, 13 y and up recommended). Syphilis (treponemal and nontreponemal tests) Hepatitis B serologic testing Hepatitis C if risk factors or history unknown Stool examination 3 times for ova and parasites	Referral to/consultation with infectious disease specialists and/or local health department for infectious disease testing/treating/reporting. Consider other testing by region, symptoms, risk factors.
Immunizations Review vaccine records if available	Per ACIP[j] guidelines	If records questionable or unavailable, may repeat series, check titers or both

Note: many of these screening tools are available free online, in multiple languages.

[a] HEADSS (Home, Education/Employment, Activities, Drugs, Sex, Suicide/Depression) from Cohen, E, MacKenzie, R.G., yates, G.L. (1991). HEADSS, a psychosocial risk assessment instrument: Implications for designing effective intervention programs for runaway youth. *Journal of Adolescent Health*. 12 (7): 539 to 544. DOI:https://doi.org/10.1016/0197 to 0070(91)90084-Y.

[b] ASQ, ASQ-SE (Ages and Stages Questionnaire, 3rd edition; Ages and Stages – social-emotional, 2nd edition) from https://agesandstages.com/about-asq/asq-development/.

[c] MCHAT – R/F (Modified Checklist for Autism in Toddlers, Revised with Follow-Up) from Robins DL, Casagrande K, Barton M, Chen CM, Dumont-Mathieu T, Fein D. validation of the modified checklist for autism in toddlers, revised with follow-up (M-CHAT-R/F). *Pediatrics*. 2014 Jan;133(1):37 to 45. https://doi.org/10.1542/peds.2013-1813.

[d] PHQ-2, 9 (Personal Health Questionnaire) from Kroenke, K., spitzer, R.L. & Williams, J.B.W. The PHQ-9. *J Gen Intern Med*. 16, 606–613 (2001). https://doi.org/10.1046/j.1525-1497.2001.016009606.x.

[e] SWYC (Survey of Well-being of Young Children) from https://www.tuftschildrenshospital.org/The-Survey-of-Wellbeing-of-Young-Children/Overview/.

[f] EPDS (Edinburgh Postnatal Depression Scale) from Cox JL, Holden JM, Sagovsky R. Detection of postnatal depression. Development of the 10-item Edinburgh Postnatal Depression Scale. *Br J Psychiatry*. 1987 Jun;150:782 to 6. https://doi.org/10.1192/bjp.150.6.782. PMID: 3,651,732.

[g] RHS-15 (Refugee Health Screener) from Hollifield M, Verbillis-Kolp S, Farmer B, Toolson EC, Woldehaimanot T, Yamazaki J, Holland A, St Clair J, SooHoo J. The Refugee Health Screener-15 (RHS-15): development and validation of an instrument for anxiety, depression, and PTSD in refugees. *Gen Hosp Psychiatry*. 2013 Mar-Apr;35(2):202 to 9. https://doi.org/10.1016/j.genhosppsych.2012.12.002.

[h] Pediatric Symptom Checklist - Jellinek MS, Murphy JM, Robinson J, Feins A, Lamb S, Fenton T. Pediatric Symptom Checklist: screening school-age children for psychosocial dysfunction. *J Pediatr*. 1988 Feb;112(2):201–9. (https://doi.org/10.1016/s0022-34768880056-8).

[i] SEEK (Safe Environment for Every Kid) from https://seekwellbeing.org/.

[j] CDC Advisory Committee on Immunization Practices (ACIP) Vaccine Recommendations and Guidelines at https://www.cdc.gov/vaccines/hcp/acip-recs/index.html.

risk groups, including internationally adopted children, because household contacts may be susceptible to infection. Hepatitis A is transmitted via the fecal–oral route and individuals with chronic liver disease and HIV-infected persons are at increased risk for severe disease from hepatitis A virus infection.[14,15,17,21]

Hepatitis B infection acquired during infancy or childhood can lead to chronic liver disease and increase the risk of developing hepatocellular carcinoma if left untreated. The risk for hepatitis B infection in an immigrant child depends on the prevalence of hepatitis B in their country of origin, as reported on the CDC website. Transmission can occur vertically, through sexual contact, or needle sharing or blood products.[14]

Infection with hepatitis C can also lead to chronic disease and increase the risk for hepatocellular carcinoma. Transmission may occur vertically as well as through needle sharing, contaminated medical equipment, blood products and via sexual contact.[14,15,17] Testing recommendations for the different types of viral hepatitis are summarized in **Table 3**.

Congenital Syphilis

The CDC recommends screening for immigrant children with nontreponemal and treponemal serology regardless of any report of treatment before arrival. Positive serologic

Table 3
Testing recommendations for hepatitis

	Populations That Should Be Tested	What to Order
Hepatitis A[14]	Routine screening not recommended Consider immunization for household contacts	–
Hepatitis B[14]	Screen arrivals born in or who have resided in countries with intermediate (2%–7%) or high (≥8%) prevalence of chronic hepatitis B virus infection For countries with chronic HBV infection prevalence of <2%, screen children/adolescents in high-risk groups[a] Household contact with HBV Pregnant adolescents	Hepatitis B surface antigen, hepatitis B surface antibody (anti-HBs), total hepatitis B core antibody (anti-HBc), IgM antibody to hepatitis core antigen (IgM anti-HBc)
Hepatitis C[14]	Unaccompanied refugee minors Children with risk factors [a] Children born to HCV-positive mothers Household contact with HCV Internationally adopted children	Anti-HCV HCV RNA testing (if anti-HCV is positive) HCV RNA testing if <18 mo of age to avoid false positives from maternal antibodies
Hepatitis D[14]	Recommended if hepatitis B surface antigen positive	–
Hepatitis E[14]	Routine screening not recommended	–

[a] High-risk groups include intravenous drug users (past/current); persons who are HIV positive; those with elevated liver function tests or other signs/symptoms of liver disease; hemodialysis patients; male children/adolescents who have had sex with males; children/adolescents with a history of sexual exploitation; history of blood/bodily fluid exposure especially requiring postexposure prophylaxis; persons requiring immunosuppressive therapy; history of female genital mutilation/cutting; history of overseas surgery, major dental work, blood transfusion; tattoos.[14]

tests should be further evaluated to determine stage of infection and to rule out differential diagnoses such as pinta and yaws. Positive results on nontreponemal tests (eg, rapid plasma reagin, Venereal Disease Research Laboratory) should be confirmed with a treponemal test (eg, fluorescent treponemal antibody absorption test, treponema pallidum particle agglutination, enzyme immunoassays, and chemiluminescence immunoassays).[14,21] Interpretation of syphilis serology test results is delineated in **Table 4**.

HIV 1 and HIV 2

Testing of refugees and immigrant children for HIV infection before arrival in the United States is no longer a requirement as of 2010.[14] The CDC recommends that all children less than 13 years of age be screened for HIV unless the biological mother's HIV status is confirmed negative and the child is at low risk for infection. In other populations of immigrant children, testing for HIV is recommended based on an individual's risk profile and the disease burden in the country of origin. Risk factors to consider include maternal drug use, a history of receiving blood products, early sexual activity, or a history of sexual abuse. Children less than 18 months of age with a positive result on HIV antibody test should undergo a DNA or RNA test to avoid false positives owing to persistent maternal antibodies. Testing for HIV should be done before the administration of live vaccines.[14,15,17,21]

Intestinal and Tissue Parasites

Testing for these parasites is typically done by performing a microscopic evaluation of a stool specimen looking for ova and parasites.[10,14] Most sources recommend 3 samples collected on separate days to increase sensitivity. Despite this practice, some of these pathogens, such as *Strongyloides* or *Schistosomes*, still only yield a sensitivity of about 50%.[10,14] Serologic testing, an elevated absolute eosinophil count, and the presence of hematuria can also be considered to increase detection for these 2

Table 4
Interpretation of Syphilis Serology Tests (table content copied from the CDC's online resource for Immigrant, Refugee, and Migrant Health)[14,23]

Nontreponemal Test (eg, Rapid Plasma Reagin (RPR), Venereal Disease Research Laboratory (VDRL))	Treponemal Test (eg, Fluorescent Treponemal Antibody Absorption Test, TPPA)	Interpretation
Nonreactive	Nonreactive	No evidence of syphilis
Reactive	Reactive	Untreated syphilis OR Previously treated late syphilis OR Other spirochetal diseases
Reactive	Nonreactive	False positive, can be seen in (1) tuberculosis, hepatitis, malaria, early HIV infection (2) autoimmune diseases (3) injection drug use (4) pregnancy (5) after vaccinations with vaccines such as MMR or smallpox vaccines
Nonreactive	Reactive	Very early untreated syphilis OR previously treated syphilis OR very late untreated syphilis After successful treatment, a positive nontreponemal test usually becomes negative whereas the treponemal test usually remains positive for life.

diseases.[10] If the stool ova and parasites examination is negative, an elevated absolute eosinophil count (>450 cells/μL) should prompt an investigation for *Strongyloides*, *Schistosomiasis*, *Toxocara canis*, and other endemic parasites, although the absence of eosinophilia does not rule them out.[10]

In regions where these parasites are endemic, empiric treatment may be administered to some populations of immigrants or refugees as part of their predeparture medical examination. Additional details can be found in the instructions from the CDC Division of Global Migration and Quarantine.[5] The clinical presentation, testing, and treatment for intestinal and tissue parasites are summarized in **Tables 5–8**.

ADDITIONAL PATHOGENS (REGION SPECIFIC)

Less commonly diagnosed infectious diseases may only need to be screened for in children coming from specific regions or with risk factors. Only refugees from sub-Saharan Africa are routinely tested or treated for malaria before departure; if not, they should receive presumptive treatment or screening within 3 months of arrival.[14] Lymphatic filariasis serologic testing (for *W bancrofti* or *Brugia* spp.) should be considered for children more than 2 years of age from endemic regions of Asia, Africa, the Caribbean, or South America. Chagas disease is endemic to most countries of Central

Table 5
Soil-transmitted helminth infections (*Ancylostoma duodenale* and *Necator americanus* [hookworm], *Ascaris lumbricoides* [ascariasis], and *Trichuris trichiura* [whipworm])[14]

Drug of Choice	Albendazole, Mebendazole
Presumptive treatment overseas	Yes, in Asia, the Middle East, Africa, Central/South America, and the Caribbean
Prevalence	Areas of the world with warm and humid climates and poor sanitation systems
Transmission	*Ascaris* and *Trichuris* infections occur through ingestion of eggs. Hookworm infections require direct contact of skin with contaminated soil and penetration of the larval worm through the skin.
Spectrum of clinical presentation	Can be asymptomatic Ascariasis: abdominal pain, cough (Loffler syndrome), intestinal obstruction, appendicitis, cholecystitis Trichuriasis: hematochezia, anemia, and rectal prolapse in rare cases Hookworm: anemia, gastrointestinal complaints, eosinophilia, and poor growth in cases of chronic infection
Recommendations for testing and treatment	Stool examination 3 times for ova and parasites Asymptomatic refugees not treated before departure may be presumptively treated at arrival; recommendation is to screen first if there are contraindications to presumptive treatment or if albendazole is unavailable.

Table 6 Giardia[14,21]	
Drug of Choice	Metronidazole, Tinidazole, or Nitazoxanide
Presumptive treatment overseas	No
Prevalence	Found worldwide
Transmission	Ingestion of contaminated water or eating uncooked food that contains organisms
Spectrum of clinical presentation	Majority asymptomatic Can present with diarrhea, nausea, anorexia, malnutrition, and abdominal distension
Recommendations for testing and treatment	Testing by direct immunofluorescence assay or enzyme immunoassay if symptomatic Presumptive treatment not recommended

Table 7 Schistosoma species [10,14,24]	
Drug of Choice	Praziquantel
Presumptive treatment overseas	Yes, for sub-Saharan African refugees
Prevalence	Endemicity in >50 countries including some in South American, the Caribbean, China, Southeast Asia, the Middle East and sub-Saharan Africa
Transmission	Via direct skin contact with schistosome-contaminated fresh water
Spectrum of clinical presentation	May be asymptomatic or present with eosinophilia. Severe manifestations of chronic *S mansoni* infections include bowel wall pathology, liver cirrhosis, and portal hypertension. *S haematobium* may cause severe genitourinary tract complications.
Recommendations for testing and treatment	Serology, presence of eosinophilia, hematuria, or urine ova and parasites (for *S haematobium*) may assist in diagnosis. Stool ova and parasites is associated with low sensitivity (approximately 50% with 3 samples).[24] Asymptomatic sub-Saharan African refugees not treated before departure may be presumptively treated at arrival; recommendation is to screen first if contraindications to presumptive treatment or praziquantel is unavailable.

Table 8
Strongyloides[14,21,24]

Drug of Choice	Ivermectin
Presumptive treatment overseas	Yes
Prevalence	25%–46% in refugee populations (especially high in Southeast Asian refugees)
Transmission	Via contact with soil contaminated with Strongyloides larvae. Can live in human host for years via autoinoculation.
Spectrum of clinical presentation	May be asymptomatic, present with eosinophilia, or often with vague gastrointestinal symptoms, dry cough, and skin manifestations.
Recommendations for testing and treatment	Serology and presence of eosinophilia may assist in diagnosis. Stool ova and parasites is associated with low sensitivity (approximately 50% with 3 samples).[24] Asymptomatic refugees not treated before departure may be presumptively treated at arrival; recommendation is to screen first if there are contraindications to presumptive treatment (eg, those from loa loa endemic areas) or if ivermectin is unavailable.

and South America and immigrant children 12 months or older from this region should undergo *Trypanosoma cruzi* serology testing.[10] Screening for sexually transmitted diseases is especially important for unaccompanied minors and other youth with history of increased risk for human trafficking, sexual assault, or sexual abuse.[10]

Other testing should be done only in the presence of specific symptoms. Children with watery diarrhea should be tested for *Cryptosporidium*. Because it may not be detected on routine examination of stool for ova and parasites, specific testing for it should be requested and may be done by direct immunofluorescence assay, enzyme immunoassay, or nucleic acid amplification testing.[10] A stool culture looking for bacterial pathogens should also be ordered for symptomatic children. Infestations such as scabies and pediculosis capitis are common; they are typically diagnosed by clinical appearance and most often treated with topical permethrin. Alternative treatments are reviewed in the Red Book.[10]

Some investigators have noted an increased burden of multidrug-resistant pathogens among refugees, associated with increased antimicrobial resistance rates in their countries of origin, especially in the Middle East, sub-Saharan Africa, and Afghanistan. The spread of these multidrug-resistant organisms within immigrant populations is facilitated by crowded living conditions and a lack of hygiene; in some populations it seems to be more prevalent among children.[25] In addition to the public health implications, this finding could impact the treatment of bacterial infections in sick immigrant children.

Assessment of Immunization Records and Recommendations for Immunizations for Immigrant Children

Evaluation of immunization status is a very important part of the medical examination of an immigrant, refugee, or internationally adopted child. Immigrants entering as legal permanent residents should have documentation of all vaccines recommended by ACIP, generally those vaccines that are age appropriate and are considered to prevent spread of a disease with the potential to cause an outbreak, or one that has been eliminated in the United States. Refugees are not required to have completed these vaccines before arriving in the United States, but will require proof of vaccination by the time they apply for permanent residency, usually 1 year after arrival. International adoptees aged 10 years and younger may obtain a waiver of exemption requiring receipt of required vaccines before departure; under certain conditions, an adoptee's parents may be required to sign an affidavit stating they will obtain recommended vaccines within 30 days of arrival in the United States.[26]

Some children, such as those with undocumented status, may not have immunization records available at all. Others, including international adoptees, may have immunization records of questionable validity. The pediatric provider may need to make their own assessment of apparent accuracy of the records. At times there are logical explanations for points of concern; for example, a date written in the order day–month–year instead of month–day–year, or all entries written in the same handwriting and same ink being due to preparing a copy for the adoption process, rather than a forgery. However, dates that do not make sense in relation to the child's age or the immunization schedule should raise concerns. It should be kept in mind that the immunization schedules of other countries often differ from that in the United States[15,27]; nonetheless, those given earlier than the recommended age in the United States (eg, measles at 9 months instead of 12) or with intervals that are too short will need to be made up according to ACIP recommendations.

Aside from the reliability of the immunization records, the concern remains that a child may have failed to develop adequate protection against disease despite apparently reliable documentation of vaccine administration. Studies examining this issue in international adoptees in the 1990s suggest that institutionalized children were more likely than those in foster care settings to have inadequate protection, possibly owing not only to falsified vaccine records but to less potent vaccines, related to improper handling and storage, as well as poor immune response related to stress, disease, or malnutrition.[16,17]

Hence, when vaccine records are unavailable or there is any concern regarding their validity, the pediatric provider is left with 2 options: repeating the entire vaccine series or checking antibody titers and administering only those vaccines for which the child does not have evidence of immunity. In fact, a combination of both may end up being the most practical approach. This is partly because serologic testing may not be readily available for all vaccines (eg, pertussis). The AAP Clinical Report on the Comprehensive Health Evaluation of the Newly Adopted Child summarizes the serologic testing for assessing immunization status.[28] It should be noted that, even if a child has serologic evidence of immunity, the vaccine series should be completed as appropriate for their age. Furthermore, a previous history of disease should not serve as proof of immunity. One consideration regarding repeating the entire series is the need to limit the number of tetanus and diphtheria toxoid doses to a maximum of 6 before the age of 7 years. If there is any uncertainty regarding immunization status in infants less than 6 months of age, vaccines should be reinitiated according to the ACIP immunization schedule. Further guidance on this topic is provided in the Red Book.[10]

For immigrant and refugee children, there are special considerations regarding the polio vaccine. With the eradication of type 2 wild poliovirus declared by the World Health Organization in 2015, and the recognition that all cases of disease associated with type 2 poliovirus were vaccine-associated paralytic polio, there was a global switch in 2016 from trivalent to bivalent oral polio vaccine containing serotypes 1 and 3 only, thus eliminating potential exposure to vaccine-associated type 2 poliovirus. Concurrently, the World Health Organization recommendation was made that at least 1 dose of the trivalent inactivated polio vaccine be included into the country's routine immunization schedule to mitigate the risk of vaccine-derived type 2 poliovirus poliomyelitis. An immigrant, refugee or internationally adopted child who has documentation of having received previous doses of OPV should complete the series using the inactivated polio vaccine; however, only trivalent OPV can count toward the series. Doses of oral polio vaccine given on or after April 1, 2016, should be assumed to be bivalent oral polio vaccine or monovalent oral polio vaccine (given during serotype-specific outbreaks) and should not be counted.[10,29] There is no serologic testing readily available for polio, so if reliable documentation is not available, the child should be revaccinated according to ACIP and Red Book guidelines.[10]

When unaccompanied minors at the United States–Mexico border are held in the custody of the Office of Refugee Resettlement of the Department of Health and Human Services, they are vaccinated per the ACIP catch-up vaccination schedule and are provided with their vaccination records when released to a sponsor.[13] The CDC has made special recommendations for vaccinating this population in response to disease outbreaks, such as the recommendation for a 1-time dose of the PCV13 pneumococcal vaccine after an outbreak of severe respiratory disease associated with pneumococcal serotype 5 among 16 adolescents in the summer of 2014.[30]

Vaccine hesitancy has been identified as a global threat to health and contributes to health disparities affecting immigrant populations.[27] Measles outbreaks disproportionately impacting Somali immigrant communities in Minnesota in 2011 and 2017 were linked to lower rates of MMR vaccine uptake. Concern that the vaccine could cause autism was identified as one of the major barriers to MMR vaccination in that population.[31] Other factors that have been associated with vaccine hesitancy or refusal in immigrant populations include an overall distrust of the health system, low health literacy, barriers to health information including lack of linguistically and culturally appropriate materials, lack of access to online information and low literacy, and fears of vaccine side effects and their impact on the ability to work or care for family. Among undocumented immigrants or mixed status families, there may be a fear of collection or sharing of personal data. Such concerns should be heard and addressed by the pediatric provider at the individual level; systems-based changes to address these issues, such as the use of community advisory boards to develop culturally and linguistically appropriate patient education materials or not requiring government-issued identification when obtaining vaccines, should also be encouraged.[32]

IMPACT OF THE CORONAVIRUS DISEASE 2019 PANDEMIC ON IMMIGRANT CHILDREN

The impact of the COVID-19 pandemic on immigrant children in North America has not been studied widely. However, immigrant families typically reside in areas with higher population densities and lower socioeconomic conditions.[11,33,34] Owing to limited resources and shared housing, many people cannot practice social distancing guidelines.[35,36] Immigrants often engage in occupations with a relatively high risk of exposure to the virus, while lacking the necessary personal protective equipment, increasing their risk of bringing the virus home. Immigrant children may also lack medical homes and access to COVID-19 diagnostic testing, treatment, or vaccination or may be unaware of opportunities to access such services.[37–39] School closures may hinder language acquisition and learning in general, thereby creating barriers to integration and advancement in their new country.[40] Increased morbidity and mortality owing to severe acute respiratory syndrome coronavirus 2 among immigrant communities in the United States has been noted, as has a decreased likelihood of receiving the COVID-19 vaccine. Part of this may be owing to factors contributing to vaccine hesitancy, as noted elsewhere in this article, but other barriers, such as an inability to schedule the vaccine owing to lack of internet access, language barriers, and transportation difficulties also play a role.[31,41]

Another striking example of COVID-related health inequities for immigrant children is seen in reports of COVID outbreaks in facilities for youth at the United States–Mexico border. There are reports of inadequate testing and an inability to properly isolate affected children and, for legal reasons, unaccompanied minors are not able to consent for the COVID-19 vaccine.[42–44]

SUMMARY

Immigrant children are a very diverse group and include refugees, asylum seekers, internationally adopted children, and unaccompanied immigrant minors. They have various infectious disease risk factors unique to the conditions within their country of origin, the journey they took, their current living conditions, and their health status. Infectious disease screening should take place within the framework of a comprehensive medical evaluation in a culturally safe and effective medical home. Certain screening is recommended for all immigrant children, including hepatitis B, syphilis, HIV, tuberculosis, and intestinal parasites; other communicable diseases can be tested for based on history and physical examination findings. Although numerous authoritative guidelines and other resources are readily accessible to the pediatric provider caring for the immigrant child, there is limited evidence supporting many practices especially regarding cost effectiveness and the interplay between infectious diseases, chronic diseases and conditions, and the social determinants of health.

CLINICS CARE POINTS

- Several clinical tools are readily available to guide the pediatric provider caring for immigrant children; these include the AAP Immigrant Child Health Toolkit, the AAP Red Book and the CDC Immigrant and Refugee Health Guidelines.
- Connecting with a medical home should be a priority for the immigrant child because this provides care that is comprehensive, and it allows for continuity of care.
- Screening for certain infections, including tuberculosis, hepatitis B and C, HIV, syphilis and intestinal parasites, should be strongly considered for every immigrant child; testing for malaria, extraintestinal parasites and other pathogens should be considered on a case-by-case basis, depending on symptomatology and country of origin.
- A complete blood count is recommended for all immigrant children; abnormalities such as eosinophilia, anemia, or an abnormal leukocyte count may suggest the need for further testing looking for specific parasitic diseases or other infections.
- When immunization records are unavailable or seem to be unreliable, the provider will need to check antibody titers and/or repeat the vaccine series per the age-appropriate immunization schedule.

DISCLOSURE

A. Abu-Shamsieh and S. Maw have nothing to disclose.

REFERENCES

1. Batalova J, Hanna M, Levesque C. Frequently requested statistics on immigrants and immigration in the United States. migrationpolicy.org. 2021. Available at: https://www.migrationpolicy.org/article/frequently-requested-statistics-immigrants-and-immigration-united-states-2020. Accessed July 7, 2021.
2. Capps R, Gelatt J, Ruiz Soto AG, et al. Unauthorized immigrants in the United States: stable numbers, changing origins. migrationpolicy.org. 2020. Available at:. https://www.migrationpolicy.org/research/unauthorized-immigrants-united-states-stable-numbers-changing-origins. Accessed July 7, 2021.
3. U.S. Annual Refugee Resettlement Ceilings and Number of Refugees Admitted, 1980-Present. migrationpolicy.org. 2013. Available at: https://www.migrationpolicy.org/programs/data-hub/charts/us-annual-refugee-resettlement-ceilings-and-number-refugees-admitted-united. Accessed July 7, 2021.
4. Intercountry Adoption Annual Reports. Available at: https://travel.state.gov/content/travel/en/Intercountry-Adoption/adopt_ref/AnnualReports.html. Accessed July 7, 2021.
5. Immigrant, Refugee, and Migrant Health | Immigrant and Refugee Health | CDC. 2021. Available at: https://www.cdc.gov/immigrantrefugeehealth/index.html. Accessed July 7, 2021.
6. Legal Immigration and Adjustment of Status Report. Department of Homeland Security. 2017. Available at: https://www.dhs.gov/immigration-statistics/special-reports/legal-immigration. Accessed July 7, 2021.
7. Refugee Processing Center. Refugee Processing Center. Available at: http://www.wrapsnet.org. Accessed July 7, 2021.
8. Unauthorized Immigrant Population Profiles. 2015. Available at: migrationpolicy.org; https://www.migrationpolicy.org/programs/us-immigration-policy-program-data-hub/unauthorized-immigrant-population-profiles. Accessed July 7, 2021.
9. Immigrant Child Health Toolkit. AAP.org. Available at: http://www.aap.org/en-us/advocacy-and-policy/aap-health-initiatives/Immigrant-Child-Health-Toolkit/Pages/Immigrant-Child-Health-Toolkit.aspx. Accessed July 7, 2021.
10. American Academy of Pediatrics. Red Book (2021): Report of the Committee on Infectious Diseases, 32nd edition. Ed. Kimberlin DW et al. Available at: https://ebooks.aappublications.org/content/red-book-2021. Accessed July 7, 2021.
11. Linton JM, Green A. Providing Care for Children in Immigrant Families. Pediatrics 2019;144(3):e20192077.
12. Centers for Disease Control and Prevention. CDC Yellow Book 2020: Health Information for International Travel. New York: Oxford University Press; 2017. Available at: https://wwwnc.cdc.gov/travel/page/yellowbook-home-2020. Accessed July 7, 2021.
13. United States Department of Health and Human Services. Key documents for the unaccompanied children program. Washington, DC: Office of Refugee Resettlement. Online publication date May 19, 2021. Available at: https://acf.hhs.gov/orr/policy-guidance/unaccompanied-children-program. Accessed July 7, 2021.
14. Guidance for the U.S. Domestic Medical Examination for Newly Arriving Refugees | Immigrant and Refugee Health | CDC. 2021. Available at: https://www.cdc.gov/immigrantrefugeehealth/guidelines/domestic-guidelines.html. Accessed June 29, 2021.
15. Eckerle JK, Howard CR, John CC. Infections in internationally adopted children. Pediatr Clin North Am 2013;60(2):487–505.

16. Miller L. The Handbook of international adoption medicine: a guide for physicians, parents, and providers. New York: Oxford University Press; 2004.
17. Barnett ED. Immunizations and infectious disease screening for internationally adopted children. Pediatr Clin North Am 2005;52(5):1287–1309, vi.
18. Committee MHI for CWSNPA. The Medical Home. Pediatrics 2002;110(1):184–6.
19. Turner C, Ibrahim A, Linton JM. Clinical Tools Working at Home with Immigrants and Refugees. Pediatr Clin North America 2019;66(3):601–17.
20. American Academy of Pediatrics. Bright Futures. Available at: https://brightfutures.aap.org/Pages/default.aspx. Accessed July 7, 2021.
21. Medical Evaluation for Infectious Diseases for Internationally Adopted. Refugee, and Immigrant Children. In: Red Book: 2021–2024 Report of the Committee on Infectious Diseases. Am Acad Pediatr 2021;158–9.
22. Shetty AK. Infectious Diseases among Refugee Children. Children (Basel). 2019; 6(12). https://doi.org/10.3390/children6120129.
23. Syphilis | Immigrant and Refugee Health | CDC. 2019. Available at: https://www.cdc.gov/immigrantrefugeehealth/guidelines/domestic/sexually-transmitted-diseases/syphilis.html. Accessed September 9, 2021.
24. Dang K, Tribble AC. Strategies in Infectious Disease Prevention and Management Among US-Bound Refugee Children. Curr Probl Pediatr Adolesc Health Care 2014;44(7):196–207.
25. Maltezou HC, Theodoridou M, Daikos GL. Antimicrobial resistance and the current refugee crisis. J Glob Antimicrob Resist 2017;10:75–9. https://doi.org/10.1016/j.jgar.2017.03.013.
26. International Adoption Simplification Act of 2010. Available at: https://travel.state.gov/content/travel/en/Intercountry-Adoption/adopt_ref/international-adoption-simplification-act-2010.html. Accessed July 7, 2021.
27. WHO vaccine-preventable diseases: monitoring system. 2020 global summary. Available at: https://apps.who.int/immunization_monitoring/globalsummary/schedules. Accessed July 7, 2021.
28. Jones V, Schulte E, COUNCIL ON FOSTER CARE. ADOPTION, AND KINSHIP CARE, Comprehensive Health Evaluation of the Newly Adopted Child. Pediatrics 2019;143(5). https://doi.org/10.1542/peds.2019-0657.
29. Marin M, Patel M, Oberste S, et al. Guidance for Assessment of Poliovirus Vaccination Status and Vaccination of Children Who Have Received Poliovirus Vaccine Outside the United States. MMWR Morb Mortal Wkly Rep 2017;66. https://doi.org/10.15585/mmwr.mm6601a6.
30. Nyangoma EN, Arriola CS, Hagan J, et al. Notes from the field: hospitalizations for respiratory disease among unaccompanied children from Central America - multiple States, June-July 2014. MMWR Morb Mortal Wkly Rep 2014;63(32):698–9.
31. Tankwanchi AS, Jaca A, Larson HJ, et al. Taking stock of vaccine hesitancy among migrants: a scoping review protocol. BMJ Open 2020;10(5):e035225.
32. Isa Álvarez PO, Rusch D. Op-Ed: vaccinate our undocumented. 2021. Available at: https://www.medpagetoday.com/infectiousdisease/covid19vaccine/92492. Accessed July 7, 2021.
33. Ludwig S, Steenhoff AP, Linton JM. Immigrant and refugee health: why this topic? Why now? Pediatr Clin 2019;66(3):xvii–xix.
34. Linton JM, Griffin M, Shapiro AJ, Council on Community Pediatrics. . Detention of immigrant children. Pediatrics 2017;139(5):e20170483.
35. Ross J, Diaz CM, Starrels JL. The disproportionate burden of COVID-19 for immigrants in the Bronx, New York. JAMA Intern Med 2020;180(8):1043.

36. Kline NS. Rethinking COVID-19 vulnerability: a call for LGBTQ+ immigrant health equity in the United States during and after a pandemic. Health Equity 2020;4(1):239–42.
37. Belue R, Degboe AN, Miranda PY, et al. Do medical homes reduce disparities in receipt of preventive services between children living in immigrant and non-immigrant families? J Immigr Minor Health 2012;14(4):617–25.
38. Kan K, Choi H, Davis M. Immigrant families, children with special health care needs, and the medical home. Pediatrics 2016;137(1). https://doi.org/10.1542/peds.2015-3221.
39. A new home, but with no medical home? Study of immigrants' kids with special health needs: One in four children in the US live in immigrant families, but many lack a true "medical home." ScienceDaily. Available at: https://www.sciencedaily.com/releases/2016/02/160209121724.htm. Accessed June 29, 2021.
40. Aguilera E. Migrant students work in fields during COVID school closures. CalMatters. 2020. Available at: https://calmatters.org/children-and-youth/2020/06/california-teens-school-closures-migrant-farmworkers-fields-coronavirus/. Accessed June 30, 2021.
41. Crawshaw AF, Deal A, Rustage K, et al. What must be done to tackle vaccine hesitancy and barriers to COVID-19 vaccination in migrants? J Trav Med 2021;28(4). https://doi.org/10.1093/jtm/taab048.
42. Child migrants: massive drop in children held by border officials. BBC News. Available at: https://www.bbc.com/news/world-us-canada-56405009. Accessed July 7, 2021.
43. Lenthang M. COVID-19 cases among unaccompanied migrant children in facilities spark concerns over crowding. ABC News. 2021. Available at: https://abcnews.go.com/Health/covid-19-cases-unaccompanied-migrant-children-facilities-spark/story?id=76788478. Accessed July 7, 2021.
44. Owermohle S. Foster and migrant kids shut out from Covid vaccinations. Politico. Available at: https://www.politico.com/news/2021/05/30/migrant-children-coronavirus-vaccine-491412. Accessed July 7, 2021.

Vaccines for International Pediatric Travelers

Vini Vijayan, MD, FIDSA[a,b,*]

KEYWORDS

• Travel health • Travel vaccines • International traveler • Pediatric traveler

KEY POINTS

- Children and adolescents travel internationally for the purpose of leisure, studying abroad, volunteerism, adventure travel, and visiting friends and relatives and are at risk of exposure to vaccine-preventable diseases.
- Pediatricians should be aware of destination-specific recommendations regarding immunization of children who are traveling abroad.
- Travelers should receive routine immunizations as well as travel-specific immunizations to reduce the risk of illness and death from vaccine-preventable diseases.

INTRODUCTION

In the United States, an estimated 2.4 million children travel internationally each year. The number of families traveling internationally continues to grow. Children and adolescents tend to travel for the purpose of leisure, studying abroad, volunteerism, adventure travel, and visiting friends and relatives (VFR).[1,2] Pediatricians are often the first to be contacted by families about plans for travel and hence should be able to effectively provide preventive education, chemoprophylaxis against malaria and traveler's diarrhea, as well as travel vaccinations to ensure a safe and healthy trip for their patients. Pediatricians may need to consult travel medicine specialists, especially when encountering travelers who are immunocompromised, have allergies to vaccine components, or are traveling to destinations that require specific vaccines because some vaccines (yellow fever [YF] vaccine, Japanese encephalitis [JE] vaccine) may be challenging to obtain and administer in a regular clinic.[3–5]

This article provides an overview of the vaccines recommended for children traveling internationally.

Financial Support: None.
[a] Division of Pediatric Infectious Diseases, Valley Children's Healthcare, Madera, CA, USA; [b] Stanford University School of Medicine, Stanford, CA, USA

* Division of Pediatric Infectious Diseases, Department of Pediatrics, Valley Children's Healthcare, Madera, CA 93636.

E-mail address: VVijayan@valleychildrens.org

Pediatr Clin N Am 69 (2022) 171–184
https://doi.org/10.1016/j.pcl.2021.08.009 pediatric.theclinics.com

PREPARING PATIENTS FOR TRAVEL

Families that are traveling with children should seek medical consultation with their pediatric or travel medicine providers at least 1 month before departure to allow for timely administration of all routine and recommended travel vaccines.[3,4] This visit also provides time to prepare the traveler for health concerns and assess vaccine requirements. Immunization requirements are determined based on the traveler's pretravel immunization status, age, medical history, and destination. Immunization needs also vary depending on the exposures during the trip, and hence clinicians should review the planned activities and detailed itinerary of the traveler. Potential exposure to water, insects, or animals as well as duration of travel will help tailor risk avoidance education and travel immunizations.[5–7]

The pretravel consultation allows for dedicated time for the provider to do the following:

- Perform an individual risk assessment based on analysis of medical history and the itinerary.
- Communicate the destination-specific anticipated health risks for the traveler.
- Manage health risks by providing risk mitigation strategies, such as immunizations, malaria, and traveler's diarrhea prophylaxis.[4–7]

When performing an individual risk assessment, it is important to note that children VFR may be at an increased risk of travel-related illness.[8,9] Travelers VFR include immigrants, refugees, migrants, students, or displaced persons who are traveling back to their country of origin for purposes of VFR.[8,9] These travelers tend to stay in the country for extended periods and do not seek pretravel advice, vaccinations, and/or prophylactic medications.[8,9] An effective consultation also includes communicating the anticipated health risks based on the destination and itinerary because activities planned during travel may inform risk mitigation strategies. Key components of risk communication include anticipatory guidance regarding prevention of insect bites, sun exposure, food and water safety, and altitude sickness when applicable. Mitigating risk involves providing prophylactic medication against malaria, altitude sickness, and traveler's diarrhea and travel immunizations.[3–7] For the purpose of this article, we review only travel immunizations.

General Principles Regarding Travel Immunizations

In the United States, travel vaccine requirements and recommendations for different countries are provided by the Centers for Disease Control and Prevention (CDC). These recommendations are available online at https://wwwnc.cdc.gov/travel/page/yellowbook-home.[4] Vaccine schedules for children and adolescents are updated annually by the CDC's Advisory Committee on Immunization Practices (ACIP) and are available at https://www.cdc.gov/vaccines/schedules/hcp/imz/child-adolescent.html.[10]

Recommendations for immunization of travelers are not always the same as routine childhood immunization recommendations.[3,4,10] Each vaccination schedule must be individualized based on factors such as the age of the traveler, allergies, and presence of any underlying medical conditions. Destination-specific factors to consider include the country of destination, length of visit in the country, season, itinerary, and planned activities. It is also important to take into account the time available before departure, because some vaccines may need booster doses. In addition, country-specific vaccination recommendations and requirements for departure and entry vary over time, such as for polio vaccine.[3,4,10]

Travel vaccines are generally categorized into

- *Routine vaccines:* These vaccines are the standard child and adult immunizations recommended by the ACIP, including vaccines such as hepatitis B virus, diphtheria, tetanus, pertussis, and *Haemophilus influenzae* type b (Hib).
- *Recommended vaccines:* These vaccines are recommended by the CDC based on the travel destination and activities, including vaccines such as the typhoid vaccine and hepatitis A.
- *Required vaccines:* Certain vaccines are required to be documented on the International Certificate of Vaccination for entry into the country, including vaccines such as YF, meningococcal, and polio vaccines.

ROUTINE VACCINES

Immunization records of the traveler should be carefully reviewed to ensure that the traveler is update on their routine vaccinations. Children should receive the ACIP-recommended childhood vaccines, including hepatitis A virus (HAV); hepatitis B virus; diphtheria, tetanus, pertussis; Hib; human papillomavirus; influenza; measles-mumps-rubella (MMR); *Neisseria meningitidis*; polio; rotavirus; *Streptococcus pneumoniae*; and varicella because vaccine-preventable illnesses are still highly prevalent in many parts of the world.[4] Routine pediatric vaccinations may need to be at accelerated schedule to complete the vaccine series before departure. The recommended minimum intervals between vaccines are available at https://www.cdc.gov/vaccines/schedules/hcp/imz/child-adolescent.html.[10]

Measles-Mumps-Rubella or Measles-Mumps-Rubella vaccine

All children aged 12 months or older should receive at least 2 doses of MMR vaccine before departure regardless of their destination but infants between 6 and 11 months may receive a single dose earlier than the routine recommendation, considering the high morbidity in young infants. Infants receiving MMR before 12 months of age should be revaccinated upon return, because immunization before 1 year of age does not reliably induce long-term immunity. Adolescents who do not have evidence of immunity against measles should get 2 doses of MMR separated by at least 28 days. Children aged 12 months or older must be given 2 MMR or MMR vaccine (MMRV) doses separated by 28 days or more.[10–13] The maximum age for use of MMRV is 12 years.[10]

Influenza

Influenza remains a common vaccine-preventable illness among pediatric travelers, and the influenza vaccine is routinely recommended for all travelers aged 6 months or older.[14,15] The risk of acquiring influenza depends on the time of year because the distribution of the types and subtypes of influenza virus varies geographically from year to year. In the Northern Hemisphere, the influenza season may begin as early as October and can extend until May, but in the Southern Hemisphere, it may begin in April and last through September. In tropical climates, influenza viruses can circulate year-round.[14,15] Travelers should be vaccinated at least 2 weeks before travel for adequate immunity to develop.[13]

Varicella

Varicella is endemic worldwide, and hence all susceptible travelers are at risk of infection during their trip because varicella can be seen more frequently in other countries. Travelers at highest risk for severe varicella are infants, adults, and immunocompromised people without evidence of immunity. All children aged 12 months or older who have no history of varicella vaccination or chickenpox should be vaccinated unless there is a contraindication to vaccination.[16] Children require 2 doses of the varicella vaccine, the first dose at age 12 through 15 months and a second dose at age 4 through 6 years. If the second dose is administered after the seventh birthday, the minimum interval between doses is 3 months for children aged less than 13 years and 4 weeks for persons aged 13 years or more. Infants younger than 6 months are generally protected by maternal antibodies.[10,13]

Polio

On May 5, 2014, the World Health Organization (WHO) Director-General declared the international spread of polio to be a public health emergency of international concern under the authority of the International Health Regulations and issued temporary polio vaccine recommendations to reduce the international spread of polio.[17] This regulation recommends that long-term travelers (staying >4 weeks) and residents departing from countries with wild poliovirus type (WPV) transmission be vaccinated against poliomyelitis. Travelers may be required to show proof of polio vaccination when departing from these countries.[17–21]

At present, the CDC recommends that all infants and children in the United States be routinely vaccinated against poliomyelitis with 4 doses of the inactivated polio vaccine given at ages 2 months, 4 months, 6 to 18 months, and 4 to 6 years. The last dose of the vaccine should be given at greater than 4 years of age and more than 6 months from the previous dose. Children traveling to areas where WPV has circulated in the last 12 months should complete the routine polio vaccine series before departure. If a child cannot complete the routine series before departure, an accelerated schedule is recommended. If the vaccines are administered outside the United States, this may still be accepted as valid doses as long as the schedule is similar to that recommended in the United States.[10,21,22] The polio vaccine must be received between 4 weeks and 12 months before departure from the polio-affected country.[10,19,20,22]

As of May 2021, countries infected with WPV include Pakistan and Afghanistan.[22] Circulating vaccine-derived polioviruses with potential risk of international spread have been reported in Malaysia, Madagascar, and Yemen.[23] However, it is important to be aware that the requirements for each country may change rapidly. The requirements for vaccination before travel can be found at https://wwwnc.cdc.gov/travel/. The list of countries where the poliovirus is currently circulating is available at https://polioeradication.org/where-we-work/.

RECOMMENDED VACCINES

Typhoid Fever

Typhoid fever, also known as enteric fever, is caused primarily by *Salmonella enterica* serotypes *typhi* and to a lesser extent serotypes *Salmonella paratyphi* A, B, and C. The disease presents with fever, malaise, diffuse abdominal pain, and constipation and if left untreated can cause delirium, intestinal hemorrhage, bowel perforation, and death. Typhoid fever is acquired through consumption of water or food contaminated by feces of an acutely infected or convalescent person or a chronic, asymptomatic carrier.[11,24] Travelers visiting countries with endemic disease and poor access to safe food, water, and sanitation are at risk of acquiring the disease, including many low- and middle-income countries in Asia, Africa, and Latin America.[4,11,24] Extensively drug-resistant *Salmonella typhi* infections have also been reported in Pakistan and recently among US residents without travel.[25,26]

Indications

Typhoid vaccination is recommended for children older than 2 years traveling to endemic areas such as the Indian subcontinent, Southeast Asia, the Middle East, Africa, and Central and South America.[27] Specific areas where the typhoid vaccine is recommended are available at www.cdc.gov/travel.

Vaccines and administration

There are 2 typhoid vaccines available for use in the United States:

- Intramuscular, Vi capsular polysaccharide vaccine (ViCPS) (Typhim Vi, Sanofi Pasteur)
- Oral live attenuated vaccine manufactured from Ty21a strain of serotype typhi (Vivotif, Emergent BioSolutions)

Vaccination with ViCPS comprises one 0.5-mL dose administered intramuscularly for children aged 2 years or older. The primary dose should be given at 2 weeks or more before travel. A booster dose is recommended every 2 years for children who remain at risk. Vaccination with the oral Ty21a vaccine consists of 4 capsules, 1 taken every other day, ideally 1 hour before a meal and 2 or more hours after a previous meal. The child must be able to swallow the capsule, thus it is recommended for those aged 6 years or older. All 4 doses should be taken at 1 week or more before potential exposure. Ty21a must be kept refrigerated at 35.6°F to 46.4°F (2°C–8°C) and administered with cool liquid no warmer than 98.6°F (37°C). As Ty21a is a live vaccine, it should not be given to immunocompromised children or those on antibiotics because this may reduce immunogenicity. Booster dose is recommended every 5 years for children who remain at risk.

Both vaccines are only 50% to 80% efficacious, and therefore the importance of clean food and water should be emphasized with the traveler.[3,5,24] The typhoid vaccines should not be given to children with a febrile illness. In addition, Ty21a is not recommended for use in people with acute gastroenteritis and immunocompromised travelers.[27]

Hepatitis A

Hepatitis A is a vaccine-preventable, highly contagious infection caused by the HAV. The infection is transmitted through the fecal-oral route, direct person-to-person contact, or ingestion of contaminated food such as unwashed vegetables or fruits or water. Hepatitis A is a self-limited illness, and symptoms include fever, headache, malaise, anorexia, nausea, vomiting, diarrhea, abdominal pain, or dark urine. Young children infected with hepatitis A are often asymptomatic but can transmit the infection to unvaccinated older children and adults.[28–30]

Indications

The ACIP recommends that all children aged 12 to 23 months receive a 2-dose series of hepatitis A vaccine as a part of their routine immunization schedule. Children aged 2 to 18 years who have not previously received the vaccine and are planning to travel to a hepatitis A endemic area should receive a single dose of the vaccine as soon as travel is planned. For infants aged 6 to 11 months who are traveling internationally, hepatitis A vaccination should be administered[10,31] at least 2 weeks before departure. However, the travel-related dose is not counted toward the routine ACIP recommended 2-dose series.[4,11]

Hepatitis immune globulin (IG) should be considered before travel for persons with special risk factors or increased risk for severe disease from HAV infection such as immunocompromised children who may not mount an immune response to the vaccine and infant travelers who are younger than 6 month and are too young to receive the vaccine.[10,31–34]

Vaccines and administration
The available vaccines in the United States include inactivated hepatitis A vaccine (HAVRIX or VAQTA) and consist of 2 doses separated by a minimum interval of 6 months. A combination hepatitis A and hepatitis B vaccine TWINRIX is available for adults.

GamaSTAN is the immunoglobulin product for infants younger than 6 months who would not be able to receive the hepatitis A vaccine. Dosing consists of 0.1 mL/kg intramuscularly (for anticipated risk of exposure up to 1 month) or 0.2 mL/kg intramuscularly (for anticipated risk of exposure up to 2 months). If the anticipated risk of exposure is greater than 2 months, a repeat dose of 0.2 mL/kg should be administered every 2 months for the duration of exposure. It is important to remember that MMRV and hepatitis A vaccine can be administered together but that the immunoglobulin cannot be administered simultaneously with MMR due to the interference of the immune response to MMR. For travelers who require both MMR and hepatitis A immunoglobulin, MMR should be given 2 weeks before administration of hepatitis A immunoglobulin. If immunoglobulin is administered within 14 days after MMR, MMR should be readministered after an interval of 6 months. This interval should provide enough time for decrease in passive antibodies to allow for an adequate response to the MMR vaccine.[4,10,31,32]

Postexposure prophylaxis
For travelers who report exposure to hepatitis A during their trip, postexposure prophylaxis (PEP) with hepatitis A vaccine or IG has been shown to effectively prevent hepatitis A infection when administered within 2 weeks of exposure. There are rare situations where both are given to the same person—immunocompromised hosts and chronic liver disease. Hepatitis A vaccine and IG must be administered in different extremities to prevent interference of antibody responses. The hepatitis A vaccine series should be completed with a second dose at least 6 months after the first dose for long-term protection.

For healthy children who have previously completed their hepatitis A vaccine series, no additional PEP is necessary.[31,32]

Rabies

Rabies is a viral disease that causes acute, fatal progressive encephalitis in humans. Nearly 99% of human rabies occurs in countries that are endemic for the diseases, including countries in Africa, Asia, and Central and South America. Children are at a higher risk for acquisition of disease because they are less likely to report bites and because facial bites are more common in children owing to their smaller stature.[35–37]

Indications
Preexposure prophylaxis is recommended for children with long-term travel to high-risk areas, especially children traveling to or living in rural areas where enzootic dog rabies is endemic or where timely PEP might not be available following an animal bite. Rabies preexposure vaccination should also be considered for adolescents traveling for the purpose of adventure such as hikers, or spelunkers. Students who are working with animal or bat conservation are also likely to encounter rabies vectors.[35,36,38]

Vaccines and administration
In the United States, preexposure vaccination consists of a series of 3 intramuscular injections given on days 0, 7, and 21 or 28 in the deltoid with human diploid cell

vaccine (Imovax, Sanofi Pasteur, SA) and purified chick embryo cell (RabAvert, Novartis) vaccine. Travelers should receive all 3 preexposure immunizations before travel, and if the series cannot be completed, they should not start the series because there are limited data on how to provide PEP when the preexposure vaccine series is incomplete. If the child is exposed to rabies during the trip, the child will need 2 more doses of rabies vaccine on days 0 and 3. These children do not need rabies immunoglobulin.

Postexposure prophylaxis

For those children who sustain an animal bite but have not received preexposure immunization, immediate cleaning of the wound and PEP significantly decreases the risk of infection. PEP includes a series of 4 rabies vaccine doses on days 0, 3, 7, and 14 and local infiltrate of the human rabies IG at the site of the bite. For immunocompromised children, a fifth dose of the rabies vaccines is recommended at day 28. The vaccine should never be administered in the gluteal area because this may result in lower antibody titers.[38]

Japanese Encephalitis

JE is a vaccine-preventable mosquito-borne infection that is endemic throughout most of Asia and parts of the Western Pacific region especially in rural agricultural areas. JE virus is a single-stranded RNA virus that belongs to the genus *Flavivirus* and is transmitted to humans through the bite of an infected Culex mosquito. Families that are traveling to countries endemic for JE should be advised of the risks of disease and the importance of personal protective measures to reduce the risk for mosquito bites.[39,40]

Indications

The JE vaccine is recommended for travelers who plan to spend greater than 1 month in endemic areas during the JE virus transmission season, including long-term travelers, recurrent travelers, or expatriates who are likely to visit endemic rural or agricultural areas during a high-risk period of JE virus transmission. The risk to short-term (<1 month) travelers and those who confine their travel to urban centers is low.[4,39]

Vaccination of short-term travelers is determined based on their accommodations, season, and activities during the trip. Vaccination may be deemed necessary if the traveler plans to travel outside an urban area and if their activities will increase the risk of JE virus exposure. These activities include camping, hiking, trekking, biking, fishing, hunting, or farming.[4,39]

Vaccines and administration

In the United States, inactivated Vero cell culture-derived JE vaccine, Ixiaro is the only licensed and available vaccine. The vaccine is approved for children aged 2 months and older. Ixiaro is given as a 2-dose series, with the doses spaced 28 days apart. The last dose should be given at least 1 week before travel.4,39 For adults and children, a booster dose (third dose) should be given at 1 year or more after completion of the primary Ixiaro series if ongoing exposure or reexposure to JE virus is expected.[4,39]

REQUIRED VACCINES

Yellow Fever

YF is a mosquito-borne disease that is caused by the YF virus. YF is endemic to tropical South America and sub-Saharan Africa. The clinical manifestations of YF range from flulike illness with fever, chills, headache, myalgia, and vomiting to catastrophic illness with coagulopathy, shock, and multisystem organ failure.[40]

Indications

The YF vaccine is recommended for children aged 9 months or more who are traveling to areas at risk for YF virus transmission in South America and Africa. In YF endemic counties, vaccination is legally required for entry, and proof of vaccination must be documented on an International Certificate of Vaccination or Prophylaxis. Some countries also require proof of vaccination if traveling through an endemic region to prevent introduction of the disease to their prevalent mosquito vectors. Infants and children with a specific contraindication to YF vaccine should obtain a waiver from a travel physician before traveling to a country requiring vaccination.[4,41] Updated recommendations on country-specific recommendations are available at http://www.cdc.gov/yellowfever/maps/.

Vaccines and administration

YF vaccine is a live attenuated virus vaccine developed in chick embryos and therefore should not be given to individuals with primary immunodeficiencies, transplant recipients, patients on immunosuppressive and immunomodulatory therapies, or patients with human immunodeficiency virus (HIV) whose CD4 count is less than 200/mL. Other contraindications include age less than 6 months, allergy to a vaccine component, and thymic disorders. Adverse reactions to the vaccine are very rare but include 2 syndromes, YF-associated neurotropic disease (YEL-AND) and YF vaccine-associated viscerotropic disease (YEL-AVD),[40] and therefore only children who are at risk of disease or who require proof of YF vaccination to enter a country should be vaccinated.[4,40–42] YEL-AND is a rarely fatal disease that can present as acute disseminated encephalomyelitis, meningoencephalitis, Guillain-Barré syndrome, and cranial nerve palsies after receipt of the YF vaccine. YEL-AVD occurs 4 days (range, 1–18 days) after the first dose of the vaccine; it presents similar to wild-type YF diseases but causes multiorgan failure and death.

The vaccine is given as a single 0.5-mL injection administered subcutaneously. A single primary dose confers lifelong immunity, and a booster is not needed. In the United States, the YF vaccine is distributed only through approved vaccinating centers.[4,40–42] These designated centers are listed in a registry at the CDC travel Web site at https://wwwnc.cdc.gov/travel/yellow-fever-vaccination-clinics/search.

Meningococcal Disease

N meningitidis is a gram-negative diplococcus and the causative agent for meningococcal meningitis. Meningococcal meningitis is a cause of significant morbidity and mortality worldwide, and despite therapy, meningococcal disease is still associated with a high mortality rate and neurologic sequelae in survivors, particularly among infants and young children.[43]

The highest incidence of *N meningitidis* occurs in the "meningitis belt" of sub-Saharan Africa wherein periodic epidemics are seen especially during the dry season (December–June). Serotype A has been the most common serotype associated with outbreaks, but more recently meningococcal outbreaks due to serogroups C, W, and X have been reported. In addition, the Hajj pilgrimage to Saudi Arabia has also been associated with outbreaks of meningococcal disease in returning pilgrims and their contacts.[44,45]

Indications

The ACIP recommends that all 11- to 12-year-old children should receive a meningococcal conjugate vaccine as a part of their routinely recommended vaccination and a booster dose at age 16 to 18 years. The booster dose provides protection during the ages when adolescents are at the highest risk of meningococcal disease. High-risk children should also be given a meningococcal conjugate vaccine earlier than the routine recommendation if they have underlying health problems that are recognized to increase the risk of acquiring meningococcal disease; this includes individuals with terminal complement component deficiency, functional or anatomic asplenia, and HIV.

In addition, vaccination is recommended for travelers who visit or reside in countries where meningococcal disease is hyperendemic or epidemic, such as the meningitis belt of sub-Saharan Africa during the dry season (December–June). Travelers to Saudi Arabia during the Hajj are required to have a certificate of vaccination with quadrivalent (A,C,Y,W-135) meningococcal vaccine before entering, issued not more than 5 years and not less than 10 days before arrival if a conjugate vaccine was administered; the vaccination certificate should specifically state that a conjugate vaccine was given.[10,46]

Children traveling to a country where a travel advisory exists for epidemic meningitis should also be vaccinated before travel. Travel advisories for these countries may be found at www.cdc.gov/travel/.

Of note, MenB vaccine is not recommended for people who live in or travel to meningitis belt countries, because serogroup B disease is extremely rare in this region. MenB vaccine is not routinely recommended for travel to other regions of the world unless an outbreak of serogroup B disease has been reported.[46–48]

Vaccines, dosing, and administration

At present, there are 3 quadrivalent meningococcal vaccine formulations licensed and available for use in the United States (MenACWY-D [Menactra], MenACWY-CRM [Menveo], and MenACWY-TT [MenQuadfi]. There are 2 serogroup B meningococcal vaccines, MenB-FHbp (Trumenba) and MenB-4C (Bexsero). The choice of vaccine given will depend on knowledge of the predominant strains causing disease in the country of travel.

Children who were previously vaccinated with a quadrivalent vaccine should receive a booster dose. For children who completed the primary dose or series at less than 7 years of age, a booster dose of MenACWY should be administered after 3 years and repeated every 5 years thereafter if they live in or travel to a hyperendemic area. For people who received the primary dose or series at age 7 years or more, a booster dose should be administered after 5 years and every 5 years thereafter if they live in or travel to a hyperendemic area.

For infants aged less than 9 months, MenACWY-CRM (Menveo) is the only licensed and available meningococcal vaccine. In children initiating vaccination at 2 months of age, MenACWY-CRM should be administered as a 4-dose series at 2, 4, 6, and 12 months of age. In children initiating vaccination at 7 to 23 months of age, MenACWY-CRM should be administered as a 2-dose series, with the second dose administered at 12 months of age or more and 3 months or more after the first dose, although it can be administered as early as 8 weeks after the first dose preceding travel. For travelers initiating vaccination at 9 months or more (ie, 9 months through 55 years), either MenACWY-CRM or MenACWY-D (Menactra) may be used. For travelers aged 9 to 23 months who receive MenACWY-D, 2 doses should be administered, with the second dose administered 12 weeks or more after the first dose.[10,43,46]

Cholera

Cholera is an acute diarrheal illness caused by toxigenic *Vibrio cholerae* O1. Cholera is endemic in many low- and middle-income countries, but primarily in Africa and South and Southeast Asia. The infection is most commonly acquired from drinking water contaminated with *V cholerae*.

At present, there is no licensed cholera vaccine available for pediatric travelers in the United States. CVD 103-HgR, a single-dose oral cholera vaccine (Vaxchora, Emergent BioSolutions), is licensed and available in the United States. According to the United States Food and Drug Administration, it is approved for those aged 2 to 64 years, but it is currently not available in the United States. Vaxchora is an oral vaccine, administered in single dose.[49,50] This vaccine is dispensed as one double-chambered sachet. Eating or drinking should be avoided for 60 minutes before and after oral ingestion of Vaxchora. Vaxchora should be taken at least 10 days before travel. Vaxchora may be shed in the stool for at least 7 days, and the vaccine strain may be transmitted to nonvaccinated close contacts. Clinicians and travelers should use caution when considering whether to use the vaccine in people with immunocompromised close contacts.[49,50] In addition, 3 inactivated vaccines are approved by WHO but are not available in the United States.

TIMING AND SPACING OF IMMUNOBIOLOGICS

When administering multiple vaccines, the timing and spacing of the vaccine doses are key to the appropriate use of vaccines. Clinicians should adhere to the ACIP vaccination schedule to ensure vaccine efficacy and stay in accordance with the minimal intervals between doses or use the recommended accelerated schedule when necessary. If a scheduled dose of the vaccine cannot be given on time or the child forgets to complete the series, the series does not need to be restarted and extra doses are not necessary. The dose may be given at the next visit. The oral typhoid vaccine and the preexposure rabies vaccines are exceptions to this rule, and if doses are missed, the vaccine series may need to be repeated to ensure protection.

Providers should pay special attention to the timing of antibody-containing blood products and live vaccines such as measles and varicella-containing vaccines, and the interval between subsequent doses of the same vaccines.[13] As a general rule, all required vaccines can be administered at the same visit with a few exceptions. The quadrivalent meningococcal conjugate vaccine (MCV4)-D (MenACWY-D, Menactra) and pneumococcal conjugate vaccine (PCV) 13 (PCV13, Prevnar 13) should not be administered simultaneously because of reduced immunogenicity. Similarly, in a child that requires both PCV13 and PPSV23, the 2 vaccines should not be administered together and PCV13 should be administered first and the PPSV23 should be given 8 weeks later. All live vaccines (MMR, varicella, live attenuated influenza, YF, and oral typhoid) can be given at the same visit if indicated. If live vaccines are not administered during the same visit, they should be separated by 4 weeks or more because the immunogenicity may be affected if administered within 28 days of another live-virus vaccine. If 2 injected or intranasal live-virus vaccines are not administered on the same day but less than 28 days apart, the second vaccine should be repeated at 28 days or more. Measles and other live-virus vaccines may interfere with the response to tuberculin skin testing and the interferon-γ release assay.[13] Tuberculin testing may be performed either on the same day that live-virus vaccines are administered or 4 to 6 weeks later.

SUMMARY

The care of the traveling child has become more complex and specialized because of vaccine developments and as destination-specific recommendations evolve. Child travelers are at risk of travel-related illnesses, and the risks of exposure to infectious pathogens vary based on their age, purpose of travel, itinerary, and destination. Families that are traveling with children should seek advice from their pediatrician and/or specialized travel medicine clinic to develop an individualized plan to ensure a safe and healthy trip. Protecting travelers from travel-related illnesses include updating routine childhood immunizations and appropriately administering itinerary-specific travel vaccines before departure. The routine childhood vaccinations may need to be accelerated for infant travelers if the standard primary vaccine series cannot be completed before departure.

CLINICS CARE POINTS

- Administering itinerary-specific travel vaccines and updating the routine childhood immunizations is essential to prevent travel-related vaccine-preventable illnesses.
- Routine childhood vaccinations should be accelerated for infant travelers if the standard primary vaccine series cannot be completed before departure.
- Vaccine requirements and recommendations vary depending on the age and medical history of the traveler and the destination country (eg, YF vaccine).

DISCLOSURE

The author denies any conflict of interest or relationship with a commercial company that has a direct financial interest in subject matter of materials discussed in this article.

REFERENCES

1. World Tourism Organization. International tourism highlights. 2020th edition. Madrid: UNWTO; 2021. Available at: https://doi.org/10.18111/9789284422456. Accessed June 2, 2021.
2. US Department of Commerce, Office of Travel and Tourism Industries. 2017 US citizen travel to international regions. Washington, DC: US Department of Commerce; 2018. Available at: https://travel.trade.gov/view/m-2017-O-001/index.html. Accessed June 2, 2021.
3. Hill DR, Ericsson CD, Pearson RD, et al. The practice of travel medicine: guidelines by the Infectious Diseases Society of America. Clin Infect Dis 2006;43:1499–539.
4. Centers for Disease Control and Prevention. Health information for international travel 2020: the yellow book. Available at: https://wwwnc.cdc.gov/travel/page/yellowbook-home. Accessed May 2, 2021.
5. Freedman DO, Chen LH, Kozarsky P. Medical considerations before travel. N Engl J Med 2016;375:247–60.
6. Hatz CFR, Chen LH. Pre-travel consultation. In: Keystone JS, Freedman DO, Kozarsky PE, et al, editors. Travel medicine. 3rd edition. Philadelphia: Saunders Elsevier; 2013. p. 31–6.
7. Kozarsky PE, Steffen R. Travel medicine education—what are the needs? J Trav Med 2016;23(5).
8. Hendel-Paterson B, Swanson SJ. Pediatric travelers visiting friends and relatives (VFR) abroad: illnesses, barriers and pre-travel recommendations. Trav Med Infect Dis 2011;9(4):192–203.
9. Monge-Maillo B, Norman FF, Perez-Molina JA, et al. Travelers visiting friends and relatives (VFR) and imported infectious disease: travelers, immigrants or both? A comparative analysis. Trav Med Infect Dis 2014;12(1):88–94.

10. Wodi AP, Ault K, Hunter P, et al. Advisory committee on immunization practices recommended immunization schedule for children and adolescents aged 18 years or younger — United States, 2021. MMWR Morb Mortal Wkly Rep 2021; 70(6):189–92.
11. Centers for Disease Control and Prevention. Epidemiology and prevention of vaccine-preventable diseases. Hamborsky J, Kroger A, Wolfe S, eds. 13th edition Washington D.C. Public Health Foundation. Available at: www.cdc.gov/vaccines/pubs/pinkbook/index.html. Accessed May 2, 2021.
12. American Academy of Pediatrics. Measles red book. In: Kimberlin DW, Brady MT, Jackson MA, editors. 2018-2021 report of the committee on infectious diseases. 31st edition. Elk Grove Village, IL: American Academy of Pediatrics; 2018. p. 537–50.
13. Kroger AT, Duchin J, Vázquez M. General best practice guidelines for immunization. Best practices guidance of the Advisory Committee on Immunization Practices (ACIP). Atlanta, GA: CDC. Available at: www.cdc.gov/vaccines/hcp/acip-recs/general-recs/downloads/general-recs.pdf. Accessed May 1, 2021.
14. Marti F, Steffen R, Mutsch M. Influenza vaccine: a travelers' vaccine? Expert Rev Vaccin 2008;7(5):679–87.
15. Grohskopf LA, Alyanak E, Broder KR, et al. Prevention and control of seasonal influenza with vaccines: recommendations of the advisory committee on immunization practices - United States, 2020-21 Influenza Season. MMWR Recomm Rep 2020;69(8):1–24.
16. American Academy of Pediatrics. Varicella. In: Kimberlin DW, Brady MT, Jackson MA, editors. Red book. 2018 report of the committee on infectious diseases. 31st edition. Elk Grove Village, IL: American Academy of Pediatrics; 2018. p. 869–83.
17. World Health Organization. WHO statement on the meeting of the International Health Regulations Emergency Committee concerning the international spread of wild poliovirus. Available at: https://www.who.int/news/item/05-05-2014-who-statement-on-the-meeting-of-the-international-health-regulations-emergency-committee-concerning-the-international-spread-of-wild-poliovirus. Accessed May 31, 2021.
18. World Health Organization. Polio public health emergency: temporary recommendations to reduce international spread of poliovirus. Geneva, Switzerland: World Health Organization; 2014. Available at: https://polioeradication.org/polio-today/polio-now/public-health-emergency-. Accessed May 23, 2021.
19. Centers for Disease Control and Prevention. Guidance to US clinicians regarding new WHO polio vaccination requirements for travel by residents of and long-term visitors to countries with active polio transmission. Atlanta, GA: US Department of Health and Human Services, CDC; 2014. Available at: http://emergency.cdc.gov/han/han00362.asp.
20. Wallace GS, Seward JF, Pallansch MA. Interim CDC guidance for polio vaccination for travel to and from countries affected by wild poliovirus. MMWR Morb Mortal Wkly Rep 2014;63(27):591–4.
21. Centers for Disease Control and Prevention. Updated recommendations of the Advisory Committee on Immunization Practices (ACIP) regarding routine poliovirus vaccination. MMWR Morb Mortal Wkly Rep 2009;58(30):829–30.
22. Elhamidi Y, Mahamud A, Safdar M, et al. Progress toward poliomyelitis eradication—Pakistan, January 2016–September 2017. MMWR Morb Mortal Wkly Rep 2017;66(46):1276–80.

23. World Health Organization. Statement following the twenty-eighth IHR emergency committee for polio. Available at: https://www.who.int/news/item/21-05-2021-statement-following-the-twenty-eighth-ihr-emergency-committee-for-polio. Accessed May 23, 2021.
24. Crump JA, Sjölund-Karlsson M, Gordon MA, et al. Epidemiology, clinical presentation, laboratory diagnosis, antimicrobial resistance, and antimicrobial management of invasive Salmonella infections. Clin Microbiol Rev 2015;28(4):90137.
25. François Watkins LK, Winstead A, Appiah GD, et al. Update on extensively drug-resistant salmonella serotype typhi infections among travelers to or from Pakistan and Report of Ceftriaxone-Resistant Salmonella Serotype Typhi Infections Among Travelers to Iraq - United States, 2018-2019. MMWR Morb Mortal Wkly Rep 2020; 69:618.
26. Centers for Disease Control and Prevention. Health alert network: extensively drug-resistant salmonella typhi infections among U.S. residents without international travel. Available at: https://emergency.cdc.gov/han/2021/han00439.asp. Accessed May 23, 2021.
27. Jackson BR, Iqbal S, Mahon B. Updated recommendations for the use of typhoid vaccine—Advisory Committee on Immunization Practices, United States, 2015. MMWR Morb Mortal Wkly Rep 2015;64(11):305–8.
28. Koff RS. Clinical manifestations and diagnosis of hepatitis A virus infection. Vaccine 1992;10(Suppl 1):S15.
29. Wasley A, Fiore A, Bell BP. Hepatitis A in the era of vaccination. Epidemiol Rev 2006;28:101–11.
30. Fiore AE. Hepatitis A transmitted by food. Clin Infect Dis 2004;38(5):705–15.
31. Nelson NP, Link-Gelles R, Hofmeister MG, et al. Update: recommendations of the advisory committee on immunization practices for use of hepatitis A vaccine for postexposure prophylaxis and for preexposure prophylaxis for international travel. MMWR Morb Mortal Wkly Rep 2018;67:1216.
32. Nelson NP. Updated dosing instructions for immune globulin (human) GamaSTAN S/D for hepatitis A virus prophylaxis. MMWR Morb Mortal Wkly Rep 2017;66:959–60.
33. Keeffe EB, Iwarson S, McMahon BJ, et al. Safety and immunogenicity of hepatitis A vaccine in patients with chronic liver disease. Hepatology 1998;27(3):881–6.
34. Rubin LG, Levin MJ, Ljungman P, et al. Infectious Diseases Society of America 2013 IDSA clinical practice guideline for vaccination of the immunocompromised host. Clin Infect Dis 2014;58(3):e44–100.
35. Gautret P, Parola P. Rabies vaccination for international travelers. Vaccine 2012; 30(2):126–33.
36. Rupprecht CE, Gibbons RV. Clinical practice. Prophylaxis against rabies. N Engl J Med 2004;351(25):2626–35.
37. World Health Organization. WHO expert consultation on rabies. World Health Organ Tech Rep Ser 2005;931:1–88.
38. Rupprecht CE, Briggs D, Brown CM, et al. Use of a reduced (4-dose) vaccine schedule for postexposure prophylaxis to prevent human rabies: recommendations of the Advisory Committee on Immunization Practices. MMWR Recomm Rep 2010;59(RR-2):1–9.
39. Hills SL, Walter EB, Atmar RL, et al. Japanese encephalitis vaccine: recommendations of the advisory committee on immunization practices. MMWR Recomm Rep 2019;68(No. RR-2):1–33.

40. Monath T, Cetron MS, Teuwen DE. Yellow fever vaccine. In: Plotkin SA, Orenstein WA, Offit PA, editors. Vaccines. 5th edition. Philadelphia, PA: Saunders Elsevier; 2008. p. 959–1055.
41. Staples JE, Gershman M, Fischer M, et al. Yellow fever vaccine: recommendations of the Advisory Committee on Immunization Practices (ACIP). MMWR Recomm Rep 2010;59:1.
42. Lindsey NP, Rabe IB, Miller ER, et al. Adverse event reports following yellow fever vaccination, 2007-13. J Trav Med 2016;23(5):10.1093.
43. American Academy of Pediatrics. Meningococcal infections. In: Kimberlin DW, Brady MT, Jackson MA, editors. Red book. 2018 report of the committee on infectious diseases. 31st edition. Elk Grove Village, IL: American Academy of Pediatrics; 2018. p. 550–60.
44. World Health Organization. Epidemic meningitis control in countries of the African meningitis belt, 2016. Wkly Epidemiol Rec 2017;92(13):145–54.
45. Halperin SA, Bettinger JA, Greenwood B, et al. The changing and dynamic epidemiology of meningococcal disease. Vaccine 2012;30(Suppl 2):B26–36.
46. Mbaeyi SA, Bozio CH, Duffy J, et al. Meningococcal vaccination: recommendations of the advisory committee on immunization practices, United States, 2020. MMWR Recomm Rep 2020;69(No. RR-9):1–41.
47. Trotter CL, Lingani C, Fernandez K, et al. Impact of MenAfriVac in nine countries of the African meningitis belt, 2010–2015: an analysis of surveillance data. Lancet Infect Dis 2017;17(8):867–72.
48. MacNeil JR, Rubin L, Folaranmi T, et al. Use of serogroup B meningococcal vaccines in adolescents and young adults: recommendations of the Advisory Committee on Immunization Practices, 2015. MMWR Morb Mortal Wkly Rep 2015; 64(41):1171–6.
49. Wong KK, Burdette E, Mahon BE, et al. Recommendations of the advisory committee on immunization practices for use of cholera vaccine. MMWR Morb Mortal Wkly Rep 2017;66:482.
50. American Academy of Pediatrics. Cholera. In: Kimberlin DW, Brady MT, Jackson MA, editors. Red book. 2018 report of the committee on infectious diseases. 31st edition. Elk Grove Village, IL: American Academy of Pediatrics; 2018. p. 883–7.

Prevention of Emerging Infections in Children

Thanyawee Puthanakit, MD[a,*], Suvaporn Anugulruengkitt, MD, PhD[b], Watsamon Jantarabenjakul, MD, PhD[c]

KEYWORDS

- Emerging infections • Prevention • Avian influenza
- Middle-East respiratory syndrome • Dengue • Chikungunya • Ebola

KEY POINTS

- Emerging infectious diseases are major health challenges affecting children globally.
- The zoonoses avian influenza and the Middle East respiratory syndrome, mosquito-borne diseases dengue and chikungunya, and Ebola have been major causes of morbidity and mortality across Asia, Latin America, and Africa in recent years.
- Multiple strategies can be employed for prevention with transmission-targeted prevention, chemoprophylaxis, and vaccination.
- Although multiple vaccines are under development for all, the dengue vaccine is the only pediatric-specific vaccine approved, with potential public health impact if scaled up.

INTRODUCTION

The prevention of emerging infections in children is a constantly dynamic arena, where substantial medical advances have enabled intervention and prevention of infection outbreaks. This article focuses on 5 infections causing significant morbidity and mortality across Asia, Latin America, and Africa in recent years. Because severe acute respiratory syndrome coronavirus 2 (SARS-CoV-2) was reviewed extensively in a previous issue of this journal, it is not addressed in this article. Avian influenza and the Middle East respiratory syndrome (MERS) are highly contagious zoonoses spread through aerosol and droplets that have predominantly affected Asia. Dengue infection and chikungunya are extremely endemic mosquito-borne viruses in tropical regions across Asia, Latin America, and Africa, with vector control and vaccination central to efforts in their management. Ebola is a highly contagious virus spread through

[a] Division of Pediatric Infectious Diseases, Department of Pediatrics, Faculty of Medicine, Chulalongkorn University, King Chulalongkorn Memorial Hospital, 9th Floor, Sor Kor Building, Rama 4 Road, Patumwan, Bangkok 10330, Thailand; [b] Department of Pediatrics, Faculty of Medicine, Chulalongkorn University, Bangkok, Thailand; [c] Center of Excellence for Pediatric Infectious Diseases, Chulalongkorn University and King Chulalongkorn Memorial Hospital, Bangkok, Thailand
* Corresponding author.
E-mail address: thanyawee.p@chula.ac.th

Pediatr Clin N Am 69 (2022) 185–202
https://doi.org/10.1016/j.pcl.2021.08.006 pediatric.theclinics.com

human-to-human contact. The latest information in clinical manifestations, infection, prevention control, chemoprophylaxis, vaccination, and other public health measures effective at controlling and preventing these infections is reviewed.

AVIAN INFLUENZA

Avian influenza is a highly contagious viral disease affecting several species of birds and occasionally affects mammals, including humans. Avian influenza is classified into 2 types, low pathogenic avian influenza and highly pathogenic avian influenza (HPAI) strains. In 1997, human infections with the HPAI virus of type A of subtype H5N1 (A[H5N1]) virus were reported during an outbreak in poultry in Hong Kong SAR, China. Since 2003, this avian virus has spread from Asia to Europe and Africa and has become endemic in poultry populations in some countries. From January 2003 to May 2021, there were 862 cases of human infection with avian influenza A (H5N1) virus, including 193 children reported from 17 countries with a case fatality rate (CFR) of 53%.[1,2] In 2013, human infections with the Asian lineage avian influenza A (H7N9) virus were reported for the first time in China. The virus since has spread in the poultry population across the country and has resulted in more than 1500 reported human cases with high mortality rates. Compared with H5N1-infected children, lower severity and greater transmission have been found in the H7N9-infected children.[3] Other avian influenza viruses have resulted in sporadic human infections, including the avian influenza virus subtypes A(H5), A(H7N7), and A(H9N2) viruses.

The route of transmission from animals to humans is direct or indirect exposure to infected live or dead poultry or contaminated environments, such as live bird markets. Human-to-human transmission is rare; there previously have been reports of transmission in family clusters.[4] Because of the possibility of transmission and severity of disease, however, droplet and contact transmission–based precautions should be considered as well as aerosol transmission–based precautions in aerosol-generating procedures in health care settings.[5]

Prevention and Control

Personal protective measures

The best prevention measure is to avoid sources of exposure.[6] Several measures may be taken to prevent animal-to-human transmission, including avoidance of poultry farms, contact with wild and domestic birds in live poultry markets, entering areas where poultry may be slaughtered, and contact with any surfaces that may be contaminated with feces from poultry or other animals. Good food safety and hygiene practices also are advisable. Prevention of human-to-human transmission can be facilitated by handwashing with soap and water or alcohol-based sanitizer; good respiratory hygiene (covering the mouth and nose when coughing or sneezing and correct use and disposal of tissues); avoidance of touching eyes, nose, or mouth if hands are unwashed; and cleaning and disinfection of surfaces and objects. In terms of managing suspected index cases, practice of early self-isolation for symptomatic persons and avoidance of close contact with symptomatic persons are advisable.

Postexposure chemoprophylaxis

According to Centers for Disease Control and Prevention (CDC) recommendations, chemoprophylaxis with influenza antiviral medications can be considered for persons with high-risk and moderate-risk exposure to avian influenza (household members, closed contact to or health care workers not protected with appropriate equipment during exposure to confirmed or probable cases).[7] Administration of chemoprophylaxis should begin as soon as possible (within 48 hours) after exposure with neuraminidase inhibitors (oseltamivir and zanamivir). Instead of the once-daily typical chemoprophylaxis dosing for seasonal influenza viruses, administration of chemoprophylaxis for avian influenza should be administered twice daily. Chemoprophylaxis should continue for 5 days to 10 days depending on exposure time. There is a role for postexposure chemoprophylaxis in children with confirmed cases in household contacts. Detail on dosage is useful.

Vaccination

The first avian influenza vaccine approved by the US Food and Drug administration (FDA) was a nonadjuvant subvirion H5N1 avian influenza vaccine in 2007. Conventional influenza vaccine platforms predominantly rely on production in embryonated chicken eggs and have low immunogenicity. In contrast, an ideal vaccine for an avian influenza pandemic should induce a robust protective immune response with minimal antigen use, provide cross-protection against viruses from different clades, and be rapidly producible if a pandemic occurs.[8] In response, new avian influenza vaccine development has expanded to several different platforms to overcome these issues. Use of adjuvants plays an important role in augmenting protective immunity by accelerating helper T-cell function. An oil-in-water emulsion (AS03)-adjuvant subvirion H5N1 avian influenza vaccine was approved for prepandemic use in the European Union (EU) in 2008 and in the United States in 2013.[9] AS03-adjuvant H5N1 vaccines not only are highly immunogenic against the homologous vaccine strain but also induce cross-clade neutralizing antibodies against circulating antigenically distinct H5N1 viruses,[10,11] including in children ages 6 months to 17 years.[12] The MF59-adjuvant tetravalent vaccine contains A/H5N1, and seasonal A/H3N1, A/H1N1, and B components also induce similar antibody responses and reactogenicity compared with administration of separate A/H5N1 and seasonal vaccines.[13] The modified vaccinia virus Ankara (MVA), a viral vector platform, also is well tolerated and immunogenic with approved use in adults by the World Health Organization (WHO) and EU.[14,15] Moreover, there are other platforms to develop avian influenza vaccines, such as virus-like particles (VLPs) and nonreplicating adenoviral vectored vaccines–stable double-stranded DNA genome and vectors, such as adenovirus (Ad5, Ad26, ChAdOx1, and BAdV-3) in clinical trials.[16]

Currently available H5N1 vaccines in children are the AS03-adjuvant vaccine for infants greater than 6 months and children and adolescents ages less than 17 years, administered 0.25 mL intramuscularly followed by a second 0.25-mL dose 21 days later, although the MF59-adjunvant vaccine can be administered as 0.5 mL intramuscularly followed by a second 0.5-mL dose 21 days later. There are no studies, however, of adjuvanted AS03-adjuvant or MF59-adjuvant vaccines among infants less than 6 months.[17]

Prepandemic vaccine production and stockpiling are important parts of preparedness planning when outbreaks occur. The limitation, however, is vaccine matching relative to actual antigenic diversity of circulating H5N1 viruses and regarding timing due to the uncertainty of when the next pandemic will occur and the shelf-life of stored bulk antigens. Another approach is prepandemic vaccination administration to specific segments of the population and single revaccination boosters in the future. The widespread use of prepandemic vaccines among the population, however, must weigh the potential risks of unexpected adverse reactions with the benefit of vaccinations. Therefore, this approach should be considered in those with high risk of exposure to pandemic influenza, such as health care workers, but not in children.

THE MIDDLE EAST RESPIRATORY SYNDROME

MERS is an emerging respiratory virus caused by the MERS coronavirus (MERS-CoV) that first was identified in Saudi Arabia in 2012 with high case fatality rates. A major outbreak occurred outside the Middle East in South Korea, and infections were reported in 27 countries in 2015.[18] MERS-CoV also occurs in children, most commonly from household contacts. Lower mortality has been observed in children compared with adults.[19,20] The mechanism of transmission from animals to humans is not fully understood, but dromedary camels are a major intermediate host for MERS-CoV and an animal source of infection in humans.[21] Strains of MERS-CoV that are identical to human strains have been isolated from dromedaries in several countries, including Egypt, Oman, Qatar, and Saudi Arabia. No history of exposure to camels, however, is present in more than half of patients with primary MERS-CoV infections.[22,23] There is evidence of human-to-human transmission from clustering of cases in hospitals and among household contacts.[24–26] Consequently, airborne, droplet, and contact transmission–based precautions are recommended for patients with suspected MERS-CoV infection by the WHO and CDC.

Prevention and Control

Personal protective measures

General prevention measures are health education to promote community awareness of the disease. There are several strategies to prevent camel-to-human transmission[21,27–29]: avoid direct contact with camels (including nasal and eye discharge, urine, and feces) and camel products (eg, milk and meat), especially with symptomatic camels and during seasons of high transmission, usually between April and July. This is the season where new camel generations become susceptible to MERS-CoV infection after the decline of their maternal protective antibodies.[30] Frequent handwashing and use of personal protective equipment while handling dromedary camels are advised for those with occupational risk, such as farmers, veterinarians, market workers, and slaughterhouse workers. Educational campaigns can be implemented to target camel owners and the general public to inform them of the risks of consuming unpasteurized camel products (eg, milk) and undercooked meat. Furthermore, disease control in camels is essential and includes strict regulation of camel movements, including a requirement for MERS-CoV infection clearance prior to importation and transport of camels between farms or to slaughterhouses, and camels with detectable MERS-CoV RNA should be quarantined and tested at regular intervals.

Prevention of human-to-human transmission, particularly in household contacts, includes observation of respiratory etiquette during sneezing or coughing in suspected or confirmed MERS-CoV–positive patients, regular mask use, and minimal touching of surfaces near MERS-CoV–infected persons. Disposable glove use is advised when in contact with bodily fluids, including urine, stool, vomit, and respiratory secretions. All waste generated in the room of a MERS-CoV–positive patient should be bagged securely. Hand hygiene with alcohol-based hand rub should be performed by both the infected patient and caregiver following any contact with the patient or their environment. Household items in the MERS-CoV–positive patient room should be cleaned regularly with Environmental Protection Agency–approved commercial solution or diluted bleach (1 part bleach to 99 parts water).

Postexposure chemoprophylaxis

Although current studies of ribavirin and lopinavir/ritonavir for 14 days after high-risk exposure to patients with severe MERS-CoV preisolation pneumonia report a 40% decrease in the risk of infection,[31] there are no recommended regimens for preexposure or postexposure chemoprophylaxis.

Vaccination

There currently are no vaccines available for the prevention of MERS, although there are several vaccines in development in camels and humans.[26,32,33] Several challenges are present in MERS-CoV vaccine development, including absence of economic incentives; because MERS-CoV infections occur only sporadically in humans and are contained mostly in 1 geographic area, no suitable animal models exist for MERS-CoV disease for testing, and neutralizing antibodies titers wane rapidly over time in humans who recover from MERS-CoV infection, leaving uncertainty on the duration of its protection.[34,35]

There are multiple investigational vaccines developed against MERS-CoV2 in humans, however, no trial studies in children. Viral S proteins and their fragments are key vaccine targets in MERS-CoV. GLS-5300, a DNA vaccine expressing a full-length MERS coronavirus S-glycoprotein antigen, is well tolerated and immunogenic in humans.[36] The recombinant MVA vaccine with MVA-MERS-S has a favorable safety profile without serious or severe adverse events.[37] It induces both humoral and cell-mediated responses against MERS-CoV. ChAdOx1 MERS, a candidate simian adenovirus-vectored vaccine expressing a full-length spike surface glycoprotein, and is safe and well-tolerated.[38] A single dose is able to elicit both humoral and cellular responses against MERS-CoV. Several platforms of MERS-CoV vaccines have been developed further in response to the SARS-CoV-2 pandemic in 2021.

DENGUE

Dengue is a global public health threat. It is common in more than 100 countries around the world, especially in endemic areas in Southeast Asia, the Western Pacific, Latin America, and Africa. Asia shares approximately 7% of the global burden of dengue.[39] There are 96 million people who have symptomatic dengue infection each year globally and an estimated 40,000 people die from severe dengue.[40,41] The number of dengue cases reported to the WHO increased more than 8-fold in the past 2 decades, from 505,430 cases in 2000 to more than 2.4 million in 2010, and 5.2 million in 2019.[39] Factors contributing to dengue infection transmission have included rapid urbanization, increased population density, globalization of trade and travel, and lack of effective prevention control methods available.[42]

Dengue is caused by dengue viruses, which are single-stranded RNA viruses with 4 serotypes: DEN-1, DEN-2, DEN-3, and DEN-4. The virus belongs to the genus *Flavivirus*, of the family Flaviviridae. Dengue virus is transmitted mainly to humans by the bite of infected *Aedes* mosquitoes, mainly *A aegypti*.[42] Its clinical manifestations vary widely, ranging from mild febrile illness to severe and fatal disease. Severe complications are plasma leakage, severe hemorrhage, and organ dysfunction. There currently are no specific antiviral agents to treat dengue infection. Treatment remains adequate fluid management and supportive treatment.

Prevention and Control

The WHO recommends integrated vector management (IVM),[43] which is a process for managing vector populations for the optimal use of resources for vector control and vaccination.

Mosquito Bite Prevention

Measures to prevent mosquito bites are (1) wearing light-colored long pants and long-sleeved shirts when spending time outdoors or when traveling to endemic areas; (2) clothing, tents, and bed nets treated with permethrin (an insecticide), especially for young children and sick or older people; (3) mosquito coils or other insecticide vaporizers, which also may reduce indoor biting; and (4) using mosquito repellents applied to exposed skin and clothing in strict accordance with product label instructions.[44] Products containing oil of lemon eucalyptus or para-menthane-diol should be avoided in children under 3 years of age, and application of insect repellent to the hands, eyes, mouth, cuts, or irritated skin should be avoided in all children.[45]

Vector control

Vector control is recommended by environmental management, chemical, and biological controls.

Environmental management is focused on elimination of potential mosquito breeding sites and reduction of standing water sites. Accumulation of stagnant water should be prevented, and containers with water necessary for use should be covered with a fine mesh to prevent mosquito entry. Emptying and cleaning of domestic water storage containers on a weekly basis should be conducted. These source reduction strategies are effective when performed regularly.[43]

Chemical control includes application of appropriate insecticides to outdoor water storage containers to kill immature larvae and use of insecticides to kill flying mosquitoes.[43]

Biological control against eggs, larvae, and mosquitoes are also essential and can be performed using larvivorous fish, such as *Poecilia reticulata* and *Mesocyclops formosanus*, and *Crustacean* to control larvae.[46] Using larvivorous fish is a cost-effective and eco-friendly strategy in controlling the population of *A aegypti*.[47] A novel method is genetic control of *Aedes* using *Wolbachia*, which is a bacterial agent genetically inserted into vectors to interfere with the reproductive system of the vector, resulting in suppression of vector populations and therefore limiting the transmission of mosquito-borne diseases.[48]

Vector surveillance includes larval surveys, adult surveys, landing/biting collections, and resting collections, which are important to prioritizing and planning areas and timing for vector control.[43]

Vaccination

To date, only 1 licensed vaccine is available (live, attenuated [recombinant] tetravalent vaccine with a yellow fever 17D backbone [CYD] tetravalent dengue vaccine [TDV], or Dengvaxia, Sanofi Pasteur Inc.). In 2015, CYD-TDV was approved for dengue prevention in persons ages 9 years to 16 years with laboratory-confirmed previous dengue infection. This recommendation was based on study results of combined analyses of phase 3 trials (CYD 14, CYD 15, and CYD 23/57).[49] Average vaccine efficacy (VE) at 25 months for virologically confirmed dengue (VCD) was 65.6% (95% CI, 60.7–69.9). Overall VEs against severe disease and hospitalization due to VCD were 92.9% (95% CI, 76.1–97.9) and 80.8% (95% CI, 70.1–87.7), respectively. Further post hoc retrospective analyses of long-term safety data revealed an increased risk of severe dengue disease in those who were seronegative at baseline.[50] In countries considering vaccination as part of their dengue control program, prevaccination screening is recommended, so only those with evidence of a past dengue infection are vaccinated.[51] The dengue vaccine also can be considered in areas with dengue seroprevalence rates of at least 80% by age 9 years.[52] A remaining important challenge is regarding vaccine implementation strategies in real-world settings. Dengue vaccination should be based on country-specific data in populations at greatest risk but can include people between ages 9 years and 45 years.[53] A recent study in 2021, a randomized controlled phase 2 noninferiority study (CYD65) among healthy individuals ages 9 years to 50 years demonstrated noninferiority of 2-dose versus 3-dose CYD-TDV for each serotype at both 28 days and 1 year among dengue-seropositive participants. A 2-dose CYD-TDV regimen may be an alternative in individuals who are dengue seropositive at baseline and ages 9 years and older.[54] Although the dengue vaccine is needed for travelers entering endemic areas, there is limited practical use for the CYD-TDV due to the limited number of seropositive travelers and the long vaccination schedule of 3 doses 6 months apart.[55] Several other dengue vaccine candidates, including live, attenuated; purified inactivated; subunit; and DNA vaccines, currently are under clinical development (**Table 1**). There are 2 live, attenuated vaccines currently under evaluation in phase 3 trials.[55,56] Although CYD-TDV does not include nonstructural proteins of dengue, TAK-003 (Takeda) contains the dengue virus serotype 2 backbone, and the TV003/005 (National Institutes of Health [NIH] National Institute of Allergy and Infectious Diseases/Butantan Institute) vaccine contains 3 full genomes of the 4 dengue virus serotypes.[55] Data up to 18 months postvaccination from an ongoing phase 3 study in healthy children ages 4 years to 16 years showed an overall VE of 73.3 (95% CI, 66.5–78.8). TAK-003 was well tolerated and efficacious against symptomatic dengue in children regardless of serostatus before immunization.[57]

CHIKUNGUNYA

Chikungunya is a mosquito-borne viral disease caused by an arbovirus. The name, chikungunya, derives from the Kimakonde language, meaning “that which bends up,” to describe the arthralgia that affected patients suffer from.[58] The first identified case of chikungunya was reported in Tanzania in 1952, and since, periodic outbreaks have occurred in Asia and Africa.[59] Since 2004, chikungunya has spread rapidly and been identified in more than 60 countries throughout Asia, Africa, Europe, and the Americas.[60] Factors held responsible for the resurgence of chikungunya include lack of herd immunity, inefficient vector control activities, and emergence of viral mutations in *A albopictus* mosquitoes as more efficient vectors.[61]

Chikungunya is caused by the chikungunya virus (CHIKV), which is a single-stranded RNA virus. The virus belongs to the genus *Alphavirus*, from the family *Togaviridae.* CHIKV is transmitted primarily to humans by the bite of infected mosquitoes, including *A aegypti and A albopictus.*[62] Less common transmission is mother-to-child transmission in mothers who acquire chikungunya infection during the second trimester or within 1 week before delivery, which can cause neonatal chikungunya infection. Chikungunya shares some clinical signs and symptoms with dengue and can be misdiagnosed in areas where dengue is common. The incubation period is 3 days to 7 days (range 1–12 days).[62] It is characterized by a triad of fever, rash, and symmetric polyarthralgia, particularly affecting small joints. Symptoms generally are self-limited and usually resolve within 7 days to 10 days, but chronic symptoms of arthralgia can occur and persist for many months to years. Children tend to have less arthralgia compared with adults and more neurologic and dermatologic manifestations, such as bullous rashes and pigment changes.[63] In areas where chikungunya is not endemic, the diagnosis should be considered in travelers recently returning from endemic areas with acute onset of fever and polyarthralgia.[64] There are no specific antiviral agents to treat chikungunya infection. Treatment is supportive care includes rest, antipyretics, and analgesics. The use of nonsteroidal anti-inflammatory drugs, corticosteroids, and physiotherapy may benefit patients with persistent joint pain.[62]

Prevention and Control

Chikungunya is a mosquito-borne disease. Prevention, therefore, is focused on mosquito bite prevention and vector control in accordance with epidemiologic surveillance similar to dengue.[46] Details on vector control are discussed previously.

Table 1
Overview of current dengue vaccine clinical trials[55–57]

Platform	Vaccine	Vaccine Structure	Doses	Clinical Trial Phase
Live, attenuated	CYD-TDV (Dengvaxia, Sanofi Pasteur)	Yellow fever backbone with prM and E proteins from DEN-1-4	3 doses (6 mo apart)	Licensed in 2015
	TAK-003 (DENVax, Takeda)	DEN-2 backbone with prM and E proteins of from DEN-1, 3, 4	2 doses (3 mo apart)	3
	TV003/T005 (Tetravax, US NIH)	Deletion of 3′UTR of DEN-1, DEN-3, DEN-4 and a chimeric DEN-2/DEN-4	1 dose	3
Purified inactivated	PIV	Purified formalin inactivated DEN-1-4 and adjuvants	2 doses (1 mo apart)	1/2
Subunit	V180	Recombinant truncated protein containing DEN-80E and adjuvants	3 doses (1 mo apart)	1
DNA	D1ME100	Recombinant plasmid vector encoding prM/E of DEN-1 and adjuvants	3 doses (0, 1, 5 mo)	1
	TVDV	Recombinant plasmid vector encoding prM/E proteins of DEN-1-4 and adjuvants	3 doses (0, 1, 3 mo)	1

Abbreviations: DENVax, live, attenuated tetravalent dengue vaccine; PIV, purified formalin-inactivated virus vaccine; TVDV, the tetravalent DNA vaccine.

Vaccination

Currently, no CHIKV vaccine has been licensed, but several are in the pipeline of vaccine research in clinical and preclinical studies: live, attenuated; VLP; inactivated; and viral vector vaccines[65] (**Table 2**). The challenge of developing a CHIKV vaccine is reduction of side effects, such as secondary arthralgia following immunization with the attenuated virus.[46] The first live, attenuated CHIKV vaccine in clinical trials was the TSI-GSD-218. The study on TSI-GSD-218 was terminated, however, due to safety concerns, with 8% of study participants developing mild arthralgia.[66]

The only CHIKV vaccine candidate to enter phase 3 clinical trials is VLA1553. The VLA1553 is a monovalent single-dose, live, attenuated vaccine based on an infectious clone (CHIKV LR2006-OPY1) vaccine candidate attenuated by deleting a major part of the gene encoding the nonstructural replicase complex protein nsP3.[67,68]

The VLP, the VRC-CHKVLP059-00-VP, is one of the most advanced technologies to date. In a 3-dose escalation phase 1 trial, the VLP vaccine was found to be safe, well tolerated, and highly immunogenic, with a 100% seroconversion rate in all dose cohorts after booster immunizations and cross-protection seen against multiple CHIKV strains.[69,70] The candidate currently has finished phase 2 clinical trials (NCT02562482), and phase 3 trials are needed to assess clinical efficacy.[71]

EBOLA

Ebolaviruses are negative-strand RNA viruses in the Filoviridae family, first identified in 1976. Of the 5 Ebola species known to date, 4, including the Sudan Ebola, Zaire Ebola, Bundibugyo Ebola, and Tai Forest Ebola viruses, are the known causes of epidemics in humans.[72] More than 20 outbreaks of Ebola disease have been identified in sub-Saharan Africa, mainly due to the Zaire and Sudan viruses. The largest outbreak occurred during 2013 to 2016 in West Africa, predominantly affecting Guinea, Sierra Leone, and Liberia.[73] Approximately 20% of Ebola virus disease (EVD) cases were reported in children.[74]

Table 2
Chikungunya vaccines in clinical trials[65–71]

Platform	Vaccine	Vaccine Type	Clinical Trial Phase
Live, attenuated	VLA1553	CHIKV with nsP3 deletion	3
	MV-CHIK	Recombinant live, attenuated measles vaccine expressing CHIKV VLP structural proteins	2
VLP	VRC-CHKVLP059-00-VP (PXVX0317 CHIKV-VLP)	VLP with plasmid expressing CHIKV structural proteins (West African strain 37997)	2
Whole-virus inactivated vaccine	BBV87	Inactivated whole-virion vaccine based on East, Central, South, African genotypea	1
Viral vector	ChAdOx1 Chik	Replication-deficient simian adenoviral vector expressing CHIKV antigens	1

EVD is a zoonotic disease, of which fruit bats are thought to be natural hosts. Humans likely are infected by handling infected forest animals or by contact with infected bats. Secondary human-to-human transmission can occur via direct contact with blood, secretions, or other body fluids from infected humans or corpses. The virus can persist in immunologically privileged sites, such as the testes, for weeks to months; therefore, sexual transmission by survivors of EVD can occur.[75]

The incubation period for EVD is 2 days to 21 days (mean 4–10 days).[76] Symptoms begin with dry symptoms, for example, fever, headache, muscle aches, and joint pain, followed by wet symptoms, for example, nausea, vomiting, and diarrhea, at approximately day 4 of illness.[76] Diarrhea can be severe, leading to severe dehydration and electrolyte imbalance, especially hyponatremia. Hemorrhagic manifestations usually occur during later stages of the disease, including epistaxis, hematemesis, and hematochezia. Laboratory findings in EVD include leukopenia, lymphopenia, and elevated transaminase levels. Persons with severe disease typically die due to multisystem organ failure by 7 days to 10 days after onset of disease.[73,77] In children, because clinical features of EVD are nonspecific, epidemiologic criteria of history of contact with patients with confirmed EVD is important. The gold standard laboratory diagnostic test is real-time reverse transcription–polymerase chain reaction from blood samples, usually 3 days to 6 days after the onset of the symptoms. Blood tests for ELISA IgM and IgG antibodies are quick laboratory methods for diagnosis or surveillance for EVD. Early supportive care with intravenous fluids, electrolyte supplementation, and nutritional support can reduce mortality rates to approximately 40%.[77–79] Isotonic intravenous fluids with or without added dextrose are recommended as marked hyponatremia is common in patients with EVD.[80] The only FDA-approved treatment of EVD caused by the *Zaire ebolavirus* in adult and pediatric patients is the triple monoclonal antibody REGN-EB3 (atoltivimab/maftivimab/odesivimab-ebgn, INMAZEB®, Regeneron Pharmaceuticals). A randomized trial of REGN-EB3 in the Democratic Republic of the Congo during 2018 to 2019 showed that patients receiving the triple monoclonal antibody REG-EB3 had lower 28-day mortality rates of 33.5% compared with 51.3% in the triple monoclonal antibody ZMapp group (P = .002).[81]

Prevention and Control

Transmission of Ebola viruses occur through direct contact with blood or bodily fluids, most often in the context of providing care to a sick family member or patient, or participation in burial rituals that involve washing and touching corpses.[82] Therefore, risk of EVD in children is attributed to contact with sick parents, caretakers, and relatives. Pediatric EVD often occurs in children younger than 5 years of age. Transmission through breast milk and congenital transmission also have been documented.[83] Practices in reducing risk of human-to-human transmission include contact isolation, wearing of gloves and appropriate personal protective equipment while taking care of ill patients, and regular handwashing after patient contact. Contact tracing of people with unprotected direct contact with patients during the symptomatic phase of illness should be monitored daily for evidence of disease for 21 days after last contact. Confinement of asymptomatic people usually is not warranted, due to low risk of transmission during the incubation period; however, those who develop signs or symptoms compatible with EVD should be isolated immediately until the diagnosis can be excluded.[84]

Vaccination

The recombinant vesicular stomatitis virus pseudotyped with Ebola Zaire Glycoprotein (rVSVΔG-ZEBOV-GP, Ervebo®, Merck & Co., Inc., USA), a replication-competent, live, attenuated vaccine, has been approved by the FDA for the prevention of EVD caused by the Ebola virus species *Z ebolavirus* (EBOV) in adults ages greater than or equal to 18 years. The rVSVΔG-ZEBOV-GP Ebola vaccine contains the vesicular stomatitis virus that has been modified to contain a protein from the *Z ebolavirus*. The vaccine is administered as a single intramuscular dose. Common adverse reactions include arthralgia, myalgia, rash, headache, fever, and fatigue. The Advisory Committee for Immunization Practices recommend preexposure vaccination with Ervebo for adults who are at highest risk for potential occupational exposure to EBOV because they are responding to an outbreak of EVD, working as health care personnel at Ebola treatment centers or as laboratorians. VE was evaluated among clusters of contacts of confirmed EVD patients in Guinea during the 2014 to 2016 Ebola outbreak in West Africa.[85] A study demonstrated that among 2108 participants vaccinated immediately, none developed EVD greater than or equal to 10 days after randomization. This is in contrast to the delayed vaccination group (21 days after randomization), where 10 of 1429 participants developed EVD greater than or equal to 10 days after randomization. VE in this study was 100% (95% CI, 63.5%–100%). The Sierra Leone Trial to Introduce a Vaccine against Ebola (STRIVE) trial, which combined phase II and phase III clinical trials to assess the safety and efficacy of rVSV-ZEBOV, found that no cases of Ebola were reported in the 7998 participants who were vaccinated.[86] rVSV-ZEBOV was used as a ring vaccination strategy during the 2016 outbreak in Guinea. There currently are 1510 individuals, including 303 children ages between 6 years and 17 years old, who have received vaccines through compassionate use. There were no secondary cases of EVD that occurred among those vaccinated. The most common adverse event was headache (12%), with myalgia (3%) and arthralgia in less than 1% in children, compared with 7% in adults.[87]

Table 3
Summary of prevention of emerging infections

	Prevention Control Measures		Vaccine/
Disease	**Community Settings**	**Hospital Settings**	**Chemoprophylaxis**
Avian influenza	Avoidance of poultry exposure during outbreaks	Droplet, contact, and airborne precautions	Oseltamivir chemoprophylaxis
MERS	Avoidance of camel exposure	Droplet, contact, and airborne precautions	Vaccines are in preclinical and clinical studies.
Dengue	Avoidance of mosquito bites Vector control and surveillance	Standard precautions	Licensed dengue vaccine approved in 2017
Chikungunya	Avoidance of mosquito bites Vector control and surveillance	Standard precautions	Vaccines are in preclinical and clinical studies
Ebola	Human-to-human transmission Burial ceremonies	Standard universal and contact precautions; in health care setting, it is important to use personal protective equipment and environmental infection control	Licensed Ebola vaccine approved in 2019

The Chimpanzee adenovirus type 3 vector vaccine (ChAd3-EBO-Z) was studied as a phase II clinical trial, using a single dose in 600 children and adolescents (ages 1–17 years) in comparison with MENACWY-TT in Mali and Senegal. The vaccine induced an anti-glycoprotein Ebola virus antibody response at day 30, which declined by 6 months postvaccination and remained relatively stable thereafter. At 12 months postvaccination, 99.7% of participants had antibody concentrations greater than 36.11 ELISA units/mL. Anti-glycoprotein Ebola virus antibody had the highest antibody geometric mean titer in those 1 year to 5 years of age. A hypothesis was made that preexisting immunity against the adenovirus vector of the vaccine could have augmented their vaccine response. The most common reactions seen were fever, which occurred with higher rates in children 1 year to 5 years of age. Future research studies plan to focus on multivalent approaches, targeting also the Sudan strain. In addition, heterologous prime-boost strategies, for example, using ChAd3-EBO-Z for priming and the MVA-based vaccines, are available.[88]

In conclusion, Ebola disease in children has lower case rates compared with adults due to lower exposure. Prevention is by avoidance of direct contact with people with confirmed EVD. The clinical diagnostic criteria include history of contact with patients with EVD and subsequent evidence of fever 2 days to 21 days after contact. Although there is a vaccine approved for Ebola disease, this is only available for adults. Children may benefit from vaccination during outbreaks using the ring vaccination strategy.

SUMMARY

Emerging infectious diseases are undergoing a global health challenge. Multiple strategies can be employed for prevention with transmission-targeted prevention, chemoprophylaxis, and vaccination (**Table 3**).

CLINICS CARE POINTS

Avian influenza

- From 2003 to 2021, there were 193 children infected with the H5N1 virus, with a CFR of 53%.[1,2]
- Avoidance of exposure to infected live or dead poultry is an important preventive measure.
- Prepandemic vaccine production and stockpiling are important preventive measures. The AS03-adjuvant subvirion H5N1 avian influenza vaccine is approved for use in the EU and the United States.[9]

The Middle East respiratory syndrome

- MERS-CoV first was identified in Saudi Arabia in 2012 with very high case fatality rates.
- MERS-CoV in children usually occurs from household contacts from human-to-human transmission.
- There are vaccines in development targeting viral spike proteins, for example, ChAdOx1 MERS, a simian adenovirus-vector vaccine expressing full-length spike surface glycoproteins.[38]

Dengue

- Dengue is public health priority, with more than 5.2 million case reports in 2019.[39]
- Prevention in children includes mosquito bite prevention with repellents, bed nets treated with permethrin, and vaccination.[44]
- CYD-TDV is a live, attenuated recombinant tetravalent vaccine with a yellow fever 17D backbone licensed in 2015. Vaccination is recommended for persons ages 9 years to 45 years with previous infection. The dengue vaccine also can be considered in areas with dengue seroprevalence rates of greater than 80% by age 9 years.[52]

Chikungunya

- Chikungunya is an emerging disease that has spread to more than 60 countries throughout Asia, Africa, Europe, and the Americas.[60]
- Prevention is focused on mosquito bite prevention and vector control.[46]
- Chikungunya vaccine development has progressed to phase 3 for the VLA1553, a monovalent single-dose, live, attenuated vaccine.[68]

Ebola

- EVD is a zoonotic disease affecting mainly West Africa.
- Human-to-human transmission occurs via direct contact with blood, secretions, or other bodily fluids. Children usually are infected from household contacts.
- Ervebo, a replication-competent, live, attenuated vaccine, is approved for use by the FDA in the prevention of EVD caused by the EBOV species in adults ages greater than or equal to 18 years. Ring vaccination strategies were used successfully during the 2016 outbreak in Guinea.

DISCLOSURE

The authors have nothing to disclose.

ACKNOWLEDGMENTS

The authors would like to acknowledge Dr Wipaporn Natalie Songtaweesin and Miss Rachaneekorn Nadsasarn for their support in the preparation of this article.

REFERENCES

1. World Health Organization. Regional Office for the Western Pacific. Avian Influenza Weekly Update. 2021. Available at: https://apps.who.int/iris/handle/10665/341148. Accessed June 11, 2021.
2. Oner AF, Dogan N, Gasimov V, et al. H5N1 avian influenza in children. Clin Infect Dis 2012;55(1):26–32.
3. Sha J, Dong W, Liu S, et al. Differences in the Epidemiology of Childhood Infections with Avian Influenza A H7N9 and H5N1 Viruses. PLoS One 2016;11(10):e0161925.
4. Ungchusak K, Auewarakul P, Dowell SF, et al. Probable person-to-person transmission of avian influenza A (H5N1). N Engl J Med 2005;352(4):333–40.
5. Centers for Disease Control and Prevention. Interim Guidance for Infection Control Within Healthcare Settings When Caring for Confirmed Cases, Probable Cases, and Cases Under Investigation for Infection with Novel Influenza A Viruses Associated with Severe Disease. 2014. Available at: https://www.cdc.gov/flu/avianflu/novel-flu-infection-control.htm. Accessed June 11, 2021.
6. Centers for Disease Control and Prevention. Prevention and Treatment of Avian Influenza A Viruses in People. 2017. Available at: https://www.cdc.gov/flu/avianflu/prevention.htm. Accessed June 11, 2021.
7. Centers for Disease Control and Prevention. Interim Guidance on Follow-up of Close Contacts of Persons Infected with Novel Influenza A Viruses Associated with Severe Human Disease and on the Use of Antiviral Medications for Chemoprophylaxis. 2015. Available at: https://www.cdc.gov/flu/avianflu/novel-av-chemoprophylaxis-guidance.htm. Accessed June 11, 2021.
8. Clegg CH, Rininger JA, Baldwin SL. Clinical vaccine development for H5N1 influenza. Expert Rev Vaccin 2013;12(7):767–77.

9. Leroux-Roels I, Borkowski A, Vanwolleghem T, et al. Antigen sparing and cross-reactive immunity with an adjuvant rH5N1 prototype pandemic influenza vaccine: a randomised controlled trial. Lancet 2007;370(9587):580–9.
10. Levie K, Leroux-Roels I, Hoppenbrouwers K, et al. An adjuvanted, low-dose, pandemic influenza A (H5N1) vaccine candidate is safe, immunogenic, and induces cross-reactive immune responses in healthy adults. J Infect Dis 2008; 198(5):642–9.
11. Langley JM, Risi G, Caldwell M, et al. Dose-sparing H5N1 A/Indonesia/05/2005 pre-pandemic influenza vaccine in adults and elderly adults: a phase III, placebo-controlled, randomized study. J Infect Dis 2011;203(12):1729–38.
12. Kosalaraksa P, Jeanfreau R, Frenette L, et al. AS03B-adjuvanted H5N1 influenza vaccine in children 6 months through 17 years of age: a phase 2/3 randomized, placebo-controlled, observer-blinded trial. J Infect Dis 2015;211(5):801–10.
13. Herbinger KH, von Sonnenburg F, Nothdurft HD, et al. A phase II study of an investigational tetravalent influenza vaccine formulation combining MF59®: adjuvanted, pre-pandemic, A/H5N1 vaccine and trivalent seasonal influenza vaccine in healthy adults. Hum Vaccin Immunother 2014;10(1):92–9.
14. Kreijtz JH, Goeijenbier M, Moesker FM, et al. Safety and immunogenicity of a modified-vaccinia-virus-Ankara-based influenza A H5N1 vaccine: a randomised, double-blind phase 1/2a clinical trial. Lancet Infect Dis 2014;14(12):1196–207.
15. European Medicines Agency. Foclivia. 2021. Available at: https://www.ema.europa.eu/en/medicines/human/EPAR/foclivia. Accessed June 11, 2021.
16. Kerstetter LJ, Buckley S, Bliss CM, et al. Adenoviral Vectors as Vaccines for Emerging Avian Influenza Viruses. Front Immunol 2021;11:607333.
17. Wilkins AL, Kazmin D, Napolitani G, et al. AS03- and MF59-Adjuvanted Influenza Vaccines in Children. Front Immunol 2017;8:1760.
18. Korea Centers for Disease Control and Prevention. Middle East Respiratory Syndrome Coronavirus Outbreak in the Republic of Korea, 2015 [published correction appears in Osong Public Health Res Perspect. 2016 Apr;7(2):138]. Osong Public Health Res Perspect 2015;6(4):269–78.
19. Memish ZA, Al-Tawfiq JA, Assiri A, et al. Middle East respiratory syndrome coronavirus disease in children. Pediatr Infect Dis J 2014;33(9):904–6.
20. Al-Tawfiq JA, Kattan RF, Memish ZA. Middle East respiratory syndrome coronavirus disease is rare in children: An update from Saudi Arabia. World J Clin Pediatr 2016;5(4):391–6.
21. Al Hammadi ZM, Chu DK, Eltahir YM, et al. Asymptomatic MERS-CoV Infection in Humans Possibly Linked to Infected Dromedaries Imported from Oman to United Arab Emirates, May 2015. Emerg Infect Dis 2015;21(12):2197–200.
22. Alraddadi BM, Watson JT, Almarashi A, et al. Risk Factors for Primary Middle East Respiratory Syndrome Coronavirus Illness in Humans, Saudi Arabia, 2014. Emerg Infect Dis 2016;22(1):49–55.
23. Centers for Disease Control and Prevention. Interim Infection Prevention and Control Recommendations for Hospitalized Patients with Middle East Respiratory Syndrome Coronavirus (MERS-CoV) Aug. 2. 2019. Available at: https://www.cdc.gov/coronavirus/mers/infection-prevention-control.html. Accessed June 11, 2021.
24. Assiri A, McGeer A, Perl TM, et al. Hospital outbreak of Middle East respiratory syndrome coronavirus [published correction appears in N Engl J Med. 2013 Aug 29;369(9):886]. N Engl J Med 2013;369(5):407–16.

25. Memish ZA, Zumla AI, Al-Hakeem RF, et al. Family cluster of Middle East respiratory syndrome coronavirus infections [published correction appears in N Engl J Med. 2013 Aug 8;369(6):587]. N Engl J Med 2013;368(26):2487–94.
26. Azhar EI, Hashem AM, El-Kafrawy SA, et al. Detection of the Middle East respiratory syndrome coronavirus genome in an air sample originating from a camel barn owned by an infected patient. mBio 2014;5(4):e01450-14.
27. Hotez PJ, Bottazzi ME, Tseng CT, et al. Calling for rapid development of a safe and effective MERS vaccine. Microbes Infect 2014;16(7):529–31.
28. World Health Organization. WHO MERS global summary and Assessment of risk 2019. Available at: https://www.who.int/publications/i/item/10665-326126. Accessed June 11, 2021.
29. Baharoon S, Memish ZA. MERS-CoV as an emerging respiratory illness: A review of prevention methods [published online ahead of print, 2019 Nov 12]. Trav Med Infect Dis 2019;32:101520.
30. Almutairi SE, Boujenane I, Musaad A, et al. Non-genetic factors influencing reproductive traits and calving weight in Saudi camels. Trop Anim Health Prod 2010; 42(6):1087–92.
31. Park SY, Lee JS, Son JS, et al. Post-exposure prophylaxis for Middle East respiratory syndrome in healthcare workers. J Hosp Infect 2019;101(1):42–6. https://doi.org/10.1016/j.jhin.2018.09.005.
32. World Health Organization. WHO Target Product Profiles for MERS-CoV Vaccines. May 7. 2017. Available at: https://www.who.int/publications/m/item/who-target-product-profiles-for-mers-cov-vaccines. Accessed June 11, 2021.
33. Overview of the types/classes of candidate vaccines against MERS-CoV. 2020. Available at: https://www.who.int/publications/m/item/overview-of-the-types-classes-of-candidate-vaccines-against-mers-cov. Accessed June 11, 2021.
34. Vergara-Alert J, Vidal E, Bensaid A, et al. Searching for animal models and potential target species for emerging pathogens: Experience gained from Middle East respiratory syndrome (MERS) coronavirus. One Health 2017;3:34–40.
35. Zhao J, Alshukairi AN, Baharoon SA, et al. Recovery from the Middle East respiratory syndrome is associated with antibody and T-cell responses. Sci Immunol 2017;2(14):eaan5393.
36. Modjarrad K, Roberts CC, Mills KT, et al. Safety and immunogenicity of an anti-Middle East respiratory syndrome coronavirus DNA vaccine: a phase 1, open-label, single-arm, dose-escalation trial. Lancet Infect Dis 2019;19(9):1013–22.
37. Koch T, Dahlke C, Fathi A, et al. Safety and immunogenicity of a modified vaccinia virus Ankara vector vaccine candidate for Middle East respiratory syndrome: an open-label, phase 1 trial. Lancet Infect Dis 2020;20(7):827–38.
38. Folegatti PM, Bittaye M, Flaxman A, et al. Safety and immunogenicity of a candidate Middle East respiratory syndrome coronavirus viral-vectored vaccine: a dose-escalation, open-label, non-randomised, uncontrolled, phase 1 trial [published correction appears in Lancet Infect Dis. 2020 May 12;:] [published correction appears in Lancet Infect Dis. 2020 Jun 8;:]. Lancet Infect Dis 2020;20(7): 816–26.
39. World Health Organization. Dengue and severe dengue. 2021. Available at: https://www.who.int/news-room/fact-sheets/detail/dengue-and-severe-dengue. Accessed June 11, 2021.
40. World Health Organization. Dengue guidelines for diagnosis, treatment, prevention and control. 2009. Available at: https://apps.who.int/iris/handle/10665/44188. Accessed June 11, 2021.

41. Bhatt S, Gething PW, Brady OJ, et al. The global distribution and burden of dengue. Nature 2013;496(7446):504–7.
42. Simmons CP, Farrar JJ, Nguyen vV, et al. Dengue. N Engl J Med 2012;366(15): 1423–32.
43. World Health Organization. Global strategy for dengue prevention and control 2012–2020. 2012. Available at: https://www.who.int/immunization/sage/meetings/2013/april/5_Dengue_SAGE_Apr2013_Global_Strategy.pdf. Accessed June 11, 2021.
44. Vairo F, Haider N, Kock R, et al. Chikungunya: Epidemiology, Pathogenesis, Clinical Features, Management, and Prevention. Infect Dis Clin North Am 2019;33(4): 1003–25.
45. Centers for Disease Control and Prevention. Chikungunya. 2020. Available at: https://www.cdc.gov/mosquitoes/pdfs/MosquitoBitePreventionUS_508.pdf. Accessed June 11, 2021.
46. Silva JVJ Jr, Ludwig-Begall LF, Oliveira-Filho EF, et al. A scoping review of Chikungunya virus infection: epidemiology, clinical characteristics, viral co-circulation complications, and control. Acta Trop 2018;188:213–24.
47. Rather IA, Parray HA, Lone JB, et al. Prevention and Control Strategies to Counter Dengue Virus Infection. Front Cell Infect Microbiol 2017;7:336.
48. Wilke AB, Marrelli MT. Paratransgenesis: a promising new strategy for mosquito vector control. Parasit Vectors 2015;8:342.
49. Hadinegoro SR, Arredondo-García JL, Capeding MR, et al. Efficacy and Long-Term Safety of a Dengue Vaccine in Regions of Endemic Disease. N Engl J Med 2015;373(13):1195–206.
50. Sridhar S, Luedtke A, Langevin E, et al. Effect of Dengue Serostatus on Dengue Vaccine Safety and Efficacy. N Engl J Med 2018;379(4):327–40.
51. World Health Organization. SAGE Evidence to recommendations framework Table 2. 2018. Available at: http://www.who.int/immunization/policy/position_papers/E2R_2_dengue_2018.pdf. Accessed June 11, 2021.
52. Dengue vaccine: WHO position paper, September 2018 - Recommendations. Vaccine 2019;37(35):4848–9.
53. de St Maurice A, Ervin E, Chu A. Ebola, Dengue, Chikungunya, and Zika Infections in Neonates and Infants. Clin Perinatol 2021;48(2):311–29.
54. Coronel-Martínez DL, Park J, López-Medina E, et al. Immunogenicity and safety of simplified vaccination schedules for the CYD-TDV dengue vaccine in healthy individuals aged 9-50 years (CYD65): a randomised, controlled, phase 2, non-inferiority study. Lancet Infect Dis 2021;21(4):517–28.
55. Wilder-Smith A. Dengue vaccine development by the year 2020: challenges and prospects. Curr Opin Virol 2020;43:71–8.
56. Thisyakorn U, Tantawichien T. Dengue vaccine: a key for prevention. Expert Rev Vaccin 2020;19(6):499–506.
57. Biswal S, Borja-Tabora C, Martinez Vargas L, et al. Efficacy of a tetravalent dengue vaccine in healthy children aged 4-16 years: a randomised, placebo-controlled, phase 3 trial. Lancet 2020;395(10234):1423–33 [published correction appears in Lancet. 2020 Apr 4;395(10230):1114].
58. Mason PJ, Haddow AJ. An epidemic of virus disease in Southern Province, Tanganyika Territory, in 1952-1953; an additional note on Chikungunya virus isolations and serum antibodies. Trans R Soc Trop Med Hyg 1957;51(3):238–40.
59. Markoff L. Alphaviruses (Chikungunya, Eastern Equine Encephalitis). In: Bennett JE, editor. Mandell, Douglas, and Bennett's Principles and practice of infectious diseases. 9th edition. Elsevier; 2020. p. 1997–2006.e2.

60. World Health Organization. Chikungunya. 2020. Available at: https://www.who.int/news-room/fact-sheets/detail/chikungunya. Accessed June 11, 2021.
61. World Health Organization. Regional Office for South-East Asia. Guidelines for prevention and control of chikungunya fever. 2019. Available at: https://apps.who.int/iris/handle/10665/205166. Accessed June 11, 2021.
62. American Academy of Pediatrics. Chikungunya. In: Kimberlin DW, Brady MT, Jackson MA, et al, editors. Red Book: 2018 report of the Committee on infectious diseases. 31st edition. Itasca (IL): American Academy of Pediatrics; 2018. p. 271–2.
63. Ward CE, Chapman JI. Chikungunya in Children: A Clinical Review. Pediatr Emerg Care 2018;34(7):510–5.
64. Centers for Disease Control and Prevention. Chikungunya Virus: Clinical Evaluation & Disease. 2018. Available at: https://www.cdc.gov/chikungunya/hc/clinicalevaluation.html. Accessed June 11, 2021.
65. Silva LA, Dermody TS. Chikungunya virus: epidemiology, replication, disease mechanisms, and prospective intervention strategies. J Clin Invest 2017;127(3):737–49.
66. Gorchakov R, Wang E, Leal G, et al. Attenuation of Chikungunya virus vaccine strain 181/clone 25 is determined by two amino acid substitutions in the E2 envelope glycoprotein. J Virol 2012;86(11):6084–96.
67. Hallengärd D, Kakoulidou M, Lulla A, et al. Novel attenuated Chikungunya vaccine candidates elicit protective immunity in C57BL/6 mice. J Virol 2014;88(5):2858–66.
68. Valneva Initiates Phase 3 Clinical Study for its Chikungunya Vaccine Candidate VLA1553. September 8. 2020. Available at: https://valneva.com/press-release/valneva-initiates-phase-3-clinical-study-for-its-chikungunya-vaccine-candidate-vla1553/. Accessed June 11, 2021.
69. Goo L, Dowd KA, Lin TY, et al. A Virus-Like Particle Vaccine Elicits Broad Neutralizing Antibody Responses in Humans to All Chikungunya Virus Genotypes. J Infect Dis 2016;214(10):1487–91.
70. Chang LJ, Dowd KA, Mendoza FH, et al. Safety and tolerability of chikungunya virus-like particle vaccine in healthy adults: a phase 1 dose-escalation trial. Lancet 2014;384(9959):2046–52.
71. Chen GL, Coates EE, Plummer SH, et al. Effect of a Chikungunya Virus-Like Particle Vaccine on Safety and Tolerability Outcomes: A Randomized Clinical Trial. JAMA 2020;323(14):1369–77 [published correction appears in JAMA. 2020 Jul 28;324(4):400].
72. Kuhn JH, Bào Y, Bavari S, et al. Virus nomenclature below the species level: a standardized nomenclature for filovirus strains and variants rescued from cDNA. Arch Virol 2014;159(5):1229–37.
73. Malvy D, McElroy AK, de Clerck H, et al. Ebola virus disease. Lancet 2019;393(10174):936–48 [published correction appears in Lancet. 2019 May 18;393(10185):2038].
74. The Lancet Child Adolescent Health. Children's needs in an Ebola virus disease outbreak. Lancet Child Adolesc Health 2019;3(2):55.
75. Rowe AK, Bertolli J, Khan AS, et al. Clinical, virologic, and immunologic follow-up of convalescent Ebola hemorrhagic fever patients and their household contacts, Kikwit, Democratic Republic of the Congo. Commission de Lutte contre les Epidémies à Kikwit. J Infect Dis 1999;179(Suppl 1):S28–35.
76. Feldmann H, Geisbert TW. Ebola haemorrhagic fever. Lancet 2011;377(9768):849–62.

77. Bah EI, Lamah MC, Fletcher T, et al. Clinical presentation of patients with Ebola virus disease in Conakry, Guinea. N Engl J Med 2015;372(1):40–7.
78. Centers for Disease Control and Prevention. 2014–2016 Ebola outbreak in West Africa. March 8, 2019. Available at: https://www.cdc.gov/vhf/ebola/history/2014-2016-outbreak/index.html. Accessed June 11, 2021.
79. Lamontagne F, Clément C, Kojan R, et al. The evolution of supportive care for Ebola virus disease. Lancet 2019;393(10172):620–1.
80. Schieffelin JS, Shaffer JG, Goba A, et al. Clinical illness and outcomes in patients with Ebola in Sierra Leone. N Engl J Med 2014;371(22):2092–100.
81. Mulangu S, Dodd LE, Davey RT Jr, et al. A Randomized, Controlled Trial of Ebola Virus Disease Therapeutics. N Engl J Med 2019;381(24):2293–303.
82. Roels TH, Bloom AS, Buffington J, et al. Ebola hemorrhagic fever, Kikwit, Democratic Republic of the Congo, 1995: risk factors for patients without a reported exposure. J Infect Dis 1999;179(Suppl 1):S92–7.
83. Bausch DG, Towner JS, Dowell SF, et al. Assessment of the risk of Ebola virus transmission from bodily fluids and fomites. J Infect Dis 2007;196(Suppl 2): S142–7.
84. Anderson M, Bausch GB. Filoviruses and Arenaviruses. In: Long SS, Prober CG, Fischer M, editors. Principles and practice of pediatric infectious diseases. 5th edition. New York: Elsevier Saunders; 2017. p. 1190–5.e2.
85. Henao-Restrepo AM, Camacho A, Longini IM, et al. Efficacy and effectiveness of an rVSV-vectored vaccine in preventing Ebola virus disease: final results from the Guinea ring vaccination, open-label, cluster-randomised trial (Ebola Ça Suffit!). Lancet 2017;389(10068):505–18 [published correction appears in Lancet. 2017 Feb 4;389(10068):504] [published correction appears in Lancet. 2017 Feb 4;389(10068):504].
86. Conteh MA, Goldstein ST, Wurie HR, et al. Clinical Surveillance and Evaluation of Suspected Ebola Cases in a Vaccine Trial During an Ebola Epidemic: The Sierra Leone Trial to Introduce a Vaccine Against Ebola. J Infect Dis 2018;217(suppl_1): S33–9.
87. Gsell PS, Camacho A, Kucharski AJ, et al. Ring vaccination with rVSV-ZEBOV under expanded access in response to an outbreak of Ebola virus disease in Guinea, 2016: an operational and vaccine safety report [published correction appears in Lancet Infect Dis. 2017 Dec;17 (12):1232]. Lancet Infect Dis 2017; 17(12):1276–84.
88. Tapia MD, Sow SO, Mbaye KD, et al. Safety, reactogenicity, and immunogenicity of a chimpanzee adenovirus vectored Ebola vaccine in children in Africa: a randomised, observer-blind, placebo-controlled, phase 2 trial. Lancet Infect Dis 2020; 20(6):719–30.

Moving?

Make sure your subscription moves with you!

To notify us of your new address, find your **Clinics Account Number** (located on your mailing label above your name), and contact customer service at:

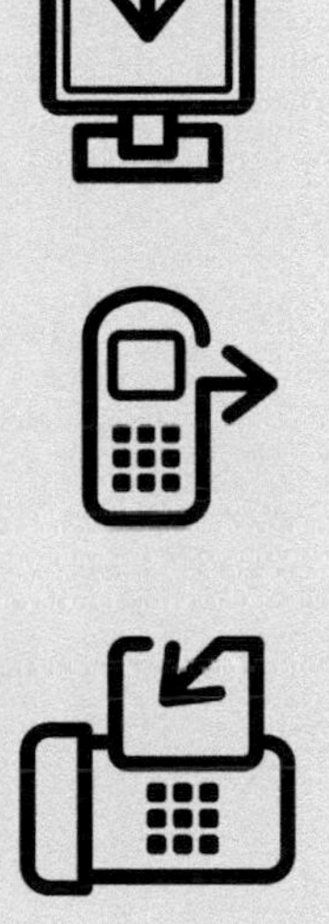

Email: journalscustomerservice-usa@elsevier.com

800-654-2452 (subscribers in the U.S. & Canada)
314-447-8871 (subscribers outside of the U.S. & Canada)

Fax number: 314-447-8029

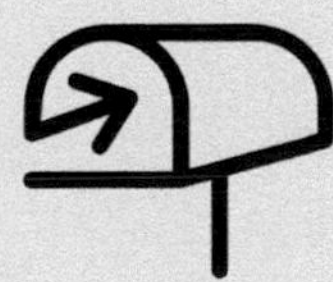

Elsevier Health Sciences Division
Subscription Customer Service
3251 Riverport Lane
Maryland Heights, MO 63043

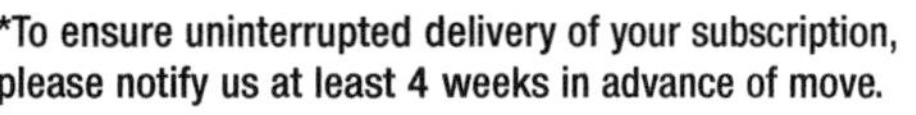

*To ensure uninterrupted delivery of your subscription, please notify us at least 4 weeks in advance of move.

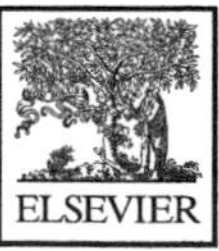

9780323848749